I0034642

Chromatin and Epigenetics

An Introduction to
Epigenetic Mechanisms

Chromatin and Epigenetics

An Introduction to Epigenetic Mechanisms

Vincenzo Pirrotta

Rutgers University, USA

World Scientific

NEW JERSEY · LONDON · SINGAPORE · BEIJING · SHANGHAI · HONG KONG · TAIPEI · CHENNAI · TOKYO

Published by

World Scientific Publishing Co. Pte. Ltd.

5 Toh Tuck Link, Singapore 596224

USA office: 27 Warren Street, Suite 401-402, Hackensack, NJ 07601

UK office: 57 Shelton Street, Covent Garden, London WC2H 9HE

British Library Cataloguing-in-Publication Data
A catalogue record for this book is available from the British Library.

CHROMATIN AND EPIGENETICS
An Introduction to Epigenetic Mechanisms

Copyright © 2023 by World Scientific Publishing Co. Pte. Ltd.

All rights reserved. This book, or parts thereof, may not be reproduced in any form or by any means, electronic or mechanical, including photocopying, recording or any information storage and retrieval system now known or to be invented, without written permission from the publisher.

For photocopying of material in this volume, please pay a copying fee through the Copyright Clearance Center, Inc., 222 Rosewood Drive, Danvers, MA 01923, USA. In this case permission to photocopy is not required from the publisher.

ISBN 978-981-125-762-9 (hardcover)
ISBN 978-981-125-890-9 (paperback)
ISBN 978-981-125-763-6 (ebook for institutions)
ISBN 978-981-125-764-3 (ebook for individuals)

For any available supplementary material, please visit
https://www.worldscientific.com/worldscibooks/10.1142/12883#t=suppl

Typeset by Stallion Press
Email: enquiries@stallionpress.com

Preface

What Is Epigenetics?

Today everybody knows that our genes reside in DNA. That is the basis of many expressions such as: "It is in our DNA", meaning it is native, instinctive, spontaneous, built-in, traditional, inherited. Of these, the only scientifically correct meaning is the last. Our genes reside in our DNA and are transmitted, in part, to our offspring through the copy of the DNA that resides in our germ cells. Genes encode the amino acid sequence of proteins that make up our bodies and the enzymes that carry out the countless biochemical transformations needed to grow our organs and bodies and to carry out the constant molecular activities that keep us alive and functioning. But the genetic material contains much more than that structural information. It spells out how each gene is to be expressed, under what conditions, at what moment, at what rate, and, critically, at what stage in the development of the organism and in response to what signals. This kind of information is often as important to what makes us human as the specific amino acid sequence of the proteins. Many proteins are highly conserved and a classical, though entirely misleading statement one often hears is that our genes are 98% the same as those of a chimpanzee. True, in a way. But a block of marble is made of 100% the same stuff as a Michelangelo masterpiece but the shape is a little different. The sequence of the proteins that make up our bodies and are contained in our cells is important and determines the proteins' functions. In this respect, the differences between a chimpanzee's proteins and human proteins are for the most part insignificant. But the instructions deploying the synthesis of those proteins, the when and where and how much are just as important. Both kinds of instructions are shaped by more than a billion years of evolution and work together to specify what we are and even who we are and what we do.

Imagine a human being with perfectly normal human genes but altered gene regulation. This could result in a very different looking beast that might even be unrecognizable as a human. It is really what is done and when it is done with those functions that is important. After all, even in the same organism, cells in different tissues have the same genes but look very different and do different things. It is true that sometimes a new gene arises or a felicitous change in an old gene provides a function not previously available. Even then it is more frequently a change in the expression of an old gene rather than a change in the protein encoded by the gene itself. Consider, for example, the acquisition of lactose utilization in adults, a mutation that has had momentous consequences for the history of human populations. The mutation (or mutations, since it happened independently in different populations) was not in the enzyme produced but in the regulation of the expression of the gene.

Regulatory elements in the DNA are sequences that recruit specific DNA-binding factors that may be specific activators or repressors to activate or silence genes, as well as general transcription factors important for the general machinery of transcription and gene expression. Many of these DNA-binding factors are enhancer proteins, produced in response to internal or external signals that determine when a set of genes should be activated. These proteins recognize particular DNA sequences that give them specificity: they regulate specific genes, not all genes or random genes. DNA-binding proteins and other nucleic acids are the only kinds of molecules that can read the nucleotide sequence of DNA and therefore they are the only regulators that can uniquely target specific genes. We know in fact that in some cases RNA molecules can serve to specify DNA targets, the genes that need to be regulated. But how does all this regulatory activity take place? To claim that it is all implicit in the DNA sequence is not helpful. This claim is either grandiosely deterministic or it ignores a great range of mechanisms that depend on the history of a system, on stochasticity, on higher order structures and myriad other features that are not immediately inherent in the amino acid sequences of the proteins encoded in the genome. It is in this vast area of genomic function that "epigenetics" lies.

There has been endless debate on what "epigenetics" means, what it should mean, what it should not mean. In principle, the word refers to what is above genetics, an overlayer, something additional (Greek "epi-" means "above"). If genetics is taken to mean the protein-coding information, there is a vast amount of additional machinery that is needed to specify how genetic information works and how it is used and implemented. Some think that the word should be restricted to mechanisms that alter the phenotype in a heritable way. Others use "epigenetics" to refer to mechanisms that involve higher order arrangements of the DNA and the way in which these arrangements affect gene expression. In practice, this means mostly chromatin structures and chromatin modifications, but genome architecture has also come to be included. For our purposes, adherence to a strict definition is not desirable. It is better to try to understand as much as possible the mechanisms that modern molecular biology has discovered to be involved in the functioning of the genome than to stick to a purist's definition. In practice, our point of view will involve all those mechanisms that acknowledge the fact that the genetic material exists in the form of chromatin folded up in a nucleus and that evolution has shaped the way these features determine how the genome works.

A common example used in describing what epigenetics is or does is the case of identical twins. They come from the same fertilized egg and therefore have the same parental genes, yet they display significant differences already since childhood. Though remarkably similar in physical and behavioral features, they are noticeably distinct. They may have slight but visible physical peculiarities, character traits, susceptibility to disease. These are often attributed in vague terms to "epigenetic" mechanisms. This is, I think, misleading. True, the parentally inherited genes are identical, but much happens during development of the embryo, let alone after birth, that is not identical.

Identical or monozygotic twins derive from a single fertilized egg, which at some early stage in development forms two separate embryos. Exactly at what stage this separation into two embryos occurs is not clear, although, to be viable, it must occur very early. Some evidence indicates that it often occurs in the course of blastocyst formation, in the first few days after fertilization. The inner cell mass, from which the actual embryo develops, may split into two inner cell masses (see the Stem Cells and Genomic Programming chapter). But the splitting need not occur at the same stage in all cases of identical twins. And the two resulting blastocysts need not have the same number of cells. So right from the causative event, the two twin embryos may have significant differences that have little to do with genetics or with epigenetics. Many more differences can occur during embryonic development. These are chance events. A very common kind of event is genetic mutation, which occurs at a certain frequency every time DNA replicates. And in embryonic development DNA replicates very frequently. Such mutations are then copied in subsequent cell divisions, leading to embryos that are genetic mosaics: they contain patches of cells with one mutation and other patches with another. Everyone of us is in this sense a genetic mosaic. Many other differences may arise in the course of the many cellular decisions that are made in the course of development. How many times a given cell will divide; how much signaling occurs among cells; how cells determine their developmental identities. And, yes, real mutations can arise in the DNA and be transmitted to all the progeny of the cell in which the mutation arose during early development. All these decisions are conditioned by the genetic information but also involve a considerable amount of chance and randomness. So it is hardly surprising that even identical twins are not exactly identical. But this is not what is really meant by epigenetics, except in the very abstract sense that it is not dictated by the genes.

The current use of the word "epigenetics" refers rather to the mechanisms that are involved in and regulate the activity and expression of the genetic material in the cell. In this sense, epigenetics includes the vast complement of proteins and molecular machinery that controls gene expression and the behavior of the genetic material. It includes the even more vast number of activities that are involved in the functioning and modifications of chromatin, the assembly of DNA and proteins that constitutes the normal structure of the genetic material. The key point here is that, during its working life in the cell, DNA is not in the form of a free-floating double helix. In eukaryotic cells from yeast to man, it is in the form of chromatin, where it is packaged into tidbits of about 150 base pairs tightly wrapped around a core of eight histone proteins. This packaging helps to fit the two meters of DNA of the human genome into a nucleus five micrometers across. But, more importantly it regulates access to the DNA sequence because the tight wrapping of DNA around the histone core makes it difficult for other proteins to bind to it and read the nucleotide sequence. It is hard to exaggerate the importance of this packaging of the genetic material and of the histones around which the genomic DNA is wound for the subtlety and complexity of the regulatory mechanisms that are based on it. A large part of the epigenetic information lies in the number and kind of post-translational modifications that can be placed on the histones and on the DNA itself. Another large part lies in the array of protein factors that read and write these modifications. This is not to belittle the importance of the sequence-specific DNA-binding proteins that read the nucleotide sequence and are ultimately the only way the cell can control the vast amount of genomic information that is stored in the DNA. But additional layers of control generated by chromatin packaging and the multitude of histone modifications create mechanisms to store memory about the way genes or even different parts of genes have been used in the recent past and provide avenues to change the way they may be used in response to external signals.

The first half of this book is devoted to describing the structure and mechanisms regulating chromatin, its architecture and its operation. In the second half we will cover some special situations that put the chromatin machinery through its paces in dealing with some of the most complex aspects of the biology of higher organisms: early embryonic development, differentiation, the problems of dealing with the genomes of two different sexes and their different demands on the genome.

For the most part I have avoided discussion of the central nervous system, memory, learning, and behavior as beyond the scope of an introductory textbook such as this. Although epigenetic mechanisms are very likely involved in these processes, in general, the level of analysis has not reached this stage yet (see, however, the accounts of nurturing and behavioral imprinting in rats in Chapter 10, for genetic imprinting).

A few words are necessary to explain the usage of names of genes and gene products. Traditionally, a specific usage has evolved for every organism, which produces confusion when budding yeast, fission yeast, nematode, *Drosophila*, mouse or human genes are discussed in the same context. I have tried to use a uniform convention according to which gene names are italicized, gene products are given with upper case initial but acronyms are all upper case. Though I have tried to be consistent, some departures from these principles have undoubtedly occurred, particularly in cases in which current usage has hardened.

In this textbook, I have not given specific references for every statement of fact or experimental finding, except in a restricted set of particularly important cases. I have also given references when specific results, figures, or models are presented in the illustrations. These attributions are combined with suggested references for more detailed accounts or for further reading and are listed at the end of each chapter.

Finally, I want to acknowledge a debt of gratitude to my wife, Donna McCabe, who has shared my research work and the functioning of my laboratory for many years. During the writing of this textbook, she succumbed to metastatic cancer, a condition in which epigenetics goes awry and cells evade regulatory mechanisms. This book is dedicated to her in loving memory.

Contents

Preface   v

Chapter 1   DNA Structure   1

Chapter 2   Chromatin   31

Chapter 3   DNA Methylation and Gene Silencing   87

Chapter 4   Genome Organization   111

Chapter 5   Heterochromatin   145

Chapter 6   Transcription   183

Chapter 7   Polycomb Mechanisms   213

Chapter 8   Genome Architecture   275

Chapter 9   Stem Cells   313

Chapter 10 Allele-Specific Expression   357

Chapter 11 X Chromosome Dosage Compensation   379

Chapter 12 Aging   407

Chapter 13 Methods   447

Glossary of Terms   479

Subject Index   495

Chapter 1

DNA Structure

Introduction

DNA (deoxyribonucleic acid) is a very long chain of repeating units, the nucleotides. There are four different nucleotides principally found in DNA: Adenosine, Guanosine, Cytidine, and Thymidine (Figure 1). They have a similar structure: each consists of an aromatic base, either a purine (Adenine or Guanine) or a pyrimidine (Cytosine or Thymine). The base is attached to a pentose sugar, deoxyribose, at position $1'$ in the pentose. In RNA, the sugar is ribose, differing from deoxyribose in having a hydroxyl at position 2 in the pentose ring. In RNA, the pyrimidine Uracil is used instead of Thymine. At the carbon at position $5'$ of the pentose is attached one or more phosphate groups through a phosphoester bond. Nucleotide triphosphates are the building blocks from which DNA is polymerized by cleaving off two of the phosphates, thus releasing the energy that powers the polymerization reaction, and attaching the remaining phosphate to the $3'$ carbon of a second nucleotide. The phosphate therefore links the $5'$ position of one ribose to the $3'$ position of another deoxyribose, forming a phosphodiester linkage. The DNA chain grows at the $3'$ end by repeating the process. The result is a long string of nucleotides with a triphosphate at the $5'$ end of the string and a hydroxyl group at the $3'$ end. This is a single strand of DNA. Note that the polynucleotide chain has a directionality. One end of the chain has a free $5'$ position (although it may be phosphorylated with one, two, or three phosphates) and the other end has a free $3'$ position, thus defining a $5'$ to $3'$ direction to the chain.

1

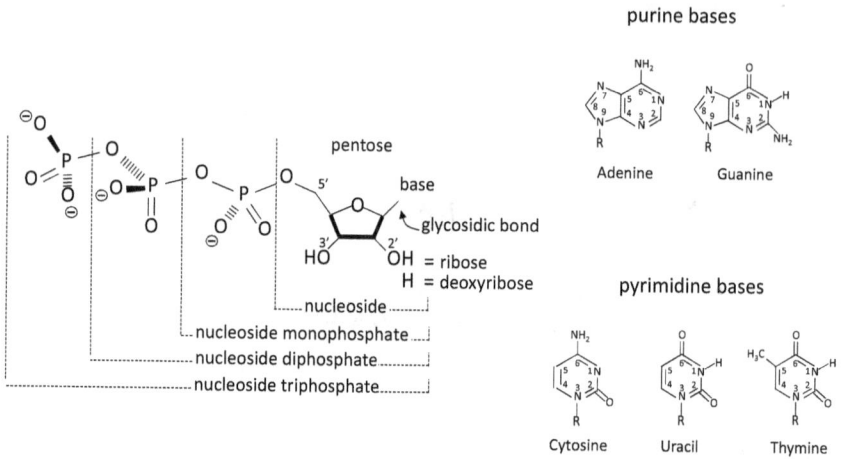

Figure 1.   Nucleotide triphosphates. The bases (purines or pyrimidines) are attached to the pentose sugar (ribose in RNA, deoxyribose in DNA) by a glycosidic bond to produce a nucleotide. The 5′ carbon of the pentose sugar is mono-, di-, or tri-phosphorylated to produce the corresponding nucleotide.

The remarkable feature of the nucleotide bases and the key to the structure of double-stranded DNA deduced by Watson and Crick in 1953 is the ability of the nucleotide bases to pair through appropriately oriented hydrogen bonds with a corresponding nucleotide base in a very specific way: Adenine pairs with Thymine and Guanine pairs with Cytosine (Figure 2). What nature discovered three or four billion years ago and what Watson and Crick understood in 1953 was that two single strands of DNA with a sequence of nucleotides that is exactly complementary will pair in antiparallel orientation (the 5′ end of one strand pairing with the 3′ end of the other strand) to form a double structure in which the two strands wind around a common axis in a right-handed double helix (Figure 3). The consequence of this structure is that this double stranded molecule can duplicate itself by separating the two complementary strands, lining up complementary mononucleotides and polymerizing them. In this way, the sequence of one strand dictates the sequence of the opposite strand and the original molecule is duplicated preserving the entire sequence information.

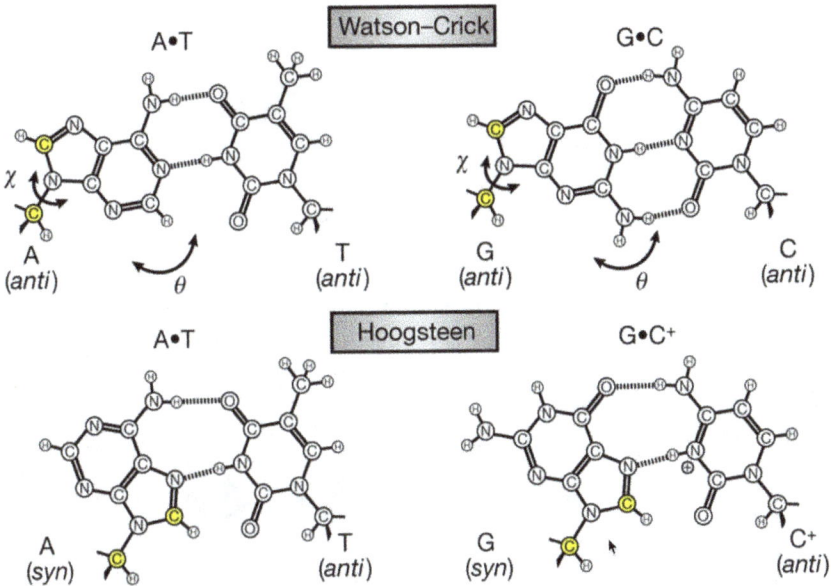

Figure 2. Base pairing. Shown above is the classical Watson–Crick base paring. A pattern of two hydrogen bonds pairs A with T while three hydrogen bonds pair G with C. The Watson–Crick pairing is found in the B form of the double helix. Other base-pairing geometries are possible, including one in which G pairs with U or A with A. One important geometry is that of the Hoogsteen pairing, found in some more unusual structures, such as triple helices.

Source: Nikolova *et al.* (2011).

This structure made immediate sense of numerous properties of DNA that had been a source of puzzlement. For example, the G content of DNA from a variety of sources was always equal to the C content; and the A content was always equal to the T content (Chargaff's Rule). Note that certain nucleotide sequences are self-complementary. For example, the dinucleotide 5'-CpG-3' is able to base pair with the same dinucleotide arranged in the antiparallel orientation. Similarly, the sequence 5'- CATG-3' can pair with the same sequence turned in the antiparallel orientation. More generally, a sequence that reads the same in the opposite strand is called a palindromic sequence. Such sequences play important roles in the structure of DNA molecules and in their interactions with proteins (Figure 4).

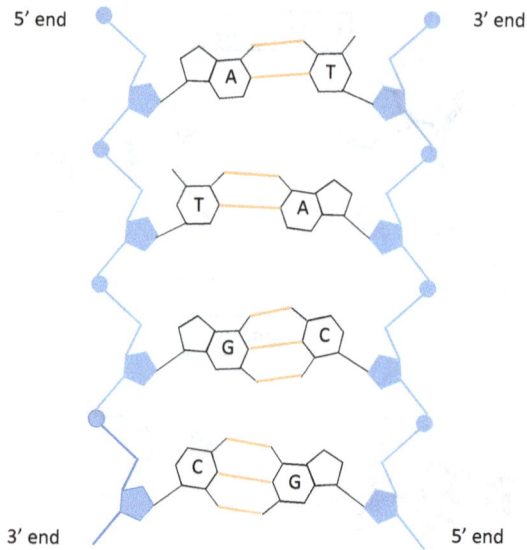

Figure 3.   Base-paired complementary polynucleotides. Nucleotides can be joined to form chains in which the phosphate at the 5′ end of a nucleotide is joined to the 3′ hydroxyl of another nucleotide by a phosphodiester bond. The formation of a phosphodiester bond usually requires that the 5′ end be di- or tri-phosphorylated. Splitting off the extra phosphates provides the energy to form the phosphodiester bond. Therefore, the polynucleotide chain grows by adding a 5′ triphosphate to the 3′ hydroxyl end of the chain, with release of a diphosphate. Two polynucleotide chains can pair along their length if they have a complementary nucleotide sequence. The two chains must be antiparallel: the 5′ end pairs with the 3′ end if the 5′ nucleotide is complementary to the 3′ nucleotide.

Alternative DNA Structures

The familiar right-handed double helix of Watson and Crick is not the only possible way in which two polynucleotide strands with complementary sequences can pair. The two chains can assume several different types of double helical structures. Three forms are found in nature, called A, B, and Z, although others can be induced to form under special conditions (Figure 5). The Z form is a left-handed helix and is relatively rare in nature. It is thought to be favored by stretches of GC sequences. The B form is believed to be most common under normal conditions. The A form is right-handed and is assumed under dehydrating conditions. An A-related

5'-CpG- 3'   5' -CATG- 3'

3'-GpG- 5'   3' -GTAC- 5'

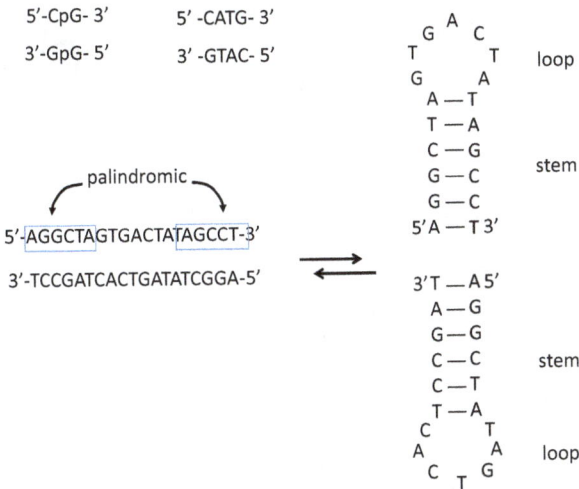

Figure 4. Palindromic sequences. Such sequences read the same on both strands. So CG on one strand pairs with a CG in the other strand. 5'CATG3' pairs with 5'CATG3'. Palindromic sequences separated by a non-palindromic sequence can form a stem and loop structure by pairing with themselves instead of with each other.

structure is formed by DNA/RNA hybrids. The predominant form *in vivo* is the B form, although local departures from this structure can occur in the presence of particular sequence features. Non-canonical structures have been shown to occur *in vivo* and *in vitro* although their function or role is not always easy to determine. Triplex structures can form by winding a third strand around a standard duplex double helix using an alternative pattern of hydrogen bonds from that used in the Watson–Crick base pairing, called Hoogsteen pairing (Figure 2). This allows the formation of triple helices such as poly(dA).2poly(dT).

Another non-canonical structure is the G-quadruplex, which can form in sequences rich in Gs. In the G-quadruplex, four Gs on four different strands assemble to form a planar square in which they bond through Hoogsteen base-pairing. DNA or RNA strands containing multiple runs of at least three Gs separated by at least one nucleotide can fold spontaneously into four-stranded structures held together by flat G-quadruplexes. Depending on the topology, such structures can be more thermodynamically stable than the double helix, particularly if stabilized by a

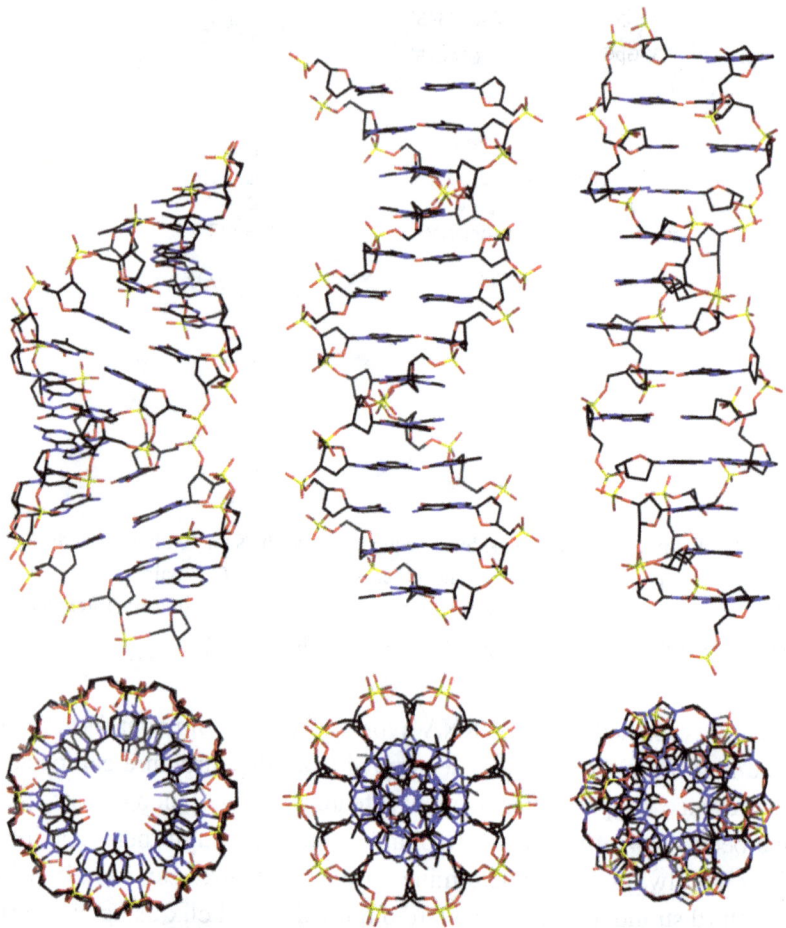

Figure 5.   DNA double helices. Two polynucleotides can pair up if they have complementary sequences as in Figure 2. When they do so, they form a double helical structure. Three
possible double helical geometries are found in nature, depending on conditions: the A, B,
and Z form, from left to right. The B form is the most common under normal conditions.
Above are side views of the helices; below are views down the helix axis.

Source: Mauroesguerroto, Creative Commons, https://commons.wikimedia.org/wiki/File:
Dnaconformations.png#filelinks.

monovalent cation like Na+ or K+. The very stability of G-quadruplexes
would pose an obstacle to DNA replication or transcription or RNA
processing and translation. In fact, sequences with high potential to
form G-quadruplexes are harmful and tend to cause DNA damage.

The introduction of such sequences in the genome is mutagenic. Helicases, such as the human WRN, BLM, and FANCJ helicases, bind to G-quadruplexes *in vitro* and unwind them. The most abundant target for G-quadruplex formation is the telomere. In most, though not all, eukaryotes, telomeres contain repeated motifs very rich in Gs. We will examine telomere mechanisms in more detail later (see the following section on telomeres). For the moment it will suffice to say that the G-rich telomere sequences tend to exist as long 3′ single-stranded overhangs. These single-strand regions must be protected against nucleases to avoid the constant loss of telomeric DNA. The G-rich single strand is particularly suited to form G-quadruplexes (Figure 6) whose structure protects them against nucleases. Unfortunately, they also prevent the activity of telomerase and must therefore be unwound to allow telomerase to elongate the 3′ single-stranded region. The WRN and BLM helicases, which are able *in vitro* to unwind G-quadruplexes, are known to accumulate at telomeres and to be required for telomere maintenance *in vivo*.

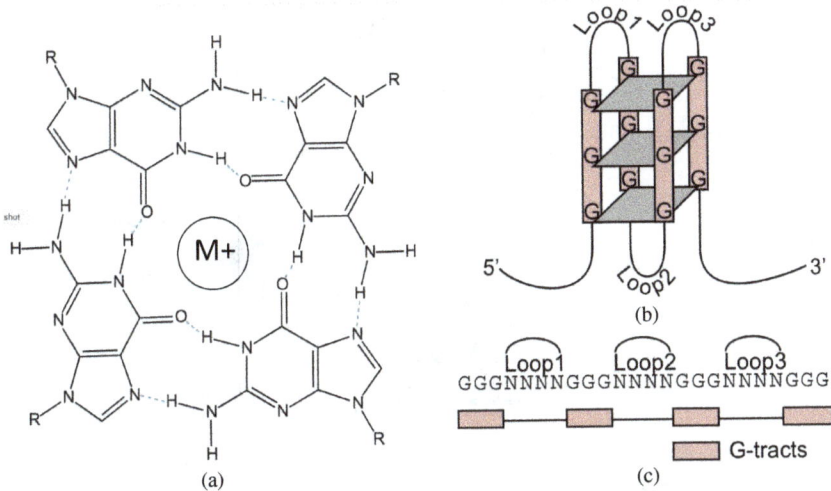

Figure 6. G-quadruplex structure. A sequence rich in Gs can loop back on itself three times and form hydrogen bonds between four stems. (a) The interactions between four planar Gs, stabilized by a monovalent cation such as Na+ or K+ in the middle. (b) Arrangement of four G tracts forming three sets of planar G interactions as in (a). (c) Ideally, the G-quadruplex requires four G tracts of three Gs each, separated by loops of at least three nucleotides each.

Source: Capra *et al.* (2010).

Properties of the Double Helix

The double-stranded DNA helix has several important structural features. The sugar–phosphate chain of each strand forms the rim of the helix and the paired nucleotide bases connect the two chains. The aromatic rings of the nucleotide bases are flat plates that lie horizontally in the middle of the helix forming a ladder-like structure. The stacking of the aromatic bases provides additional stabilization for the double helix through interactions of their π electrons. The helix twist or pitch is such that it makes a complete turn approximately every 10 base pairs, increasing the helix length by 34 angstroms or 3.4 nanometers. The width of the double helix is approximately 2.4 nm (depending on buffer conditions) (Figure 7).

Since the backbone of each single strand consists of alternating sugar and negatively charged phosphate, the formation of the double helix

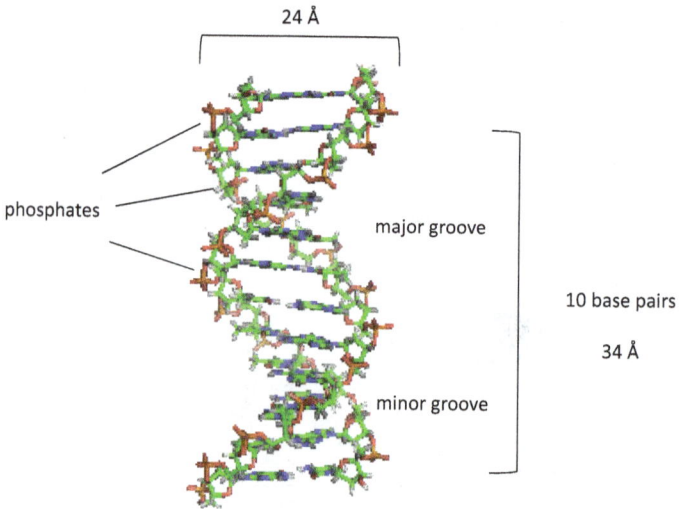

Figure 7.   DNA double helix. The rim of the double helix is formed by the sugar–phosphate chain (phosphates shown in red, sugars in green) and is therefore strongly negatively charged. The bases in the middle are aromatic and tend to avoid water. Bringing close together two negatively charged chains requires stabilization by positive ions in the solution. At high ionic strength the double helix is more stable. At very low ionic strength the two chains of the double helix will repel one another enough that they will separate or "melt" even without heat.

requires bringing close together many negative charges. The repulsion between the negative charges can be alleviated by positively charged ions in the solvent (ionic strength), but it must be overcome by strong interactions between the bases that hold the two strands together. These interactions are of two sorts. One is due to the hydrogen bonds between the complementary bases on the two strands. Hydrogen bonds are relatively weak individually, but there are very many hydrogen bonds holding the two strands together. Another contribution is made by the stacking interactions between the bases. Each base, whether purine or pyrimidine, is a flat aromatic molecule whose π orbitals above and below the flat rings can interact with those of another base stacked above it. This interaction is maximal if the two bases lie flat, one directly above the other. Both hydrogen bonds and stacking interactions can in turn be overcome by heat energy, breaking the base pairs and denaturing the double-stranded DNA. The temperature at which heat energy breaks the bonds (hydrogen bonds and stacking interactions) between the two single strands and makes the double helix come apart is called the melting temperature (Figure 8). This melting depends on the ionic strength of the solution. At very low ionic strengths, the double

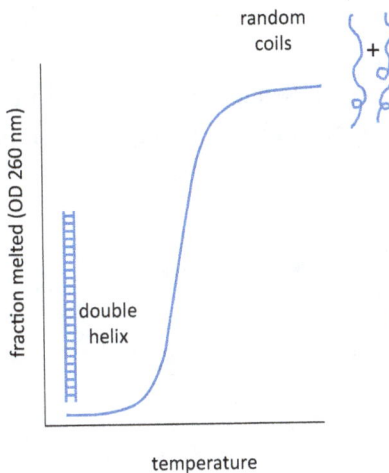

Figure 8.   Melting curve. Initially all the molecules are in the double helix form. As the temperature increases, an increasing fraction melts and separates into two single-stranded random coils. This is followed using the absorption spectrum or optical density at 260 nm wavelength. Double-stranded DNA absorbs less than the separated single strands. The melting temperature is defined as the temperature at which half the double helices have denatured.

helix becomes much easier to denature due to the repulsion between the phosphates. The pH of the solution is also important: at both extremes, the bases ionize and lose ability to form hydrogen bonds, resulting in melting. Certain organic molecules, typically formamide or urea, are powerful denaturing agents because they compete for hydrogen bond formation. The higher their concentration, the lower the melting temperature.

The G–C pairing involves three H-bonds, A–T pairing, two H-bonds. Therefore GC pairs contribute more to the binding of the two single strands than AT pairs. GC pairs require more energy to be broken and therefore contribute more to the melting temperature of the double helix. Stretches of the double helix particularly rich in AT base pairs are more readily melted than regions rich in GC pairs. The melting of a single base pair is facilitated by the melting of flanking base pairs so that when one goes, the neighbors also dissociate. This cooperativity has three important consequences. First, melting begins with ends, where there are no cooperative base pairs on one side. Another is the dependence on length. A short double-stranded DNA molecule melts more easily than a long one and tends to melt in an all-or-none way. Beyond a certain length, the ends make a proportionally small contribution and the length is no longer an important factor. So, for a double helix longer than some 20 base pairs, the base composition is the predominant factor. In a long DNA molecule, the sequence is also important. Sequence regions that are rich in AT will start to melt earlier than regions rich in GC (Figure 9). Plotting the fraction of

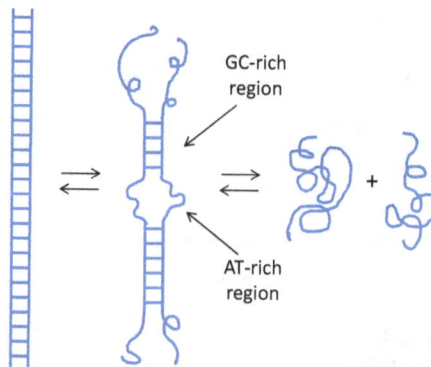

Figure 9.   Melting of a long DNA molecule with complex sequence goes through stages in which first the ends melt, then internal regions with higher AT content, until even the regions with high GC content melt and the double helix separates into two single random coil strands.

the molecules that are denatured versus the temperature produces an S-shaped melting curve, as shown in Figure 8. The rise of the curve would be sharpest for a relatively short double helix but shallower for a long DNA molecule with a complex sequence. The melting process is most commonly followed using the optical density (absorption spectrum). Double-stranded DNA has an absorption peak for ultraviolet light of 260 nm wavelength. This is mostly due to the nucleotide bases. Stacking of the bases in the double-stranded B-form DNA decreases their ability to absorb light. Therefore, the more melting occurs, the more the absorbance at 260 nm increases.

Bending and Twisting

The double helix has three degrees of freedom: bending, twisting, and compression (Figure 10). The double helix is relatively stiff and hard to bend over short regions but is easy to bend over long regions. This stiffness is described by a parameter called the persistence length: the length above which the fiber can be considered to be freely flexible. The stiffness of the double-stranded DNA helix depends on the base composition.

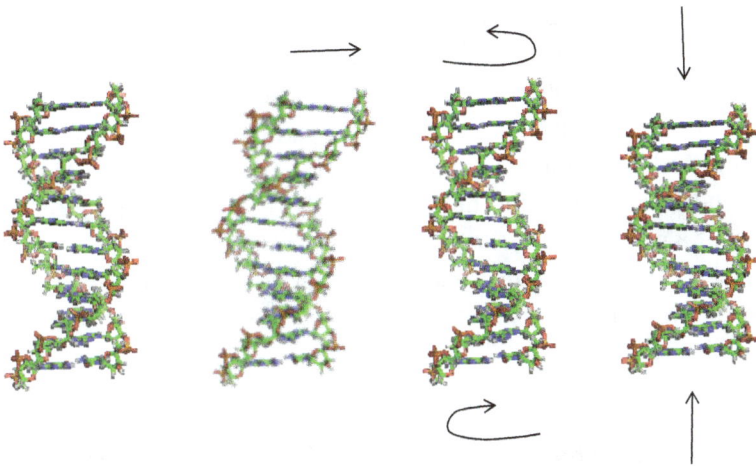

Figure 10. Degrees of freedom of the double helix. The helix can be bent, twisted, or compressed. Each of these degrees of freedom or their combinations have important relevance for the behavior of DNA.

Certain dinucleotides such as AA are slightly tilted relatively to one another. If such dinucleotides were to occur with a period close to the 10.5 base pair pitch of the B double helix, this slight tilt would add up to produce a curved structure. On the average, however, the B helix is straight over short distances and the persistence length is about 50 nm or 150 base pairs. This means that a piece of double helical DNA longer than 150 base pairs can be bent double. Long double-stranded DNA molecules can be readily bent to form circles. The stiffness of DNA clearly resists the bending when the length becomes shorter. Surprisingly, however, DNA molecules as short as 60 bp can be circularized although this length is far less than the persistence length. The explanation for this is that a certain probability exists for the double helix to develop a kink, most likely by breaking one base pair. Calculations based on the energy of base pairing indicate that one such kink/70 bp can be statistically expected to occur at physiological temperature, pH, and ionic strength. Obviously, this will depend on the base composition and GC-rich DNA will be stiffer than AT-rich DNA.

To a good approximation, the bending rigidity of DNA is mainly dependent on the properties of adjacent base pairs and can be calculated from the number of each dinucleotide base pair present in the sequence. The contribution to rigidity is not the same as the strength of the hydrogen bonds between the base pairs or the stacking interactions between adjacent base pairs. Thus, while a CG dinucleotide makes a strong contribution to stiffness, a GC dinucleotide is considerably more flexible and a CC/GG is very flexible. Short tracts of A, particularly when repeated with 10 bp periodicity, impart a structural bend to the double helix. These features and their distribution in a sequence have a strong influence on the ability of a particular DNA region to wrap around a nucleosome core (see Chapter 2). In addition, these properties can be enhanced or exploited by DNA-binding proteins, which can produce sharp kinks by a variety of mechanisms.

Torsional Stress can Facilitate the Breaking of Base Pairs

Under normal conditions, the B form of the double helix makes one complete turn every 10.4 base pairs. This normal pitch can vary if the helix is twisted or subject to torsion either increasing or decreasing the number of turns. A helix with additional turn density is said to be positively super-coiled and one with fewer turns is negatively supercoiled. Separating the strands in the middle of a DNA double helix will unwind the helix locally at the expense of adding twists to the rest of the helix. These extra turns can be transmitted along the DNA and released at the ends. But if the DNA is constrained either at the ends or at any point in the middle, the extra twists cannot be released and the molecule accumulates excess turns. Extra twists may accumulate simply because the DNA is too long and tangled to release the torsional strain. Biological processes such as tran-scription and DNA replication involve unwinding the double helix and therefore accumulate torsional stress in the rest of the DNA. So does the binding of many proteins or small molecules, particularly those that insert between base pairs. *In vivo*, proteins called topoisomerases can release the torsional strain. They do so by transiently producing a break in one DNA strand and passing the other strand through the break to change the wind-ing number and release the torsion (Figure 11). Type I topoisomerases open one strand; type II topoisomerases open both strands and pass a whole DNA duplex through the gap. Other proteins called helicases help various DNA processes by breaking the base pairs and separating the strands of the double helix using ATP hydrolysis to provide the energy. For example, DNA replication requires the help of a helicase to separate the strands in front of the replication fork. This accumulates torsion fur-ther ahead and therefore requires a topoisomerase in front of the helicase to release the extra helical turns.

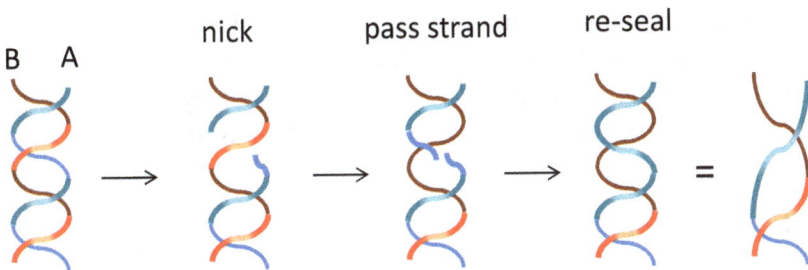

Figure 11.　Topoisomerase I changes winding number. Topoisomerase I transiently opens strand A, passes strand B through the break and re-forms the bond to close strand A. In the illustration, this results in one less turn of one strand about the other.

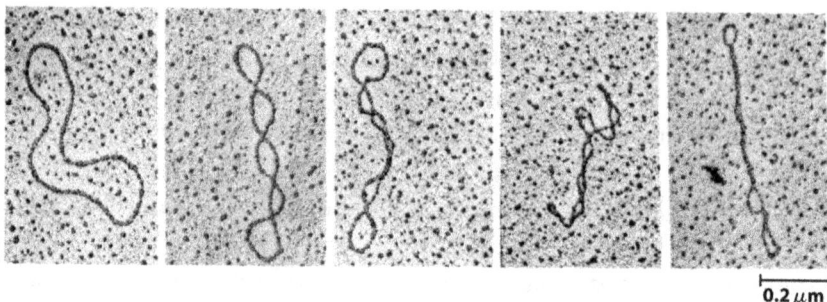

0.2 μm

Figure 12.   Supercoiled circular plasmid. These electron microscope images show a circular plasmid DNA molecule with different degrees of supercoiling. From left to right, completely relaxed circle with no superhelical turns, increasing numbers of superhelical turns.

Source: A graduate student presentation, Brian Bahnson, https://www1.udel.edu/chem/bahnson/chem645/websites/Sapra/pic14.

The problem of supercoiling is of particular concern in circular DNA double helices such as those found in plasmids and many viruses. The circular structure locks in the total torsional state because there are no free ends to release extra positive or negative turns. Only a topoisomerase can release the positive or negative torsional stress. A circular DNA molecule can convert the excess positive or negative turns in the helix into higher order turns of the helix around itself. These are called superhelical turns. The relationship between the turns of the helix (twist) and the higher order superhelical turns (writhe) is given by: $L = T + W$

Circular, double-stranded DNA molecules, such as plasmids, are often seen as tightly collapsed and twisted circles (Figure 12). This is because, *in vivo*, they may have many proteins bound, or, if eukaryotic, nucleosomes, but, when purified, these are removed. This means that the unwinding that had been caused by the bound proteins is now taken up by the rest of the circular molecule. Since the double helix tends to keep strain to a minimum, the shortage of turns is taken up by the writhe of the circular molecule, which now becomes twisted on itself.

Intercalating Dyes

The shape of the DNA double helix presents three outstanding structural features: the major and minor grooves formed by the sugar–phosphate chains and the flat, stacked aromatic bases of the nucleotides in the middle of the helix. Molecules that fit in or along these structural features are likely to bind well to DNA. One class of small molecules that can slide in between the flat aromatic rings of the base pairs includes polycyclic aromatic molecules such as ethidium bromide, proflavine, thalidomide. Such molecules have usually a positively charged group that facilitates the initial approach to the negatively charged sugar–phosphate backbone, but the flat, aromatic rings then slide or intercalate in between the aromatic base pairs where their π electrons interact with the π electrons of the base pairs. This electronic interaction lowers the energy required to absorb or emit light and therefore changes the color of the complex. Such intercalating molecules are therefore often good dyes. A typical example is ethidium bromide (Figure 13).

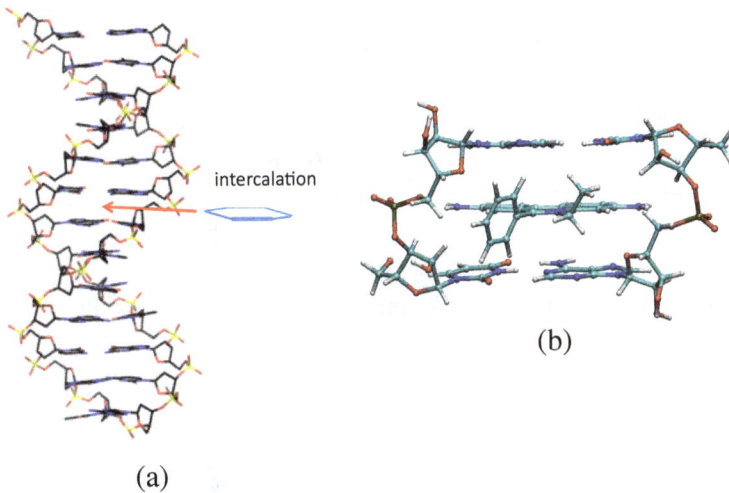

intercalation

(a)

(b)

Figure 13.   Intercalation. Flat, aromatic molecules bind strongly to DNA by intercalation between the flat, aromatic base pairs in the center of the double helix. (a) Intercalation in the double helix. (b) Here, a DNA-binding dye called ethidium bromide is shown intercalated between two base pairs. Intercalation pushes the two base pairs slightly further apart, causing a slight unwinding of the double helix.

Source: Karol Langner, Public Domain, https://commons.wikimedia.org/wiki/File:DNA_intercalation2.jpg.

However, by intercalating, these compounds also push apart two adjacent base pairs, therefore locally unwinding the double helix. In a circular plasmid DNA, this means increasing the number of turns in the rest of the DNA. *In vivo*, the distortion of the double helix can interfere with transcription or DNA replication. Because the intercalated dye simulates a base pair, it can induce the replicating machinery to insert or delete a base pair, resulting in frameshift mutations. The increased ability to absorb light also means that intercalating dyes can become energized by light of the appropriate wavelength and damage DNA. Intercalating dyes are therefore mutagenic and carcinogenic.

DNA-binding Proteins

Ultimately, all specific regulation of individual genes requires identification and specific action upon particular nucleotide sequences. To do this, proteins have had to develop ways to recognize specific sequence tracts. Many DNA-binding proteins exploit the shape of the DNA double helix to bind by fitting a part of their amino acid chain into the major or minor groove and by electrostatic binding of suitably placed basic amino acids to the negatively charged phosphates. Most important, however, are those DNA-binding proteins that can reach sufficiently into the major or minor groove to interact with specific base pairs. Such proteins see different interacting groups on the base pairs depending on which side they approach from (Figure 14). A minority of DNA-binding proteins bind

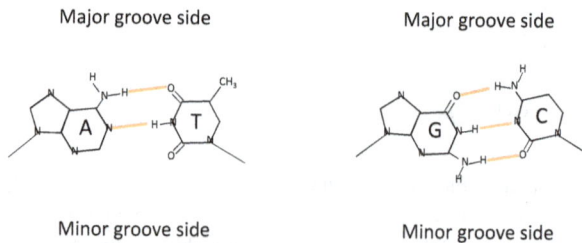

Figure 14.   Major and minor groove views of the base pairs. Each base pair has one side facing the major groove and one facing the minor groove. Proteins that interact with the base pairs see not only a broad or a narrow access, but they face different interacting groups on the base pairs.

DNA in the minor groove. An example is the TATA-box binding protein TBP (see Chapter 6, for role in transcription). In most cases known, it appears that minor groove binding results in a major distortion of the DNA and a widening of the minor groove producing a distinct bend toward the major groove. Most DNA-binding proteins bind in the major groove, which is larger and where it is easier to reach the edges of the bases and interact with them specifically without major distortion. Most sequence-specific DNA-binding proteins use one of three common structural motifs: basic leucine zipper, helix-turn-helix, and zinc finger.

The basic leucine zipper: This structural domain can be used for protein–protein as well as protein–DNA interactions. It consists of an alpha helical amino acid domain with a leucine at every seventh position. Due to the pitch of the alpha helix, this means that all the leucines face the same side (Figure 15), creating a hydrophobic surface that often mediates protein dimerization. Basic-region leucine zipper (b-ZIP) DNA-binding proteins use the leucine zipper as a dimerization motif, aligning 60–80 amino acid long helical domains in parallel by adhesion of the aligned leucines, or at times another small hydrophobic amino acid, placed at every seventh position. A basic region at the end of each α-helix fits in the major groove and forms specific interactions with several bases (Figure 16).

Helix-turn-helix: This DNA-binding motif was the first to be characterized and is an excellent example of how proteins can read the DNA

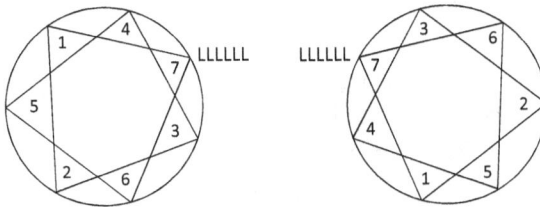

Figure 15. Leucine zipper interaction. The diagram represents two alpha helices seen down the axis of the helices. The numbers represent the first seven amino acids, the seventh is a leucine. Continuing down the helix, the eighth amino acid would be again in position one and the 14th would be in position 7. If leucines occur every seventh amino acid, they would all line up on the same side of the helix, forming a hydrophobic ridge. Two such helices would then pair lengthwise and adhere through hydrophobic interactions.

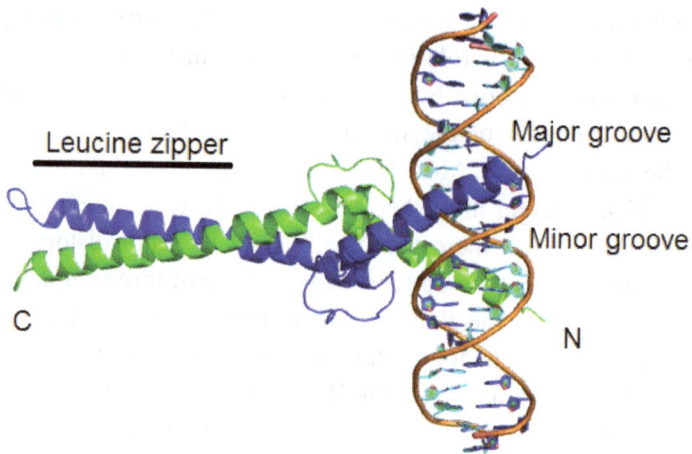

Figure 16. DNA binding by a b-ZIP factor. Two monomers of a basic leucine zipper protein pair their alpha helices. At one end of each helix, a basic helical segment fits in the major groove of the DNA and interacts with the bases.

Source: Latacca, Creative Commons, https://commons.wikimedia.org/wiki/File:Bzip_wikimedia_ modified.tif.

sequence. It consists of two alpha helical stretches joined by a loop or turn. One of the two helices, the recognition helix, fits deeply in the major groove and contacts the edges of the bases, making base-specific interactions that require a specific nucleotide sequence (Figure 16). The other helix is positioned across the recognition helix, interacting non-specifically with the sugar–phosphate chains that form the major groove and locking in the recognition helix inside the groove. Typical examples of this binding structure are the Hox proteins, the lac repressor, or the lambda repressor (Figure 17). Dimerization of the HTH unit allows recognition of a more extensive DNA sequence and therefore increases the sequence specificity as well as the stability of the binding. It also explains why so many DNA-binding sequences are repeats, often inverted repeats (palindromic) of a shorter sequence motif. Still another advantage of dimer binding to inverted repeat sequences is that it allows binding to occur when the dimer approaches the DNA from either direction along the double helix.

Zinc fingers: A third common DNA-binding motif is a combination of zinc fingers. The zinc finger motif is a fold held together by cysteines and histidines coordinating with a cation, most commonly zinc. Many varieties of zinc fingers are now known, but the principle is similar and

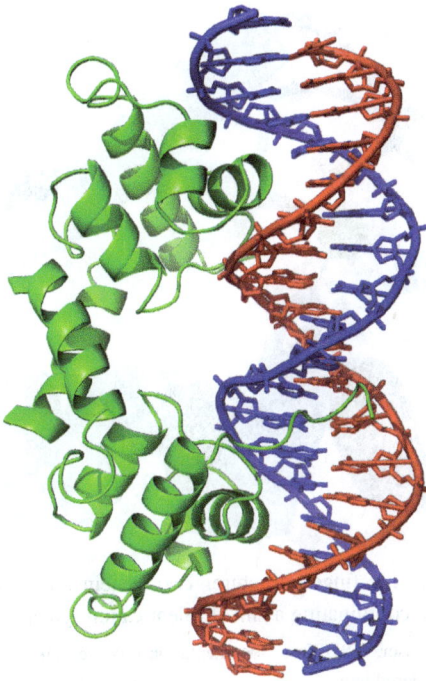

Figure 17.   DNA binding of a helix-turn-helix dimer. The image represents the lambda repressor in the form of a helix-turn-helix dimer binding to DNA. The DNA-binding helix of each monomer fits in the major groove and interacts with the bases, while a second helix of each monomer holds it in place. The third helix mediates interactions between the two monomers.

Source: Richard Wheeler (Zephyris), Creative Commons, https://commons.wikimedia.org/wiki/File:Lambda_repressor_1LMB.png.

exemplified by the Cys2His2 zinc finger found in many DNA-binding factors, although zinc finger motifs can be used for protein–protein, protein–RNA, and other kinds of interactions. This zinc finger has the structure X_2-Cys-X_{2-4}-Cys- X_{12}-His-$X_{3,4,5}$-His (Figure 18). Such a zinc finger binds DNA by fitting its α-helix in the major groove and contacting three or four bases (Figure 19). In most cases, a DNA-binding factor will contain several zinc fingers, often regularly spaced to contact DNA at intervals of three base pairs. The CTCF DNA-binding protein, an important component of chromatin architecture, contains 11 zinc fingers. Using combinations of zinc fingers with known DNA-binding specificity, it has been possible to design proteins with any desired binding specificity.

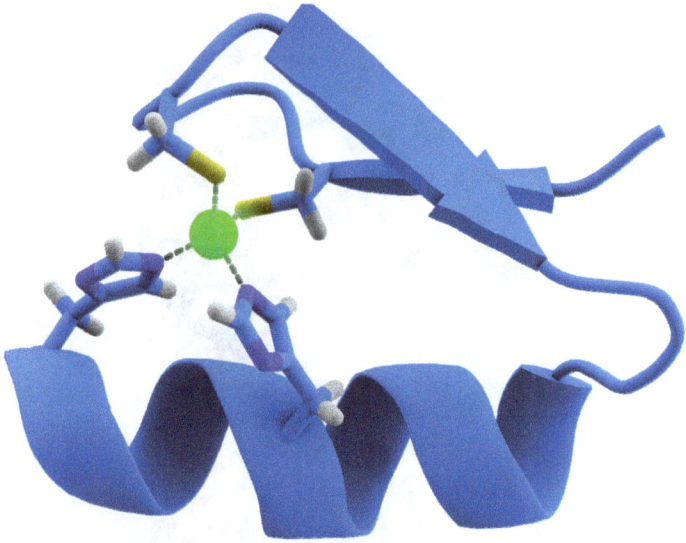

Figure 18.   Cys2His2 Zinc finger structure. Two cysteines (above) and two histidines (below) are shown here coordinating a zinc divalent cation (green).

Source: Thomas Splettstoesser, GNU Free Documentation License, https://commons.wikimedia.org/wiki/File:Zinc_finger_rendered.png.

Telomeres and How to Replicate DNA Ends

Small genomes such as plasmids or even bacterial genomes are most often circular and are relatively straightforward to replicate. Eukaryotic genomes generally consist of a number of chromosomes, each of which contains a linear DNA molecule often tens or hundreds of megabases in length. We will treat DNA replication in Chapter 2, in the context of chromatin, but here we discuss the problem of linear chromosomes and the DNA ends. The linear structure of the chromosome raises the problem of what happens at the ends, called telomeres (from Greek for "end-part"). There are two main difficulties to contend with. One is that the end of a DNA molecule looks like a broken piece of DNA to the cellular repair mechanisms that have evolved to deal with DNA damage. To avoid producing genomic rearrangements by attempting to repair telomeres, special structures are needed to protect the ends. The other major problem has to do with DNA replication. DNA polymerases operate by adding nucleotides at the 3′ end of a polynucleotide. Synthesis initiates from a short RNA primer laid down by a Primase enzyme. A DNA polymerase elongates the primer, which is eventually removed and replaced by DNA. This is fine for copying the strand, called the leading strand, where replication elongates a 3′ end continuously in the direction of the advancing replication fork. Replicating the opposite strand, which ends with a 5′ (lagging strand), requires multiple starts and stops, synthesizing small tracts in the direction away from the replication fork (Figure 20). These short segments, called Okazaki fragments, are then ligated together. At telomeres, the 3′ end is really the end and there is no space for priming an Okazaki fragment. Telomeres would therefore lose nucleotides every round of replication, progressively shortening the chromosome. The last successful Okazaki fragment generally erases 70–100 nucleotides from

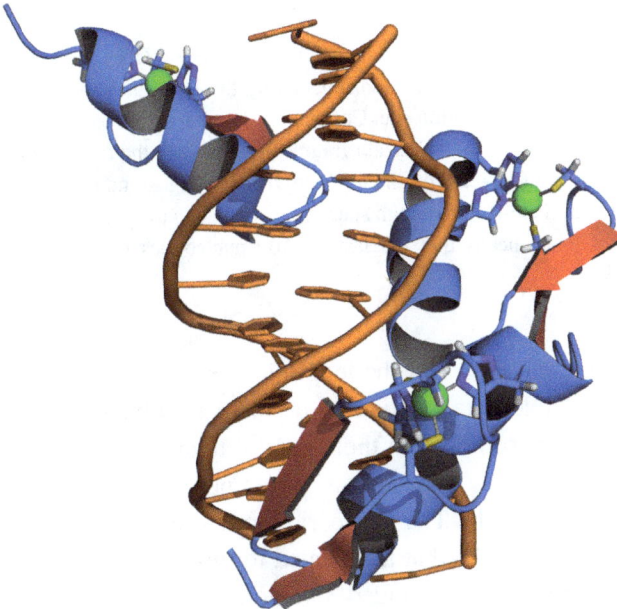

Figure 19. Structure of the zinc finger protein Zif268 bound to DNA. The protein contains three zinc fingers (blue) which fit their alpha-helices in the DNA major groove. The zinc finger ions are in green.

Source: Thomas Splettstoesser, GNU Free Documentation License, https://commons.wikimedia.org/wiki/File:Zinc_finger_DNA_complex.pn.

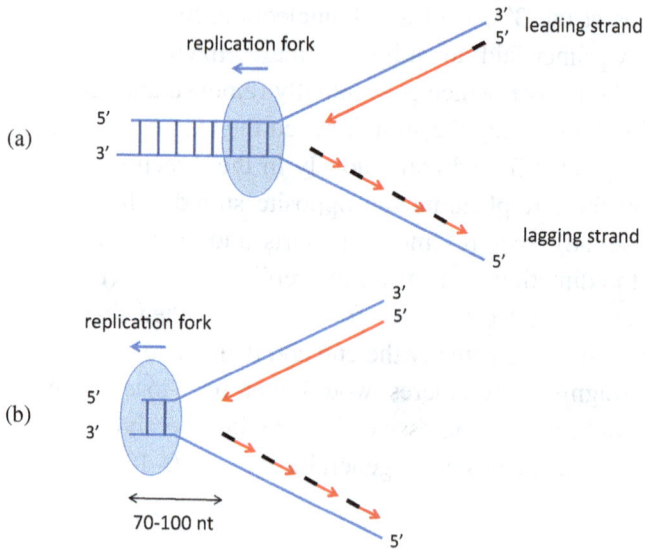

Figure 20.   Replicating the ends of a linear chromosome. (a) DNA synthesis starts with a short RNA primer (short black segment). Copying the leading strand requires only one primer at the replication initiation site. Copying the lagging strand can only be done piece-meal in short fragments, called Okazaki fragments. (b) When the replication fork reaches the chromosome end (depicted on the left side), the leading strand can be copied right to the end. However, there is not enough space near the 3′ end to synthesize a primer for the lagging strand. This means that the last 70–100 nucleotides of the 3′ end cannot be replicated.

the 3′ end and this is in fact the length lost every round of replication in the absence of telomeres. This end-problem is solved in eukaryotes by ending the chromosomes with thousands of tandem copies of a repeating motif and by providing a telomerase machinery to replicate these telomeric repeats (Figure 21). The telomeric motif is a short, G-rich sequence, in vertebrates TTAGGG, that is repeated for up to 15 kilobases in humans and extends into a single-stranded 3′ region of a few hundred nucleotides. As described above, such a sequence is a good substrate to fold and form a G-quadruplex, a stable configuration resistant to nucleases. Another mechanism to protect the 3′ end and hide it from DNA repair mechanisms is to form a T-loop (Figure 21(b)). To form this structure, the single-stranded 3′ end is guided by a protein complex called Shelterin to invade

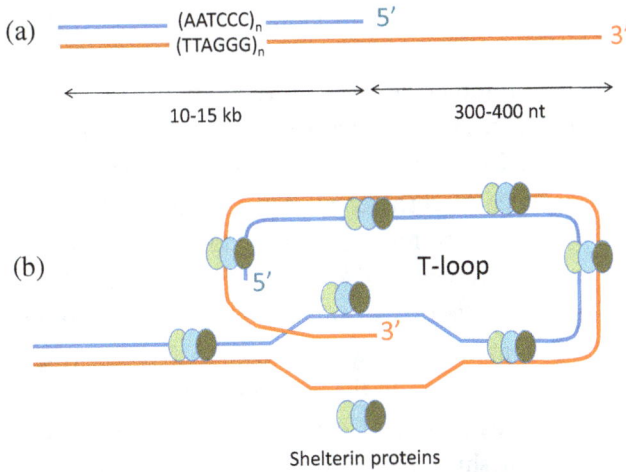

Figure 21.   Vertebrate telomeres. (a) Telomeres in vertebrates consist of TTAGGG telomeric repeats for up to 15 kb, ending with 300–400 nt single-stranded 3′ end. (b) Shelterin component proteins protect the telomeric ends by binding to the telomeric repeats and inducing the single-stranded 3′ overhang to invade the double-stranded region, forming a T-loop. This hides the 3′ end and at the same time provides an alternative method to extend the 3′ end overhang.

the double-stranded region, displacing the paired strand, which forms a displacement loop or D-loop. This shelters or hides and protects the telomeric 3′ end. The Shelterin complex includes six proteins: TRF1, TRF2, TIN2, POT1, TPP1, and RAP1 that bind to the telomeric repeat sequences. TIN2 further recruits the heterochromatin protein HP1γ, which is required for normal protection and function of telomeres and mediates their association with the nuclear envelope (see Chapter 5). Telomeric chromatin is in fact marked with heterochromatic histone H3K9 methylation (see Chapter 5) and this state is important for telomeric maintenance and for suppression of recombination between repeats, which would cause telomere shortening. In the absence of Shelterin, telomeres are recognized as DNA damage sites, and repair mechanisms attempt to heal telomeres, resulting in genomic instability, telomere fusions, senescence, or apoptosis. Absence of HP1 can lead to similar results

In principle, the T-loop could also provide a mechanism to extend the 3′ end by simply elongating it using the 5′ strand as template. In practice, this does not appear to be effective and the telomerase-dependent elongation is required in normal cells to extend the 3′ end single-stranded telomeric overhang. Telomerase is a reverse transcriptase. That is, it synthesizes a DNA strand using an RNA template. The telomerase complex includes an RNA molecule that serves as a template to prevent the erosion of the 3′ ends of chromosomes. The human telomerase complex contains two copies of the reverse transcriptase itself, called TERT, and two copies each of dyskerin (DK) and the telomerase RNA (TERC). Human TERC, also called hTR, (Figure 22) is a non-coding RNA 451 nucleotides long, containing a sequence 3′-CAAUCCCAAUC-5′ that acts as a template, base pairing with the 3′ chromosome end and allowing the telomerase to elongate it, adding one more telomeric repeat 5′-GGTTAG-3′. The telomerase then shifts position by one repeat unit and synthesizes another repeat (Figure 23). This mechanism compensates for the loss of telomere sequence that fails to be fully copied every round of DNA replication. Telomerase is strictly rate-limiting for telomere elongation. There is usually not enough to go around every cell division so only some of the telomeres are elongated every cell cycle. Telomerase preferentially binds to and elongates the shortest telomeres.

Telomerase is active in embryonic stem cells and in tissues that maintain cell proliferation, but it is not produced in most somatic cells. In most proliferating cells in the human body, although telomerase is produced, it is insufficient to maintain telomere length, so telomeres shorten in most tissues, even proliferating hematopoietic cells. The only cells in which telomerase do not shorten are embryonic stem cells and human male germ cells. The length attained in these cells is likely to set maximum telomere length for all body tissues. If dividing cells were to stop producing telomerase, telomeres would shorten until, after some 50–60 cell divisions, they would reach the so-called Hayflick limit, named after the man who discovered it in 1961. At this point, the cells would stop dividing and become senescent (see Chapter 12). It has been thought that organismal aging was due to telomere shortening. Though sorting out cause and effect is a complex matter, telomere shortening is certainly a component of cellular aging. The strict controls that limit the availability and function of telomerase appear to be part of the general control on cell proliferation, to avoid the risk of uncontrolled replication. These control mechanisms are the targets of

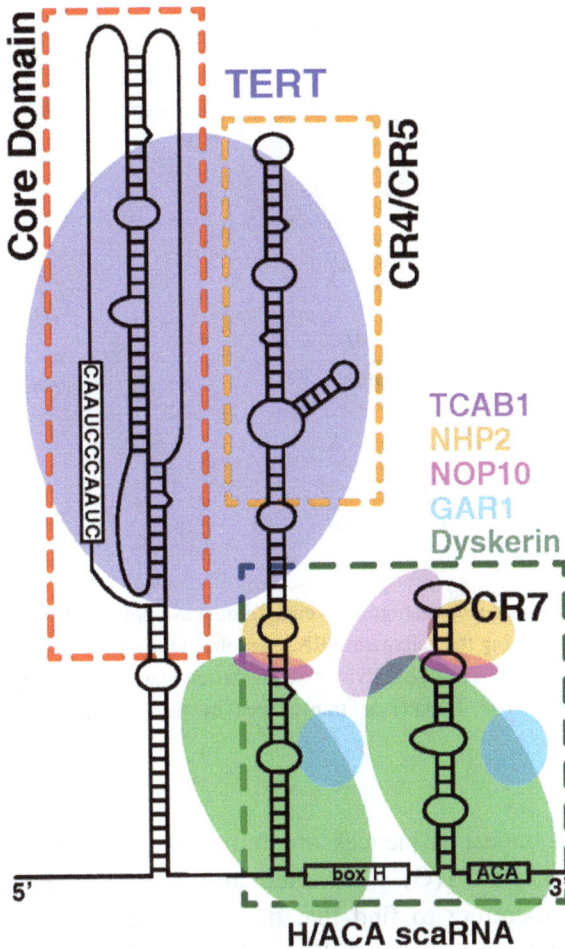

Figure 22. Human telomerase RNA, TERC or hTR. The core domain and the CR4/CR5 domains bind to telomerase, TERT, in blue. Dyskerin (green) is an RNA-binding protein of which two copies bind the H/ACA scaRNA region, stabilize the TERC RNA, and are required for effective telomerase function. The region of the TERC RNA that pairs with the telomeric 3′ end is just a short sequence CUAACCCUAAC (boxed).

Source: Zhang *et al.* (2011).

mutations found in cancer cells, without which they cannot proliferate. It is true that cancer cells reactivate the production of telomerase. This question will be raised again when we come to discuss aging (see Chapter 12).

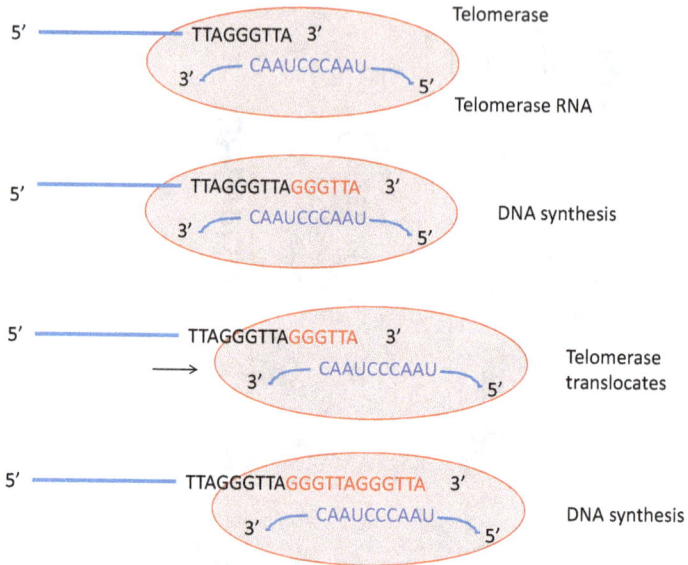

Figure 23.   Telomerase elongation of 3′ end. Telomerase binds to the end of the single-stranded 3′ end, aligning the Telomerase RNA template sequence with the telomere 3′ end. Telomerase reverse transcriptase activity extends the telomere 3′ end using the Telomerase RNA as template. The Telomerase translocates by one repeat unit and repeats the process.

Telomeric repeat sequences are remarkably similar from budding yeast, where they are $T(G)_{1-3}$, to vertebrates, where they are TTAGGG. It is surprising therefore to find that there are exceptions, organisms in which neither the sequence nor the mechanism of telomere maintenance is at all conserved. Many plant and animal species lack telomerase and use different mechanisms of which the best studied is the one found in *Drosophila*. *Drosophila* telomeres consist of a number of copies of three transposable elements that have been evolutionarily recruited to serve the purpose of telomeric maintenance. The three transposable elements, called *HeT-A, TART,* and *TAHRE,* are non-LTR retrotransposons (see Chapter 8 for these terms). They are transcribed to RNA, which is exported to the cytoplasm, where it is translated to produce reverse transcriptase and GAG protein that helps re-importing the RNA to the nucleus. The RNA is targeted to the telomeres, where the reverse transcriptase uses the 3′-OH end of the DNA to prime reverse transcription of the RNA. No telomerase enzyme is involved nor any RNA primer as in mammals. Telomere maintenance mechanisms are a striking example of the way in which billion-year-old conservation can coexist side by side with radical innovation in carrying out a fundamental process.

Centromeres

Centromeres are the chromosomal sites where the kinetochore assembles. This is the structure to which the microtubules that form the spindle attach to separate chromosomes when cells divide. A centromere holds together two sister chromatids and, during mitosis, ensures that one of the two segregates to each daughter cell so that each cell receives one complete set of chromosomes. Each chromosome needs one and only one centromere. A chromosome without centromere would segregate randomly to a daughter cell and a chromosome with two centromeres would be pulled apart at mitosis. Unlike telomeres, centromeres do not involve a specific DNA sequence, except in lower eukaryotes like budding yeast, *Saccharomyces cerevisiae*, where a DNA sequence specifies the binding site of the kinetochore. In the fission yeast *Saccharomyces pombe*, centromeres and numerous other features resemble instead those of higher eukaryotes: they form in a particular region of the chromosome but are not determined by a specific sequence. While local sequence features are preferred sites, centromere formation is epigenetically determined: it is the site where a previous centromere was assembled. If this site is deleted, a new centromere will form in the region. Some organisms such as the nematode *Caenorhabditis elegans* or insects like lepidopterans (butterflies and moths) have no specific centromere site. Rather, the centromere forms all along the length of the chromosome. This points out once again that even basic, fundamental structures such as centromeres and telomeres are not necessarily conserved in all organisms and remarkable innovations can occur in evolution even within a phylogenetic branch.

During interphase, the sister chromatids formed by the replication of chromosomal DNA are held together all along their lengths by the cohesin complex (more about cohesin in Chapter 8). During mitosis, however, cohesin is lost along the chromosome except in the centromere region, where the two sister chromatids continue to be held together as the chromosomes compact under the action of condensin, a large protein complex related to the cohesin complex.

Centromere assembly is initiated by the formation of modified nucleosomes containing a variant of histone H3 (called CENP-A in humans). This occurs in the regions containing protein components of the preceding centromere (see Chapter 2). CENP-A-containing nucleosomes recruit inner kinetochore components CENP-C, CENP-H, CENP-I. Numerous additional components form different layers of the kinetochore.

Further Reading

Alberts B, Johnson A, Lewis J, Raff M, Roberts K and Walter P (2014). *Molecular Biology of the Cell* (6th ed.). Garland. Chapter 4: DNA, Chromosomes and Genomes.

Armanios M and Blackburn EH (2012). The telomere syndromes. *Nat Rev Genet.* **13**, 693–704.

Capra JA, Paeschke K, Mona S and Zakian VA (2010). G-quadruplex DNA sequences are evolutionarily conserved and associated with distinct genomic features in *Saccharomyces cerevisiae*. *PLOS Comput Biol.* **6**, e1000861.

Casacuberta E (2017). *Drosophila*: Retrotransposons making up telomeres. *Viruses.* **9**, 192.

Champoux JJ (2001). DNA topoisomerases: Structure, function, and mechanism. *Annu Rev Biochem.* **70**, 369–413.

Geggier S and Vologodskii A (2010). Sequence dependence of DNA bending rigidity. *Proc Natl Acad Sci USA.* **107**, 1542–15426.

Landschulz WH, Johnson PF and McKnight SL (1988). The leucine zipper: A hypothetical structure common to a new class of DNA binding proteins. *Science.* **240**, 1759–1764.

Maeder ML, Thibodeau-Beganny S, Osiak A, Wright DA, Anthony RM, Eichtinger M *et al.* (2008). Rapid "open-source" engineering of customized zinc-ninger Nucleases for highly efficient gene modification. *Mol Cell.* **31**, 294–301.

Nikolova EN, Kim E, Wise AA, O'Brien PJ, Andricioaei I and Al-Hashimi HM (2011). Transient Hoogsteen base pairs in canonical duplex DNA. *Nature.* **470**, 498–502.

Perrini B, Piacentini L, Fanti L, Altieri F, Chichiarelli S, Berloco M *et al.* (2004). HP1 controls telomere capping, telomere elongation, and telomere silencing by two different mechanisms in *Drosophila*. *Mol Cell.* **15**, 467–476.

Rhodes D and Lipps HJ (2015). G-quadruplexes and their regulatory roles in biology. *Nucleic Acids Res.* **43**, 8627–8637.

Struhl K (1989). Helix-turn-helix, zinc-finger, and leucine-zipper motifs for eukaryotic transcriptional regulatory proteins. *Trends Biochem Sci.* **14**, 137–140.

Tomaska L, Nosek J, Kar A, Wilcox S and Griffith JD (2019). A new view of the T-loop junction: Implications for self-primed telomere extension, expansion of disease-related nucleotide repeat blocks, and telomere evolution. *Frontiers Genet.* **10**, 792.

Zhang Q, Kim NK and Feigon J (2011). Architecture of human telomerase RNA. *Proc Natl Acad Sci USA.* **108**, 20325–20332.

Chapter 2

Chromatin

Introduction

Genomic DNA in eukaryotes is not readily accessible to the transcriptional or the regulatory machinery. It is organized into chromatin, so named by Flemming in 1879 because it stains brightly with a dye that we now know stains DNA. The same material condenses into the well-known rod-like chromosomes during mitosis. At the end of mitosis most of this material decondenses to occupy the nucleus, but some part of it remains highly condensed and strongly staining in interphase nuclei. This was called heterochromatin: a different kind of chromatin that did not decondense. Whether condensed or decondensed, chromatin contains DNA and protein, most of which is represented by the histones. Histones are a set of small and highly basic proteins, closely related to one another and very highly conserved among eukaryotes. Although this was well known by the mid-20th century, it was not until 1974, with the publication of the structural and biochemical studies of Kornberg and Thomas (1974) that the organization of the four core histones H2A, H2B, H3, and H4, plus the linker histone H1, was understood to form a repeating structure combined with DNA to form chromatin. The repeating unit that is the basis of chromatin is called the nucleosome, first observed by electron microscopy (Olins and Olins, 1974) (Figure 1). Strings of nucleosomes were proposed to constitute a flexibly jointed chromatin fiber (Kornberg, 1974), with the typical "beads on a string" appearance.

31

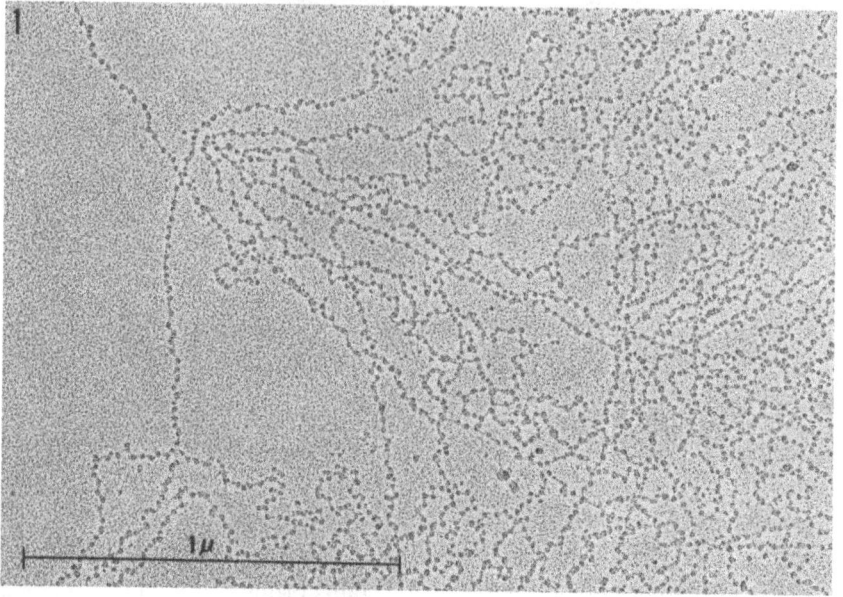

Figure 1. Nucleosome fibers. In this electron micrograph, chromatin appears in the "bead-on-a-string" form of extended nucleosome fibers.

Source: McKnight and Miller (1976).

Partial digestion of chromatin with nucleases confirms the repetitive nature of chromatin structure. Nucleosomal DNA is in fact more resistant to micrococcal nuclease, a small enzyme that cuts preferentially in the linker region between nucleosomes, releasing the more nuclease-resistant nucleosomal core. Partial micrococcal digestion produces oligonucleosomes: strings of two, three, four, or more nucleosomes still connected by linker DNA (Figure 2). Longer digestion reduces the larger fragments to shorter ones and eventually to mononucleosomes. The nucleosome consists of 147 bp of DNA wrapped 1.7 turns around a core formed by a heterooctamer of the four core histones (Figure 3). The octamer in turn can fall apart into a (H3-H4)$_2$ tetramer and two H2A-H2B dimers. The (H3-H4)$_2$ tetramer is the most stable intermediate and the core of the nucleosome.

The histones are evolutionarily ancient proteins, first clearly detectable in all branches of *Archaea* where they play a similar role, forming a

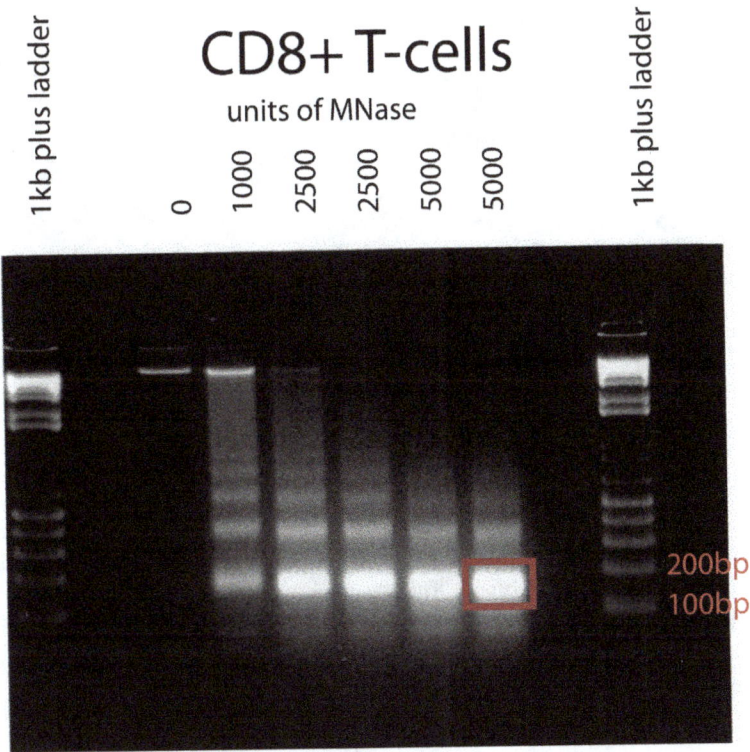

Figure 2. Micrococcal nuclease nucleosome ladders. Chromatin partially digested with increasing amounts of micrococcal nuclease and analyzed by agarose gel electrophoresis shows a ladder of bands representing DNA more resistent to digestion. The ladder corresponds to nucleosome monomers, dimers, trimers, and higher.

Source: Valouev *et al.* (2011).

core around which genomic DNA is wrapped. Among eukaryotes, the sequence of the four core histones is exceptionally highly conserved. This indicates that their amino acid sequence is so highly adapted for the complex roles they play that very little change can be tolerated without losing functional fitness. Structurally, all four core histones are small proteins, between 102 and 135 amino acids in length (Figure 4). All four have a globular central domain flanked by a C-terminal tail and a longer N-terminal tail particularly rich in the basic amino acids lysine and arginine. The globular part consists of three alpha-helical segments connected

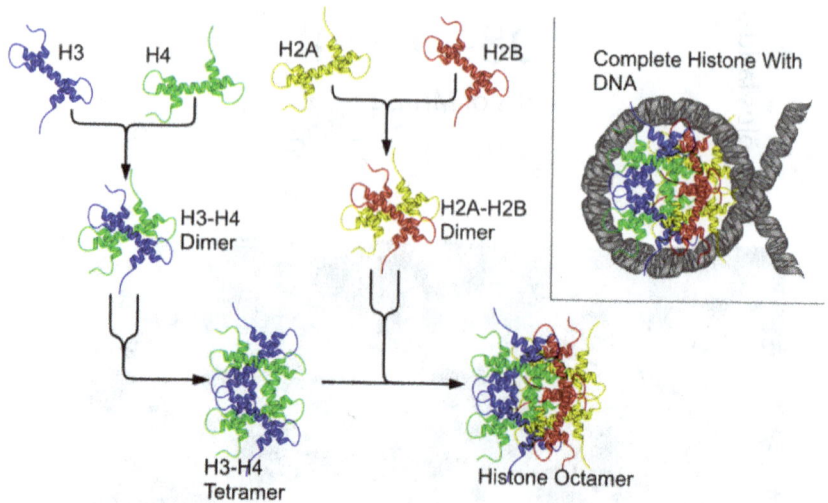

Figure 3.   The nucleosome. It consists of 147 bp of double-stranded DNA wrapped 1.7 turns around a core of eight histones. The octamer in turn has a stable heterotetramer core consisting of two h3-H4 dimers. To this core are associated two H2A-H2B heterodimers.

Source: Richard Wheeler (Zephyris), Creative Commons, https://commons.wikimedia.org/wiki/File:Nucleosome_structure.png.

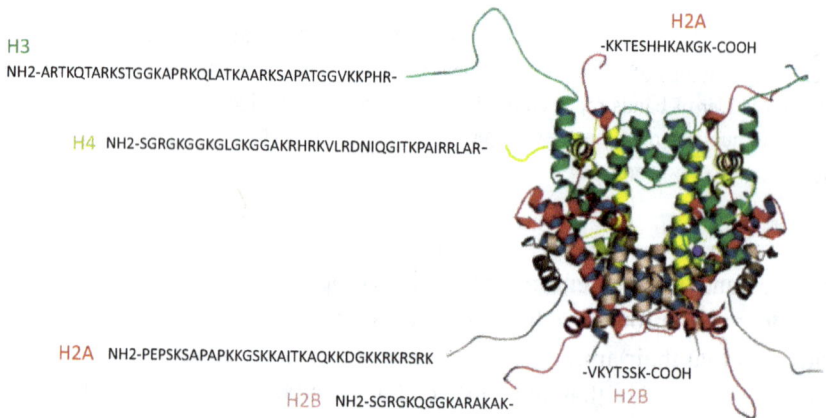

Figure 4.   The core histones. The histones are shown in the structural representation of the core octamer with two copies of each: H3 (green), H4 (yellow), H2A (red), and H2B (orange). The sequences of the N-terminal and C-terminal tails are shown. Adapted from Khorasanizadeh (2004).

by short loops that fold the helical segments into a characteristic histone fold that mediates histone–histone interactions. Two histone globular domains align in antiparallel orientation to form the characteristic "handshake" structure (Figure 5). The H3-H4 heterodimeric interaction is much more favored than the H3-H3 or H4-H4 interaction and two H3-H4 heterodimers assemble further to form a stable heterotetramer (H3-H4)$_2$. The evolutionary precursors of histones found in *Archaea* are either a single histone-like protein or multiple related proteins that correspond to the histone fold domain of eukaryotic histones. The archaeal monomers form both homo-dimers and heterodimers with the characteristic "handshake" interaction. These assemble into tetramers that protect about 60 bp of DNA from nuclease digestion, instead of the 147 bp of the eukaryotic nucleosome.

The H2A and H2B histones also form heterodimers through their histone fold domains. Interactions between the H2B component and the H4 component of the (H3-H4)$_2$ tetramer result in one H2A-H2B heterodimer binding to each side of the H3-H4 tetramer to form the histone octamer. Each of the paired histone fold domains can further interact with phosphates of the double-stranded DNA backbone folded around the

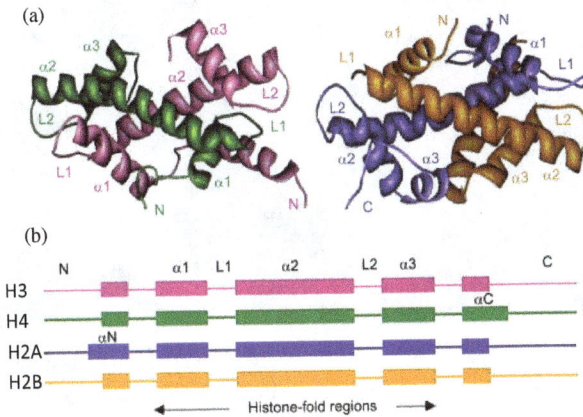

Figure 5. The histone fold and handshake motifs. (a) The H3–H4 "handshake" interaction and H2A–H2B "handshake". (b) Schematic representation of the globular domains of the four core histones with the alpha helices that constitute the histone fold.

Source: Ramaswamy and Ioshikhes (2013).

histone octamer. As a result, each pair is in close contact with a segment of 27–28 base pairs, separated by four base pairs. Overall then the core histone octamer is wrapped by 1.7 turns of double-stranded DNA to produce a disk-like particle roughly the shape of a hockey puck about 11 nm in diameter and 6 nm thick (Figure 6). The rounded edge of the disc is largely made up of DNA, but the flat site also gives access to the histone core surrounded by the DNA. It should be noted that the DNA is not smoothly curved around the histone core but is more sharply bent or kinked at the points of contact with the histones. The double helix needs to be bent or deformed to form a nucleosome and, in fact, some sequences are better suited than others. In general, there is a preference for GC dinucleotides to be on the outer edge of the DNA at 10 bp intervals, and AA,

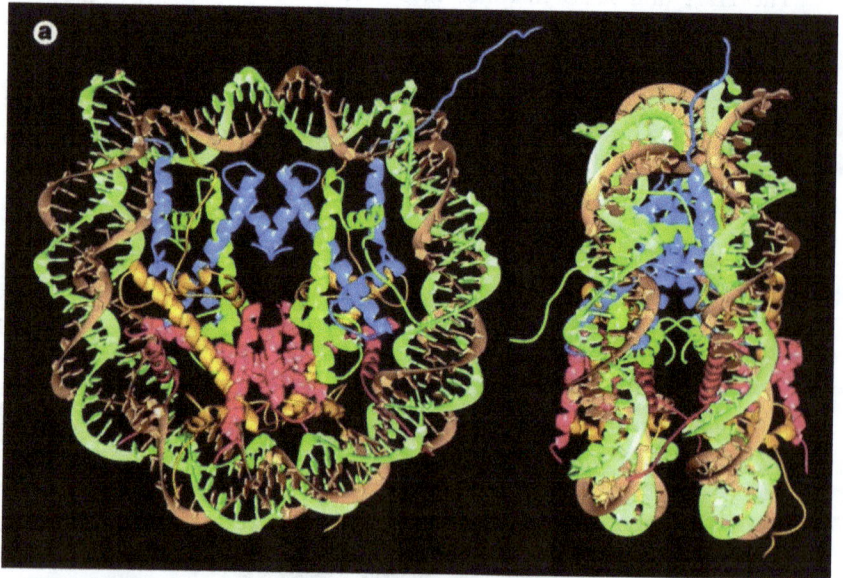

Figure 6.   The nucleosome particle. The DNA enters top left and exits near top right. This defines an axis of pseudo-symmetry also with respect to the histone octamer and its interactions with the DNA (H3, blue; H4, green; H2A, yellow; H2B, red). The image on the right represents the same nucleosome rotated around the axis of pseudo-symmetry to be viewed sideways. The histone tails, particularly the longer N-terminal tails protrude through the DNA and wave loosely.

Source: Luger *et al.* (1997).

TT, or TA dinucleotides to be on the inner side at 10 bp intervals out of phase with the GCs. This configuration facilitates the sharp bends required. In contrast, the linker DNA between nucleosomes shows preference for sequences, such as poly(A:T), that make the helix stiffer and less easy to bend around the histone core.

Nucleosome Stability

When viewed in a space-filling model, the nucleosome appears as a solid disk-shaped structure with the DNA so tightly wrapped that only the outer edge of the double helix is accessible from the outside. The histone N-terminal tails protrude between the DNA loops and are readily accessible (Figure 7). With the high number of lysines and arginines, the

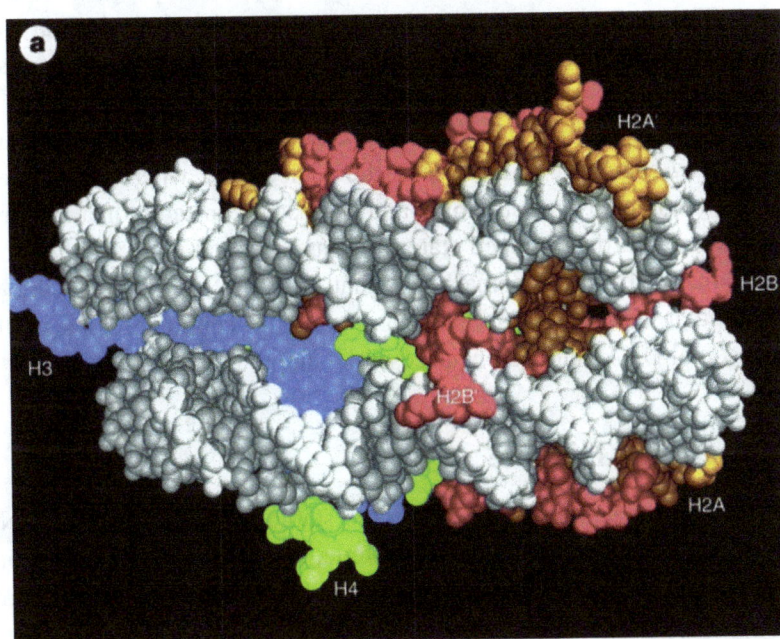

Figure 7. Histone tails protrude through the DNA. The H2B (red) and H3 (blue) N-terminal tails pass through channels in the DNA superhelix (white) formed by aligned minor grooves. They are therefore available for interactions with proteins or with other nucleosomes.

Source: Luger *et al.* (1997).

N-terminal tails are normally positively charged and tend to associate with the negatively charged phosphates of the DNA backbone, tightening the nucleosome structure. Structural requirements for histone fold and histone interactions, on the one hand, and interactions with the DNA wrapped around the histone core, on the other, account for much of the extreme sequence conservation in the globular part of the four histones. The N-terminal tails are not so structured, but they are also very highly conserved. The reason for this is the large number of specific interactions with the machinery that regulates chromatin structure and function.

Wrapping around the histone core protects DNA from interactions with proteins, from enzymes that degrade DNA, from small molecules that might damage DNA and cause mutations. The reason for this protection is that most proteins that interact with DNA need to see more than just one edge of the double helix. The tight winding prevents productive interactions. The nucleosome structure is very stable under physiological conditions, but it can of course unwrap and does so occasionally spontaneously if left to itself. The half-life of a nucleosome under these conditions is of the order of one hour, remarkably stable for a biological structure. Unwrapping begins from the ends of the nucleosome, where DNA enters or leaves the nucleosome structure, and can occur constantly in a dynamic equilibrium with the wrapped state. The nucleosomal ends are therefore the regions of the nucleosomal DNA that are more readily accessible to proteins that bind to DNA. However, even the central regions of the nucleosomal DNA can become accessible, due to thermal fluctuations.

H1, the Fifth Histone

The nucleosome can be made even more stable by tying down the DNA extremities. This is done by the H1 histone, also called the linker histone because it binds to the DNA as it enters and as it leaves the nucleosome to join with the next nucleosome in a nucleosome array. Electron micrographs show that, in the presence of H1, the two DNA ends remain associated for 3–5 nm as they leave the nucleosome core, giving the chromatin fiber a characteristic zig-zag appearance (Figure 8) The length of the linker DNA between two nucleosomes varies somewhat from one region of the genome to another or from one tissue to another but ranges from

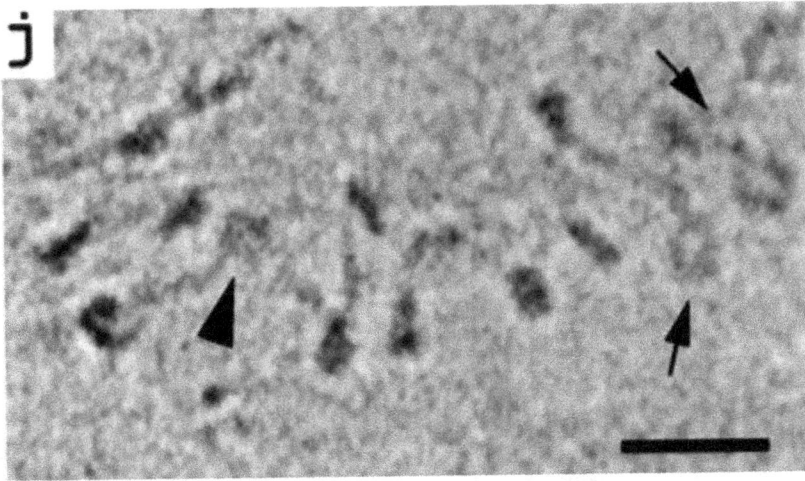

Figure 8.   Chromatin containing H1 histone. Chromatin released from nuclei and imaged without staining often shows a typical zig-zag conformation. This is caused by the binding of the H1 linker histone to the DNA ends as they enter and leave the nucleosome. When the nucleosome is appropriately oriented, lying flat, this H1-dependent stem conformation can be seen as indicated by the arrows. The arrowheads indicate nucleosomes that clearly lack the H1 histone.

Source: Bednar *et al.* (1998).

30 bp in the presence of H1 linker histone to 80 bp in its absence. Histone H1 appears to bind near the dyad axis of the nucleosome and protect additional 15–30 bp of DNA (Figure 9).

Histone H1 is evolutionarily the most ancient of the histones, with a recognizable homolog found in bacteria. It is also less well conserved than the core histones, although its globular domain is better conserved than its C- and N-terminal tails. H1 is loosely and dynamically bound to the nucleosome, but it is so closely associated with chromatin that it rebinds rapidly and spends most of its time in the bound state. There are several H1 variants in the human genome, with different levels of expression in different tissues and developmental stages. In addition, histone modifications (methylation, phosphorylation) and binding of proteins such as HP1 or p53 can modulate the role of H1 variants so that, although predominantly associated with chromatin condensation and repression, some forms can actually promote transcriptional activity.

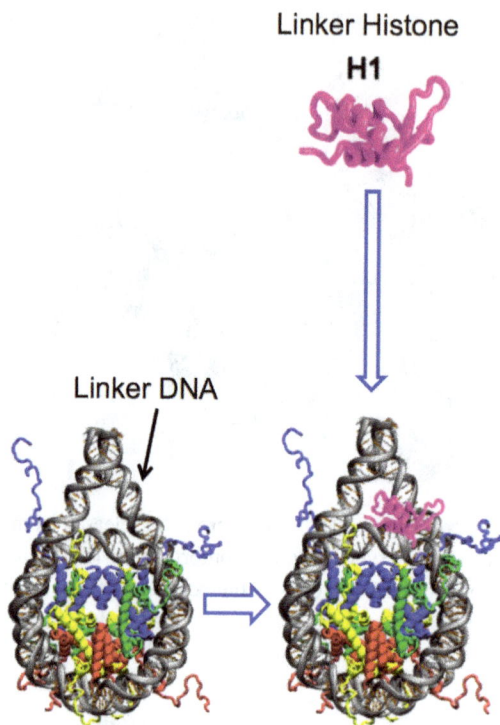

Figure 9.   Histone H1 binding to nucleosome. The linker histone H1 binds to the DNA as it enters and leaves the nucleosome, holding the two together and stabilizing the nucleosome in a form sometimes called the chromatosome.

Source: Draizen *et al.* (2016).

Reconstitution of Nucleosomes on DNA *in vitro*

The reassembly of nucleosomes from purified histones and DNA has been an important tool in the study of histones, their modifications and their effects on nucleosomes and their interacting factors. Histones can now be expressed in bacteria with or without specific mutations. Purified histones can assemble into histone H3+H4 tetramers and H2A+H2B dimers by refolding the proteins and dialysing them from high to low salt concentrations. Alternatively, the core histones can be co-expressed in bacteria and the octamers directly purified from the bacterial extracts. To assemble on DNA, almost any DNA sequence can be used. However, there are distinct preferences for sequences that best accommodate the sharp bends and twists required for wrapping around the histone core. Thus, AT-rich motifs, which favor bending, are found preferentially at 10 bp intervals and at the sharp bends, while GC motifs, which favor stiffness, are found in between the AT-rich motifs. Certain sequences in the genome are therefore optimal while other sequences tend to form less stable nucleosomes. This is exploited in the genome so that, for example, transcription start sites in genes have sequences less favorable for nucleosome formation and are therefore more readily available for transcription initiation. (see also Chapter 6). One of many commonly used DNA fragments whose sequences bias the positioning of the histones is the Widom 601 (Lowary and Widom, 1998). To reconstitute the nucleosome, the purified histone octamer is incubated with the DNA fragment of choice in a high salt concentration, usually 2M NaCl. This is necessary to overcome the intrinsic repulsion of the DNA phosphates and therefore the reluctance to fold into a tight volume. Progressive dialysis against lower salt concentrations allows the DNA folding to occur gradually, finding the energy-optimal wrapped configuration. The assembled nucleosome is then purified from the free octamer and assembly intermediates using gel electrophoresis, gradient centrifugation, or gel filtration.

Higher Order Structures

Decondensed chromatin during interphase when spread for imaging by electron microscopy has the appearance of a series of beads connected by a string of DNA. The DNA can be seen to enter and leave the nucleosome at an angle, but the average thickness of such a string of nucleosomes is roughly 10 nanometers (Figure 10). Fully decondensed chromatin is therefore said to form a 10 nm fiber, in the absence of salt to screen the repulsion between the phosphates of the DNA wrapped around each nucleosome. However, in the presence of salt (positive metal ions) to screen the charges, nucleosomes tend to be sticky and interact easily with one another to form higher order assemblies. *In vitro*, the addition of the linker histone H1 to 10 nm fibers at appropriate buffer conditions can induce the formation of a more condensed form of chromatin in which nucleosomes stack to form a fiber 30 nm thick (Figure 10). This regular

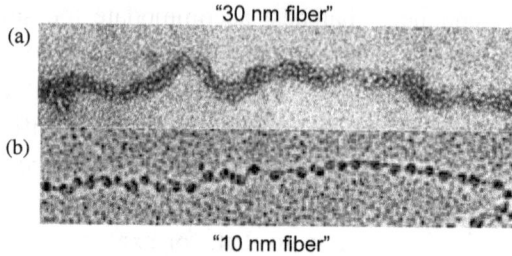

Figure 10.   Chromatin fibers. The chromatin fiber visualized by the electron microscope. The lower image is the beads-on-a-string open chromatin fiber. *Source*: McKnight and Miller (1976). The upper image is the 30 nm fiber, which forms in vitro in the presence of Mg++. *Source*: Barbara Hamkalo. This was thought to be the conformation of condensed chromatin in heterochromatin or repressed genomic regions.

stacking is stabilized by the regular interactions between nucleosomes and prevents the access of proteins to the underlying DNA. The progressive condensation of chromatin from 10 nm fiber to 30 nm fiber to higher order coiling of the 30 nm fiber into 120 nm fibers, 300 nm fibers, and eventually to a condensed mitotic chromosome has been assumed by textbooks for 40 years. Chromatin fibers isolated from cells do in fact appear in the electron microscope as regular fibers about 30 nm thick, much like *in vitro* reconstituted fibers. It seems clear that some such structure is a stable configuration that tends to be assumed by isolated nucleosome strings in the presence of magnesium ion sufficient to screen the phosphate charges so that the nucleosomes interact with their nearest neighbors. Regardless of the precise structural configuration of the nucleosomes, it seems evident that a 30 nm fiber arrangement would make it very difficult for proteins to access the DNA and was therefore the structure thought to be prevalent in heterochromatin (see Chapter 5). This makes it particularly important to determine the structural bases of chromatin in condensed states that occur *in vivo*. Over the years much work has gone into determining the arrangement of nucleosomes in a 30 nm fiber. At the same time, many studies looking at chromatin in the nucleus have failed to detect evidence of a 30 nm fiber structural organization, beginning with the foundational work in cryo-electron microscopy of Jacques Dubochet. Most recently, cryo-electron microscopy, electron microscopy combined with tomography, superresolution optical imaging, and other advanced techniques have been brought to bear. It appears that a 30 nm fiber structure rarely occurs *in vivo* for stretches of chromatin of any significant length. Electron microscopy approaches indicate instead that in interphase cells chromatin is organized in disordered nucleosome chains with diameters ranging from 5 to 24 nm (Figure 11). In more highly condensed regions such chains are more densely packed together but without assuming regular higher order structures (Figure 12). The question of how chromatin is folded and arranged in the nucleus, the genomic architecture at different scales, will be taken up in more detail later in this book (see Chapter 8).

DNA-binding Proteins

Free DNA is available to interact with DNA-binding proteins that can read the sequence and therefore bind specifically to their corresponding site. This is essential for the regulated expression of the information contained in the DNA sequence. To read the DNA sequence, specific DNA-binding proteins must be able to probe inside the double helix through one of the two deep grooves in the helix and interact specifically with the bases of the nucleotides.

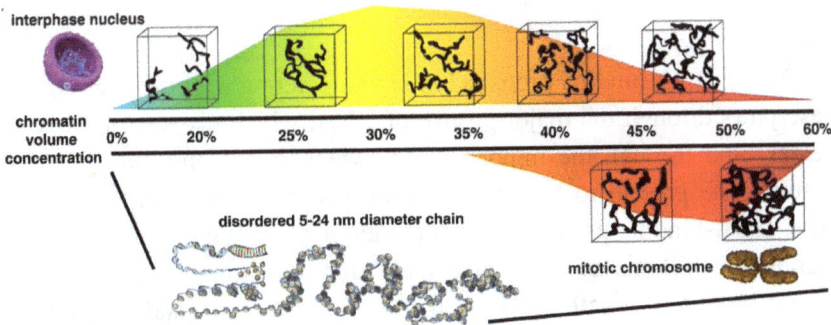

Figure 11.   High resolution Electron Microscope tomography visualization of chromatin. This novel technique reveals chromatin as a lumpy fiber of variable thickness without higher order structure but with increasing concentration from interphase euchromatin, to heterochromatin, and even in mitotic chromosomes.

Source: Ou *et al.* (2017).

Beads on a string

Euchromatin

Heterochromatin

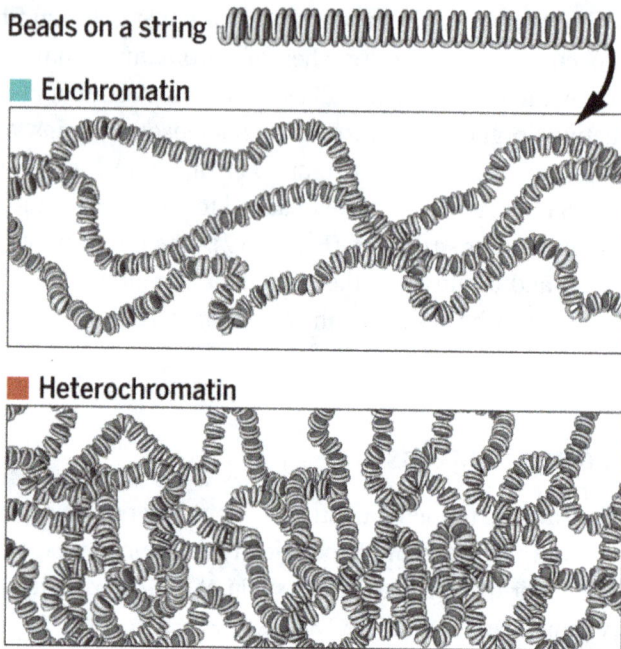

Figure 12.   New view of chromatin packaging. An interpretation of the results in Figure 43. In the upper image, euchromatin appears as a variable thickness but basically linear beads-on-a-string fiber. In the lower image, corresponding to heterochromatin, the fiber structure is the same but more fibers are packed per unit volume.

Source: Larson and Misteli (2017).

Many DNA-binding proteins bind by interacting with the edges of the base pairs through the major groove of DNA, which gives easier access. Fewer bind through the minor groove, which is not only narrower but requires the protein to bypass the sugar–phosphate backbone. In either case, DNA-binding proteins must find their appropriate binding sequence among the billions of nucleotide pairs that constitute a genome. This would be a very lengthy process if the protein had to randomly hit the DNA until the appropriate sequence is encountered. Instead, DNA-binding proteins also bind weakly and non-specifically to the exterior of the double helix, interacting with the sugar-phosphate backbone. This enables a protein to slide along the DNA sampling the nucleotide base pairs, pausing when it meets a sequence close to the optimal, then moving on until it finds the exact recognition sequence, which provides the most stable interaction. To read the base pairs, a DNA-binding protein must be able to delve deep enough into the DNA groove to interact with the several base pairs that constitute the binding site.

It is clear from this description that a nucleosome would create a formidable obstacle to the ability of a DNA-binding protein to scan and bind to its recognition sequence. The nucleosomal DNA is bent and twisted. More importantly, the interactions of the DNA with the core histones make it difficult for a DNA-binding protein to reach into the groove to interact effectively with the base pairs. This brings us to one of the most important roles of the nucleosomal organization of chromatin. It is often said that the wrapping of DNA in nucleosomes is necessary to make the enormous length of genomic DNA fit in a microscopic cell nucleus. The total length of human genomic DNA in a somatic cell is just under two meters, while the diameter of the nucleus in such a cell is around 5 micrometers or 5 millionths of a meter. Clearly, the DNA must be well folded to fit in the nucleus. However, as we have seen, the persistence length of naked DNA is around 50 nanometers, meaning that the double helix could be doubled up in a space 100 times shorter than the diameter of the nucleus. Folding into nucleosomes is highly orderly, but not the only way to fit the DNA in the nucleus.

The Nucleosome and DNA Accessibility

In fact, the major function of the nucleosomal organization of genomic DNA is not packaging to fit large amounts of DNA in the nucleus. More important is the imperative to hide the DNA so that it is less easily accessible to the protein machinery that needs to act on it. To turn on or repress a specific gene, transcription factors must be able to read the DNA sequence that alone distinguishes one gene from another. To do this job effectively, they have to bind to DNA with sufficient specificity to minimize the noise that would result from binding to inappropriate sequences. Most DNA-binding proteins recognize sequences around 12 nucleotides long. This is far from sufficient to guarantee that the sequence will be unique in a genome of over 10^9 base pairs such as the human genome. A key feature of the nucleosome is that it renders access to the DNA very difficult. Even if individual base pairs may be read, the wrapping of the DNA around the histone core interferes with interaction with and recognition of the entire binding sequence. Nucleosomes hinder the binding of most of the DNA-binding proteins that act upon the genome and express its genomic information. Only certain types of factors, called pioneer factors (see Chapter 6, for Enhancers) can overcome this difficulty and bind to nucleosomal DNA. They do this in different ways. Some, like FoxA1, have a winged-helix DNA-binding domain that resembles that of histone H1. Others, can bind successfully to a partial sequence on the outer surface of the nucleosome. Nucleosomes in effect hide much of the DNA sequence. This is important because the concentration of DNA in the cell nucleus is extremely high and DNA-binding proteins have a significant non-specific affinity for DNA. Instead of enabling the proteins to find their optimal binding sequence, this affinity would oblige DNA-binding proteins to spend most of their time interacting with the wrong regions of the genome. The nucleosomal organization of the DNA therefore reduces the amount of DNA sequence that DNA-binding proteins need to scan.

The density of nucleosomes is known to be important for correct gene expression. If insufficient histones are produced, nucleosomal density is reduced. This happens, for example, in *Drosophila* when about half of the histone genes are removed by a deletion. The result is not an explosion of the nucleus due to decondensation of the DNA. Rather, what happens is the derepression or random expression of many genes, which have become too easily accessed by transcription factors. RNA polymerase, in particular, no longer needs the help of many transcription factors or nucleosome remodeling machines to access the DNA. The formation of heterochromatin is greatly reduced.

So nucleosomes are needed to mask the DNA. At the same time, however, packaging up the DNA so that most of the genomic sequence cannot be read would render the genome undifferentiated. Somehow, some nucleosomes need to be differentiated from others or marked to distinguish them as more appropriate for attention in any particular cell. As we will see in the rest of this book, much of epigenetics consists of mechanisms and strategies to differentiate certain nucleosomes and selectively expose certain DNA sequences to facilitate the binding of appropriate DNA-binding proteins to the genes that need to be expressed at any one time in a given cell.

Histone Modifications as Signals

If the sequence of nucleosomal DNA cannot be read, one nucleosome would look much the same as another, seen from the outside. Chromatin would then become a string of identical particles. How can individual nucleosomes or whole sets of nucleosomes be modified or tagged to differentiate them from the rest and favor their interactions with different chromatin machineries? Nucleosomes have several important variables associated with them that serve to distinguish their features and how they impact the behavior of chromatin. One is their positioning: what sequences are wrapped up and what sequences form the linkers between nucleosomes. Another is what histone variants are recruited to form a nucleosome (we will deal with this aspect further down in this chapter). A very important set of variables consists of a number of post-translational modifications that can occur on histones after they are assembled into a nucleosome.

The N-terminal tails of the core histones protrude between the DNA gyres wound around the histone core (see Figure 7) and are, in principle, readily available for interactions with the solvent and with other proteins that act upon chromatin. The histone tails are rich in the basic amino acids lysine and arginine. At neutral pH, the basic tails are positively charged and will interact with the DNA phosphates, lying flat against the DNA and contributing to the stabilization of the nucleosome. The N-terminal tails, particularly the two longest, the H3 and H4 tails, are the targets of a large number of enzymes that add post-translational modifications that alter the behavior of the tails and, more importantly, that are recognized by a variety of protein factors that interact with chromatin.

A large number of post-transcriptional histone modifications have been identified in chromatin, some rare, some very frequent and well-characterized. Table 1 reports some of the most important, but by no means all, modifications that have been reported. These include acetylation, methylation, phosphorylation, ubiquitylation, to mention just the better known. Figure 13 displays most of those affecting the histone tails. Most of these modifications involve lysine residues (acetylation, methylation, ubiquitylation); methylation can also affect arginine; phosphorylation can modify serine and threonine. Several modifications (to different amino acids) can be present at the same time on one histone and a

Table 1.   Histone modifications.

Modification	Histone	Site	Enzyme	Associated function
Acetylation	H2A	K5	Tip60	Transcription activation
			p300/CBP	Transcription activation
			Esa1	Transcription activation
	H2B	K5	ATF2	Transcription activation
		K12	p300/CBP	Transcription activation
		K15	p300/CBP	Transcription activation
			ATF2	Transcription activation
		K20	p300	Transcription activation
	H3	K4	Esa1	Transcription activation
		K9	Gcn5	Transcription activation
			SRC-1	Transcription activation
		K14	GCN5, PCAF	Transcription activation
			Esa1, Tip60	Transcription activation
				DNA repair
			SRC-1	Transcription activation
			Elp3	Transcription elongation
			hTFIIIC90	RNA Pol III transcription
			TAF1	RNA Pol II transcription
			P300	Transcription activation
			Sas3	Transcription activation
		K18	GCN5	Transcription activation
				DNA repair
			p300/CBP	Transcription activation
				DNA replication
		K23	GCN5	Transcription activation
			Sas3	DNA repair
			p300/CBP	Transcription activation
		K27	p300/CBP	Transcription activation
	H4	K5	Hat1	Histone deposition
			Esa1, Tip60	Transcription activation
				DNA repair

Table 1. (*Continued*)

Modification	Histone	Site	Enzyme	Associated function
			ATF2	Transcription activation
			p300	Transcription activation
		K8	Gcn5, PCAF	Transcription activation
			Esa1, Tip60	Transcription activation
			DNA repair	
			ATF2	Transcription activation
			p300	Transcription activation
		K12	Hat1	Histone deposition
				Telomeric silencing
			Esa1, Tip60	Transcription activation
				DNA repair
		K16	Gcn5	Transcription activation
			MOF	Transcription activation
			Tip60	DNA repair
			ATF2	Transcription activation
Methylation	H3	R2	PRMT6	Me2a, Transcription repression
		K4	Set9	Me3, Transcription activation
			MLL1,2, Trx	Transcription activation
			Ash1, ASH1L	Transcription activation
		R8		
		K9	SUV39H	Transcription silencing
				Me3, DNA methylation
			G9a	Transcription silencing
			SETDB1	Me3, Transcription repression
		R17	CARM1	Me2s, Transcription activation
		R26	CARM1	Me2s, Transcription activation
		K27	EZH1,2	Transcription silencing
				X inactivation
		K36	SET2	Transcription elongation, splicing, deacetylation
			ASH1L	Transcription activation

(*Continued*)

Table 1.   (*Continued*)

Modification	Histone	Site	Enzyme	Associated function
		K79	DOT1L	Open chromatin, D?NA repair
	H4	R3	PRMT1	Me2s, Transcription activation
		K20	PR-Set7	Me1, Transcription silencing
			SUV4-20H	Me3, Heterochromatin
Phosphorylation	H2A	S1		Mitosis
		T119	NHK-1	Mitosis
	H2B	S14	MST1	Apoptosis
		S33	TAF1	Transcriptional activation
	H3	T3		Mitosis
		S10	Aurora-B	Mitosis
			MSK1,2	Transcription activation
		T11	DLK/ZIP	Mitosis
		S28	Aurora-B	Mitosis
			MSK1,2	Transcription activation
	H4	S1		Mitosis
Ubiquitylation	H2A	K119	HR6A,B	Spermatogenesis
			PRC1	Polycomb repression
	H2B	K120	HR6A,B	meiosis
			RNF20	Transcription activation, DNA damage repair
			BRCA1/BARD1	DNA damage repair

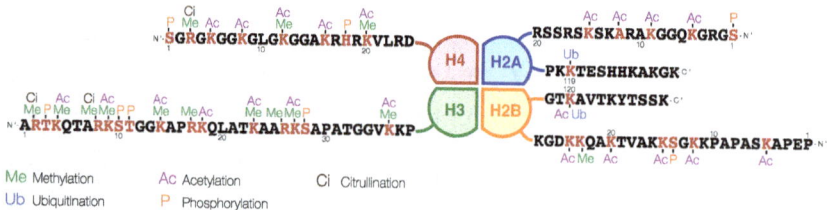

Figure 13.   Histone tail modifications. The principal post-transcriptional modifications are shown. A few modifications are also found in the globular domains (not shown).

Source: Mariuswalter, Creative Commons, https://commons.wikimedia.org/wiki/File:Histone_modifications.png.

modification at one position can occur on one or both copies of that histone in a nucleosome. In addition, lysine can accept one, two, or three methyl groups and the three degrees of methylation occur in different circumstances (Figure 14). Arginine has two equivalent nitrogens that can be methylated so dimethylation presents two choices: both methyl groups on the same nitrogen (asymmetric) or one on each nitrogen (symmetric) (Figure 15). Here also the two configurations occur in different chromatin

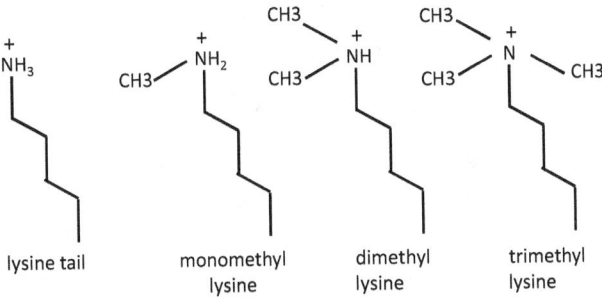

lysine tail   monomethyl lysine   dimethyl lysine   trimethyl lysine

Figure 14. Lysine methylation. Lysine can be mono-, di-, or tri-methylated, the last by acquiring a permanent positive charge. Only the lysine sidechain is shown (compare with Figure 16). A variety of lysine metyltransferases can catalyse this modification, each generally specific for particular lysine residues. The donor is the universal methyl donor S-adenosyl methionine, also used as the methyl donor for DNA methylation (see DNA methylation chapter).

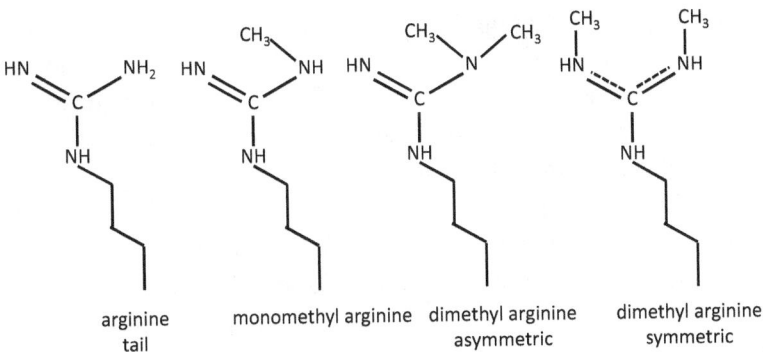

arginine tail   monomethyl arginine   dimethyl arginine asymmetric   dimethyl arginine symmetric

Figure 15. Arginine methylation. The arginine sidechain shown can be mono- and di-methylated. The latter has two possible forms: symmetric and asymmetric. The symmetric and asymmetric forms are produced by different enzymes and are read by different reader proteins.

contexts. With so many different ways of marking a nucleosome, the number becomes astronomical if we consider all the combinations (assuming all marks are independent), the potential for differential marking of nucleosomes and therefore of chromatin regions is enormous. There are in fact different enzymes and protein complexes responsible for producing these modifications. These have been called the "writers" of the histone marks. There are also, in most cases, chromatin proteins able to recognize the different marks. These have been called "readers". Much discussion and debate has taken place about whether these marks could be taken to constitute a "histone code", with different marks or perhaps even different combinations of marks conveying different instructions for chromatin proteins to carry out specific functions. Histone code? Perhaps not in the same sense as the genetic code, where the base triplets play no other role than to connect the DNA sequence information with the amino acid sequence information. At least some of the histone modifications change the physical properties of the nucleosomes that carry them and are therefore more than carriers of information. However, it is certainly true that many histone marks occur in particular chromatin contexts and their presence can be shown to have specific effects on chromatin activities. Their role is code-like in the sense that at least some of the histone modifications convey signals whose value assignment is in some way arbitrary, that is it is not dependent on the physico-chemical properties of the modification, and is read by specific machinery that has evolved to recognize that signal. In the sense that different marks have definite associated functions, I think that we are justified in saying that the set of histone marks constitute a "code" of sorts that is "written" by specific chromatin complexes in certain situations and is "read" by other chromatin complexes with certain resulting effects on that chromatin region. Much of this textbook is an account of the different chromatin activities and the role played by the histone marks. You, the reader, may decide whether it is useful to call the rules governing these activities a "code", at least in a limited sense.

In some cases, however, the specific lysine or pattern of lysines that is acetylated is important for the effect it has on chromatin. This is particularly true for histone methylation, as we will see. The reason is that many of these modifications act not so much by modifying the charge or chemical properties of the histone tails but as signals that are specifically detected by specialized proteins that bind to them in a position-specific manner. Such proteins are commonly called the **readers** of the signals while the proteins that create the histone modification signals are called the **writers**. By extension of this concept, the enzymes that remove the signals when they are no longer needed are called **erasers**.

Histone Acetylation

Some histone modifications might be thought to alter the physical properties of the nucleosome and therefore of the chromatin containing them. Histone acetylation is an example. Lysine is a basic amino acid. That is: its side chain, four carbons long, terminates with an amino group attached to the last or epsilon (ε) carbon (Figure 16). At neutral pH this amino group tends to bind a proton and therefore takes up a positive charge. Acetylation of this amino group neutralizes the charge and therefore the acetylation of lysines in the histone tails releases them from binding back to the negatively charged sugar-phosphate backbone of the DNA wrapped around the nucleosome and allows them to float freely in the solvent. This was thought to make the nucleosome less tight and the histone tails more able to interact with chromatin proteins in the nucleus. More detailed

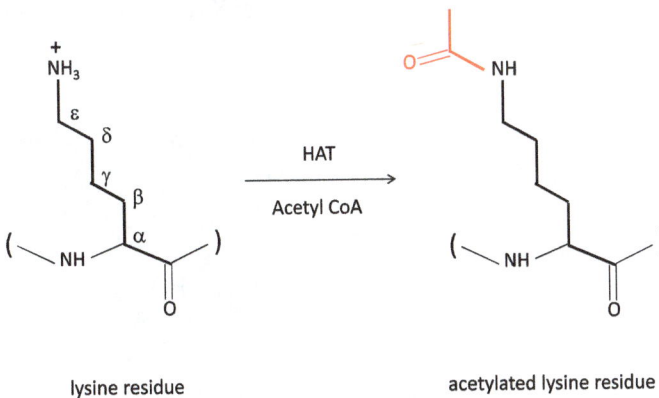

lysine residue   acetylated lysine residue

Figure 16.   Lysine acetylation. The nitrogen on the lysine sidechain can be acetylated by a variety of histone acetyl transferases (HATs), in most cases using acetyl-CoA as the acetyl donor. Note that acetylation removes the positive charge that would be on the terminal nitrogen at neutral pH.

study, however, has belied the view that histone acetylation alters the physical structure of chromatin: no changes could be detected in the association of the histone tails with nucleosomal DNA. In effect, the histone tails have large numbers of positively charged amino acids and neutralizing the charge of a few of them could not cause much change in their interaction with DNA. Nevertheless, acetylation of the histone tails is one of the first steps in the process of opening up chromatin and rendering it more accessible to DNA-binding proteins, nucleosome remodeling machines, transcription factors. Much evidence, as we shall see, shows that acetylation of specific residues in the histone tails changes their interactions with specific factors that recognize individual histone marks. Overall, however, histone acetylation has nearly always a positive effect on chromatin accessibility and on transcriptional activity, regardless of which histone or which lysine is acetylated. It might be thought of as a lubricant or softener that makes nucleosomes more pliant to further manipulation.

Histone acetyltransferases (HATs), often called histone acetylases, transfer an acetyl group from Acetyl-CoA (Figure 17) to a lysine epsilon amino group (Figure 16). While the acetylation of lysines in the N-terminal tails affects primarily the binding of factors to the tails themselves, in some cases the effects of strategically placed acetylations are structurally more profound. Histone H4 lysine 16, or H4K16 in the commonly used

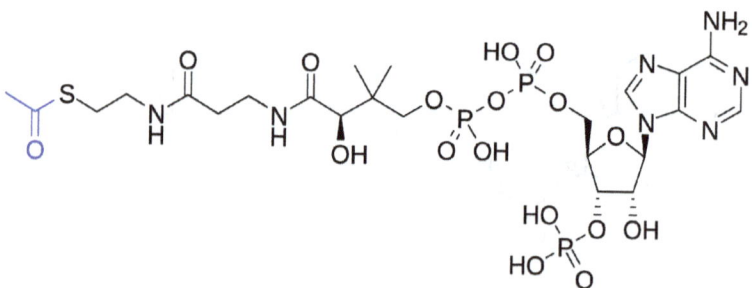

Figure 17.   Acetyl CoA. Acetyl coenzyme A is a common acetyl donor in metabolic pathways. The acetyl (in blue on the left) is linked by a high-energy thioester bond which is highly reactive and drives acetylation reactions.

Source: Bryan Derksen, public domain, https://commons.wikimedia.org/wiki/File:Acetyl-CoA-2D_colored.svg.

abbreviation, is in a region of H4 involved in interactions between nucleosomes that mediate tighter packing of chromatin. Acetylation of histone H4K16 blocks these interactions and therefore prevents compaction. It promotes instead the loose, beads-on-a-string chromatin conformation that facilitates access of chromatin proteins and gene expression.

Many HATs are known and are usually classified according to sequence homologies. The two major HAT superfamilies are the GNAT (GCN5-related HATs, named after GCN5) and the MYST family, named after its original members MOZ, Ybf2, Sas2, and Tip60. Most HATs have a variety of possible targets but often some specific histones or lysines are preferred. Thus, MOZ is particularly known for acetylating H4K16. p300/CBP acetylate most lysines, but they are particularly important since they are the only HATs that acetylate H3K27 (see Chapters 6 and 7). Many HATs are associated with complexes that require acetyltransferase activity to carry out more complex operations and may favor particular targets, including certain non-histone target proteins. For example, components of general transcription factors TFIIIC and TFII250 have HAT activities tightly associated with transcription. PCAF (p300, CBP-associated factor) is a HAT that is often associated with p300/CBP, two closely related HATs that have often interchangeable roles. PCAF itself is acetylated either by itself or by p300/CBP, thereby becoming activated to acetylate histones as well as many non-histone proteins. p300 and CBP bind to a large number of transcription factors, which bind to regulatory sites and recruit these acetylases to activate their target genes.

In the case of histone acetylation, readers of the acetylation mark most often contain a structural domain called the bromodomain (Figure 18). The name is unrelated to the element bromine but was derived from Brahma, the name of the protein in which it was first identified. The bromodomain includes approximately 110 amino acids arranged in a bundle of four alpha helices connected by loops that form an accessible hydrophobic pocket that provides a binding site for acetyl-lysine. Additional contacts with the histone sequence often provide specificity for binding to a particular acetylated lysine. Proteins containing a bromodomain bind to acetylated lysines, often to specific acetylated lysines, and help to recruit other chromatin proteins that remodel or disassemble nucleosomes or target other specific modifications that generally promote transcriptional

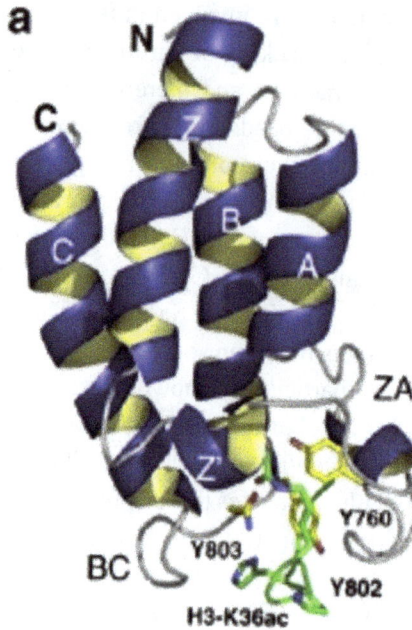

Figure 18.   Structure of bromodomain. This structural motif formed by four helices, here labeled Z, A, B, C, is found in most bromodomains. Here is shown the bromodomain of the HAT PCAF binding to histone H3K36ac.

Source: Mujtaba *et al.* (2007).

activity. Some proteins have two or more bromodomains, which allows them to recognize acetylations on multiple nucleosomes or to bind to nucleosomes that have more than one acetylated sites. Significantly, many HATs contain bromodomains, which means that one acetylated lysine favors recruiting HATs and acetylating additional lysines.

Acetylation of certain lysines in the histone tails, such as H4K5 and H4K12, occurs in the cytoplasm and is required for importing the histones into the nucleus and for the process of assembling nucleosomes by enzymes known as histone chaperones (see following section on chromatin replication). These positions will therefore be found acetylated in newly assembled chromatin and they are referred to as deposition acetylation marks.

Histone Deacetylases

Removing acetylation marks from a nucleosome erases the marks and is an effective way to prevent that nucleosome from recruiting chromatin activating factors. This is usually the prelude to transcriptional silencing. Histone deacetylases (HDACs) are now often called lysine deacetylases because they often deacetylate also non-histone proteins. There are many HDACs, classified by sequence homology but, more importantly, we can divide them into those that have a zinc-dependent active site and are inhibited by butyrate or trichostatin A (TSA) and those that require NAD^+ (Nicotinamide Adenine Dinucleotide), a key metabolic cofactor. Butyrate is a common metabolite produced by intestinal bacteria. Its activity as an inhibitor of histone deacetylases plays an important role in suppressing harmful inflammatory immune responses to normal intestinal flora. It also reduces cell proliferation and promotes differentiation. Butyrate and other inhibitors of histone deacetylases help to protect against the development of cancer in intestinal tissues.

NAD-dependent deacetylases utilize a completely different mechanism to deacetylate histones. They transfer the acetyl group from the histone lysine to the adenine ribose of NAD+, releasing nicotinamide. NAD^+ is an important oxidizing agent that accepts electrons in energy–producing reactions, becoming NADH, which in turn can produce ATP. It is therefore a key sensor of the energy availability in the cell. NAD-dependent deacetylases are also called sirtuins because of their homology to the budding yeast Sir2 protein. Sirtuins have been the focus of much attention because of their proposed role in aging, inflammation, and stress resistance, as well as histone deacetylation, but in higher eukaryotes their targets appear to be non-histone proteins.

Histone Methylation

The signaling value of histone modifications is nowhere as clear as when we consider histone methylation. The two methylatable amino acid residues are lysine and arginine. Lysine has a free amino group $-NH_2$ in which the two hydrogens can be replaced by methyl groups, which share electron pairs with the nitrogen. A third methyl group can also be added, in which case the nitrogen acquires a permanent positive charge (Figure 14). There are several lysines in the histone N-terminal tails, but the most important targets for methylation are lysines 4, 9, 27, and 36 of histone H3 and lysine 20 of histone H4. The function of methylation at each of these positions is different: H3K4 methylation is often associated with H3 acetylation and has a generally positive effect on DNA accessibility and transcription. Methylation of H3K9 or H3K27 tends to reduce accessibility and inhibit transcriptional activity. Furthermore, monomethylation has a different significance from dimethylation and dimethylation in turn has a different role from trimethylation. Acetylation and methylation both target lysine residues and are mutually incompatible. Therefore, acetylation protects a lysine from methylation and *viceversa*. An acetylated lysine must be deacetylated before it can be methylated. Similarly, a specific demethylase must remove the methyl groups before a lysine can be acetylated.

Lysine methylation is carried out by specific enzymes or enzyme complexes that share a conserved catalytic domain called the SET domain, named after the first three lysine methyltransferases characterized, which shared this conserved domain, Su(var)3–9, E(z) and Trithorax. In all cases the methyl group comes from the universal methyl donor S-adenosyl methionine (SAM). The methionine in SAM is the methyl donor for these and many other methylation reactions, including DNA methylation (see DNA Methylation chapter). In turn, methionine receives its methyl group when 5-methyltetrahydrofolate adds a methyl to homocysteine. Folate, also known as vitamin B9, is therefore essential for the synthesis of SAM and must be supplied in the diet. Levels of SAM affect histone methylation, not just because of its reduced availability but also because when it donates a methyl group for a methylation reaction, it turns into S-adenosyl homocysteine, which is a powerful inhibitor of all methylases. Low SAM levels reduce the extent of both histone and DNA methylation, in both cases facilitating the derepression of genes. The opposite is true of high SAM levels. This has implications for cancer since malignant transformations often result from the inappropriate expression of genes.

Unlike histone acetylation, which was thought to neutralize the positive charge on the lysine and release the histone tails from DNA and therefore facilitate access to the nucleosomal DNA, histone methylation has no obvious physical relation to its epigenetic effects. The functional consequences of histone methylation depend entirely on the factors that recognize and bind to the modified histone. Methylation of histone H3 at lysine 4 has the general effect of promoting access to DNA and favoring transcriptional activity, although mono-, di-, and tri-methylation of H3K4 play somewhat different roles in the process. In contrast, methylation of H3K9 is firmly associated with chromatin condensation, transcriptional silencing, and heterochromatin formation (see Chapter 5). Methylation of H3K27 is carried out by Polycomb Repressive Complex 2, PRC2 (see Chapter 7) and has a repressive effect on access and transcriptional activity. Here, mono-, di-, and tri-methylation have quite distinct consequences or outcomes. H3K27me3 is the mark characteristic of chromatin silenced by Polycomb mechanisms. H3K27me2 is associated with chromatin that is transcriptionally silent, though not necessarily repressed. H3K27me1 is associated with transcriptionally active chromatin, though it is not clear whether it plays any specific role in transcription.

Some histone positions are accessible to modifying enzymes although far from the histone tails. H3K79 is an example. It lies in a loop of the H3 globular domain that is accessible to the solvent and near the interface between H3/H4 and H2A/H2B. H3K79 methylation is carried out by DOT1 (mammalian DOT1L), the only lysine methylase that does not use a SET catalytic domain. DOT1 can mono-, di-, or tri-methylate H3K79, but in this case the three degrees of methylation appear to have the same function. DOT1 associates with the transcribing RNA pol II and favors transcriptional elongation. This is a typical example of interaction between different histone marks: DOT1 action depends on ubiquitylation of H2BK123 and H4K16 acetylation, which lie close to H3K79 in the nucleosome. H3K79 methylation is also important for DNA damage repair by helping to recruit the repair protein 53BP.

Methylation of H3K36 is usually classified as an "active" mark, that is a mark associated with transcriptional activity and therefore often assumed to favor transcription. The major source of H3K36 methylation is the SETD2 methylase, which is recruited by the RNA pol II when in the elongating stage and deposits H3K36me3 throughout the transcribed region (see Chapter 6). In yeast, this mark recruits a histone deacetylase complex, which is important to remove the abundant histone acetylation that accompanies transcription and would encourage binding of new RNA polymerase, and inappropriate transcription starts in the middle of the transcription unit. In mammals, the complex recruited by H3K36me3 does not deacetylate but includes the *de novo* DNA methylase DNMT3B (see Chapter 3) and a H3K4me3 demethylase. These activities accomplish the same objective of preventing inappropriate transcription starts. H3K36me3 has important additional roles in helping to recruit the co-transcriptional splicing factors. In fact, H3K36me3 is enriched in exons, compared to introns and, depending on which factors it recruits, it can favor splicing or retention of alternative exons. A very different and less well understood function is that of H3K36me2, which is deposited by ASH1 (ASH1L in mammals). This mark in some way recruits or collaborates with Trithorax/MLL complexes to antagonize the effects of H3K27me3 and Polycomb repression (see Chapter 7). In fact, H3K36 methylation antagonizes the methylase activity of PRC2, and H3K36 demethylases help to recruit PRC1.

H4K20 can also be mono-, di-, or tri-methylated with different effects. PR-Ser7 (also called SET8) produces H4K20me1, and SUV4-20H1 and-SUV4-20H2 can further methylate this to H4K20me2 and me3. Mitotic chromosomes are highly enriched in H4K20me1 in the chromosome arms, with H4K20me3 localized in the heterochromatic region surrounding the centromere. This is important to prevent premature decompaction of chromatin and widespread DNA replication, which would cause DNA damage. In proliferating cells, most of histone H4 is dimethylated by SUV4-20 and promotes DNA damage repair. H4K20me3 is found primarily in heterochromatin where it is an important agent for chromatin compaction and heterochromatic silencing.

Although these are the major histone methylases, the human genome contains a large number of SET domain proteins that have methyltransferase activity but have not been studied. Several target H3K4, others H3K9 in different tissues or circumstances. Some other lysines in the histone tails are also methylated but their role in chromatin activities is not well characterized.

Arginine Methylation

Arginine residues can also be methylated by a number of protein arginine N-methytransferases (PRMT) that target many proteins, including histones. The PRMT enzymes target preferentially amino acid motifs rich in glycines and arginines (GAR) to transfer a methyl group from the universal donor SAM to the guanidine nitrogen on arginine (Figure 15). The most important targets of arginine methylation are H3R2, H3R8, H3R17, H3R26, and H2R3. However, arginine can be mono- or dimethylated, but dimethylation can occur in two different configurations: symmetric (Rme2s) and asymmetric (Rme2a). These are produced by different enzymes and have very different outcomes. The asymmetric dimethylation of H4R3 by PRMT1 is read by factors that result in transcriptional activation, while the symmetric dimethylation of the same arginine residue by PRMT5 recruits DNA methylation and causes repression. Similarly, asymmetric dimethylation of H3R2 by PRMT6 represses transcription by interfering with methylation of the adjacent H3K4, but symmetric dimethylation of H3R2 by PRMT5 stimulates methylation of H3K4 and promotes transcription.

PRMTs also target many non-histone proteins in the nucleus and cytoplasm. These often collaborate with other histone-modifying factors and result in complex cross-talk among histone marks. For example, PRMT1 acts as a transcriptional co-activator recruited to promoter regions by several transcription factors. It methylates H4R3 producing H4R3me2a, which stimulates p300/CBP acetylation of H4 at K5, K8, K12, and K16. This facilitates the asymmetric dimethylation of H3R17 and R26 by PRMT4/CARM1. PRMT4/CARM1 is also recruited by steroid receptors and other transcription factors to methylate non-histone activators such as p300/CBP to stimulate transcription.

Readers of Histone Methylation

A well-studied type of reader of histone methylation is a structural element known as the chromodomain, first identified by comparing the sequence of the heterochromatin binding protein HP1 and the Polycomb

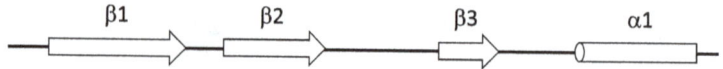

β1	β2	β3	α1

dmHP1   EYAVEKIIDRRVRKGKVEYYLKWKGYPETENTWEPENNLDCQDLIQQYEASR

dmPc   VYAAEKIIQKRVKKGVVEYRVKWKGWNQRYNTWEPEVNILDRRLIDIYEQTN

Figure 19.   Chromodomains of dmHP1a and dmPc. The dm preceding the protein name signifies that this is the form of the protein found in *Drosophila melanogaster*. In red, the amino acids forming the aromatic cage that binds the three methyl groups of the trimethyl lysine.

component of the Polycomb Repressive Complex 1 (PRC1) (Figure 19). The chromodomain forms a pocket lined with hydrophobic residues, into which the methylated nitrogen of the methyl lysine locks in (see Chapter 5, Figure 11 and Chapter 7, Figure 40). The size of the pocket determines whether mono-, di-, or tri-methyl is bound. A suitable groove accommodates the histone tail, providing specificity for the methyl lysine residue. So in HP1, the groove positions H3K9me3 in the pocket while in Polycomb, it is H3K27me3 that is positioned in the pocket. In both HP1 and Polycomb, the chromodomain binds the trimethylated nitrogen well but binds appreciably also the dimethylated nitrogen. The monomethylated nitrogen fits too loosely for tight binding.

Chromodomains are found in many methyl–lysine binding proteins. A very different methyl–lysine binding pocket is found in the Esc/Eed component of the Polycomb Repressive Complex 2 (PRC2). This pocket is not produced by a specific protein domain but by residues coming from different parts of the protein amino acid sequence. The Esc/Eed protein is a WD40 domain protein, so-called because it contains multiple copies of a structural domain of approximately 40 amino acids that often ends with tryptophan and aspartate (W and D). Each of these domains consists of four antiparallel beta sheets and is arranged like the blades of a propeller, forming a conical structure with a hollow center (see Chapter 7, Figure 33). In Esc/Eed, residues from different WD40 "blades" protrude toward the center of the cone, forming a hydrophobic pocket that binds the methyl lysine. This has important consequences because Esc/Eed is a key component of the PRC2 complex, whose enzymatic component, E(z), methylates

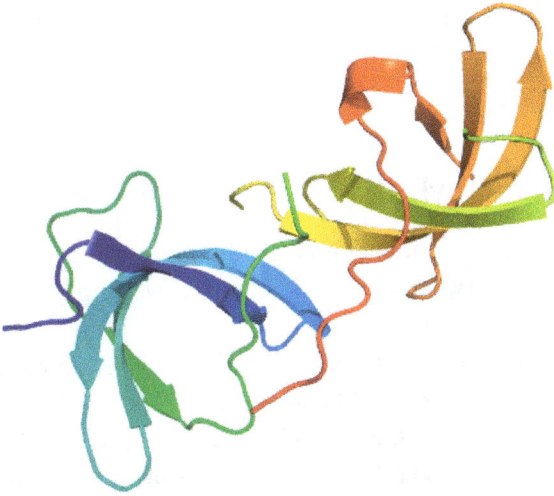

Figure 20. A double Tudor domain. The image shows the two Tudor domains of the human fragile X mental retardation protein FXR2. The Tudor domain is formed by four beta-strands in a barrel structure.

Source: Lasko (2010).

H3K27. Thus, the methylase recognizes its own product (see Chapter 7). WD40 domain proteins are often found among histone- or nucleosome-binding proteins. Another example is RbAp48, found in many complexes involved in histone methylation, histone deacetylation, chromatin remodeling, nucleosome assembly, and transcriptional silencing.

Two other readers of methyl lysines should be mentioned because of their frequent occurrence. The Tudor domain is a structure of approximately 60 amino acids folded in a five-stranded antiparallel beta-barrel (Figure 20). It forms a binding pocket lined by four or five aromatic amino acids that accommodates a methyl lysine or methyl arginine residue. The size of the pocket determines the degree of binding specificity for mono-, di-, or tri-methylated lysines or for methyl arginine.

The PHD finger is a structural motif approximately 50–80 amino acids in length, containing a Cys_4-His-Cys_3 motif with two coordinated zinc ions. It was named originally after a Plant HomeoDomain protein in which it was first identified. It is found in many chromatin-associated proteins, some of which have been shown to bind trimethylated lysines such as H3K4me3. KDM5C has a PHD finger that binds to H3K9me3 but acts as a H3K4me3 demethylase, helping to establish heterochromatic silencing.

Histone Demethylases

Compared to acetylation, which is rapidly reversed, histone methylation seemed at first a very stable modification and was thought to be irreversible. Chemically, it is more difficult to remove a methyl group, which requires its oxidation. The first histone demethylase to be characterized was LSD1, which uses FAD (Flavin Adenine Dinucleotide) as the oxidizing agent to hydroxylate the methyl group and remove it in the form of formaldehyde. LSD1 and related demethylases act on H3K4me1 and me2 (Figure 21).

Another type of demethylase based on a structural domain called Jumonji C (JmjC) uses instead coordination with Fe(II), α-ketoglutarate,

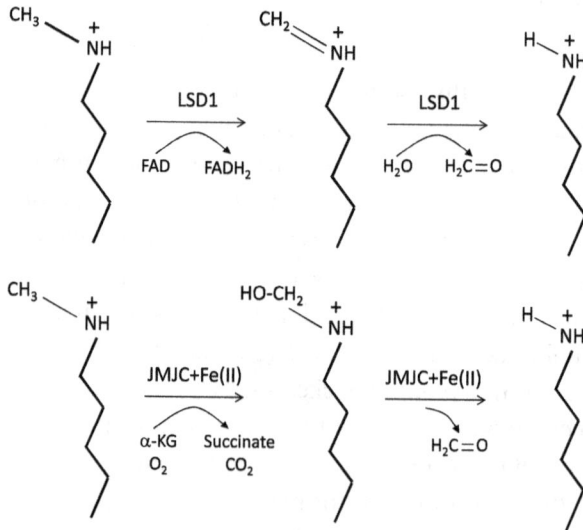

Figure 21. Lysine demethylation. Removal of methyl groups from lysine residues requires their oxidation. The first lysine demethylase studied, LSD1, uses FAD to oxidize mono- or di-methylated H3K4. A more versatile class of demethylases contains a Jumonji C domain, uses iron Fe(II) and alpha-ketoglutarate, and can demethylate mono-, di-, and tri-methyl lysines.

and molecular oxygen to mediate oxidation of the methyl groups. This type of demethylase also has names such as JHDM or JMDM referring to the Jumonji domain and seems to have a greater range. KDM2A for example can act on H3K4me3 and on H3K36me1,2. KDM3A acts on H3K9m1,2. KMD4 enzymes act on di- and trimethylated H3K9 and H3K36. The histone demethylases are often components of larger multifunctional complexes and contain domains that target them to specific chromatin environments. KDM2A, for example, contains a domain that binds to CpG islands (provided they are not DNA-methylated).

Nomenclature

In 2007, a number of workers in the chromatin field proposed a new nomenclature for the enzymes that modify histones. The names now begin with the amino acid targeted, followed by the enzymatic reaction, and by a number and letter designation. Thus, the historical names, which often derived from the context of their discovery, from the gene name, from the structural domain of the protein, etc., are now replaced by a systematic generic name that is based on the enzymatic reaction. Thus, LSD1 is now called KDM1 (lysine demethylase 1); Su(var)3–9 is now KMT1 (lysine methyltransferase1), and the mammalian homolog SUV39H1 is KMT1A (Table 2). This was a praiseworthy initiative that has created much confusion and an alphabet soup of very similar names in place of an older alphabet soup with much more diverse names. The benefits of the new nomenclature have been limited in practice and 15 years later, the old names seem to be still the names most commonly used.

Histone Phosphorylation

Although less multifarious than methylation, histone phosphorylation has complex and perplexing roles. Like acetylation, phosphorylation adds negative charges to the histone tails, repelling them from the DNA wound around the nucleosome. This is consistent with its role in promoting transcription. The most common targets of phosphorylation are serine, threonine, and tyrosine, although lysine, arginine, cysteine can also be phosphorylated. Phosphorylation of serines 10 and 28 of H3 and serine 32

Table 2.   Histone demethylase nomenclature.

Revised name	Former name	Substrate
KDM1A	LSD1	H3K4me1,2
		H3K9me1,2
KDM1B	LSD2	H3K4me1,2
KDM2A	JHDM1A	H3K4me3
		H3K36me1,2
KDM2B	JHDM1B	H3K36me1,2
KDM3A	JHDM2A	H3K9me1,2
KDM4A	JMDM3A	H3K9me2,3
KDM4B	JMDM3B	H3K36me2,3
KDM4C	JMDM3C	H1K26me2,3
KDM4D	JMDM3D	
KDM5A	JARID1A	H3K4me2,3
KDM5B	JARID1B	
KDM5C	JARID1C	
KDM5D	JARID1D	
KDM6A	UTX	(H3K27me1)
KDM6B	JMJD3	H3K27me2,3

of H2B are associated with transcriptional activation and probably also phosphorylation of H3 threonines T6 and T11. Some evidence suggests that these modifications help to recruit acetylases. An important effect of phosphorylation has to do with its relationship with lysine methylation. The phosphorylation of a serine or threonine adjacent to a lysine produces a large negatively charged phosphate, which can prevent access of a methylation reader such as a chromodomain or Tudor domain protein because it repels the hydrophobic pocket. It is probably not a coincidence that the major sites of methylation, H3K4, H3K9, H3K27 are flanked by a serine or threonine. So phosphorylation of H3S10 or H3S28 can prevent H3K9 or H3K27 methylation from being detected by the reader protein. This has been called the "phospho-switch" because it allows a rapid response to external signals without removing the methyl mark altogether. The phospho-switch is a different kind of interaction between histone marks from the incompatibility of lysine methylation and lysine acetylation, which are simply mutually exclusive. Entirely different is also the effect of methylation of H3K4 or H3K36 in inhibiting the methylation of H3K27. This is not due to a direct physical antagonism but to a regulatory effect. The PRC2 complex, responsible for methylation of H3K27 has acquired the ability to sense the methylation of H3K4 and H3K36 and respond by an allosteric change in conformation that affects the catalytic domain and inhibits its methylation activity.

H3T3 is adjacent to H3K4 and plays a similar phospho-methyl switch role. While the H3K4me3 mark in active promoters is retained during mitosis, H3T3 becomes phosphorylated, resulting in the dissociation of TFIID and the general transcription factors. At the end of mitosis, H3T3 is dephosphorylated, resulting in rapid reassembly of the promoter-associated transcriptional machinery. Although histone phosphorylation often promotes transcriptional activity, paradoxically, it is best known as a mark of mitotic chromatin. H3S10, H3S28, H3T3, and H3T11 are all associated with mitotic chromosome condensation and segregation. The first three are clearly useful to remove bound proteins, but it is not clear what role they play in chromosome condensation. Phosphorylation of H3T3 in late mitosis is due to the Haspin kinase and is necessary for the correct alignment of chromosomes at metaphase.

Histone phosphorylation plays an important role in DNA damage repair. The primary responder is the H2AX variant of histone H2A. H2AX constitutes a small percentage of the total H2A in chromatin but acts as a sensor of DNA double-strand breaks. The protein kinase ATM is activated by autophosphorylation in the presence of double-strand breaks and in turn phosphorylates H2AX at serine-139. This recruits a number of DNA damage repair proteins and more extensive H2AX phosphorylation, forming prominent foci called γH2AX foci.

Histone Ubiquitylation

Unlike most of the histone modifications, ubiquitylation involves the attachment of a large molecule. Ubiquitin is a small protein of 76 amino acids, only slightly smaller than the histones themselves. The attachment of ubiquitin to lysine residues of other proteins is a basic cellular process to tag proteins for destruction by the proteasome machinery. This generally involves many ubiquitin molecules at multiple sites, often forming chains of ubiquitins. A different type of ubiquitylation attaches a single ubiquitin at a well defined position and is found in many nuclear factors as well as histones. Mono-ubiquitylation does not target for destruction but acts as a signal, often serving as a framework for the assembly of multiprotein complexes. It can be reversed by specific deubiquitylases. Major targets for histone ubiquitylation are H2A at position 119 near the C-terminal and H2B at position 120. As might be expected, attachment of such a bulky molecule to a nucleosome would prevent close packing of nucleosomes. In fact, H2BK120ub is required for methylation of H3K4 and is therefore important for transcriptional activation. H2AK119ub is closely associated with the binding of Polycomb complexes and often leads to transcriptional repression. The DNA damage response involves the ubiquitylation of histones H1K63, H2AK13, and H2AK15. These are important to recruit multiple factors of the DNA repair mechanism.

Ubiquitylation is carried out by a series of reactions in which ubiquitin is first activated by binding to a E1 enzyme, then transferred to a E2 ubiquitin conjugating enzyme, and finally attached to the target protein by a E3 ubiquitin ligase. The last of these contains the target specificity. In the case of H2AK119ub, the E3 ligase is RING2, a core component of the Polycomb repressive complex itself (see Chapter 7).

Histone Chaperones

Assembly of nucleosomes on DNA is energetically favored. Given free histones and DNA, nucleosomes can assemble *in vitro* spontaneously in the presence of high salt in the medium to make the DNA more flexible. *In vivo*, nucleosome assembly occurs very rapidly without need of high salt, but with the help of histone chaperones. These are protein complexes that bind the appropriate histones and help them to make the right DNA contacts necessary to wind the DNA around the core histones while avoiding inappropriate DNA contacts that would slow down the process of reaching the best set of interactions. Histone chaperones are involved in many processes but the most important of these is in disassembling and reassembling nucleosomes during chromatin replication. This is a very complex process, although *in vivo* replication forks can advance at a rate of the order of 2000 bp per minute in rapidly dividing cells. We will focus here on the aspects relevant to chromatin and epigenetics.

Chromatin Replication

The key feature of DNA replication is unwinding the DNA double helix and synthesizing a new DNA strand complementary to each of the two separated old strands to produce two daughter double-stranded DNA molecules. This is intrinsically an asymmetric process because DNA synthesis proceeds only by adding nucleotides to the 3′ end of an oligonucleotide. This is a straightforward elongation in the case of one strand, in which the new strand is growing at the 3′ end, toward the replication fork, but not in the case of the other strand, which has the opposite orientation and would need to grow at the 5′ end. The problem is solved by discontinuously synthesizing short fragments (so-called Okazaki fragments) using short RNA primers to initiate synthesis in the direction away from the replication fork. In subsequent steps, the RNA primers are removed, the gaps between Okazaki fragments are filled, and the fragments ligated together (Figure 22). This complicated process means that, while one daughter DNA molecule can be synthesized immediately as soon as the parental double helix is unwound, synthesis of the other daughter DNA needs to

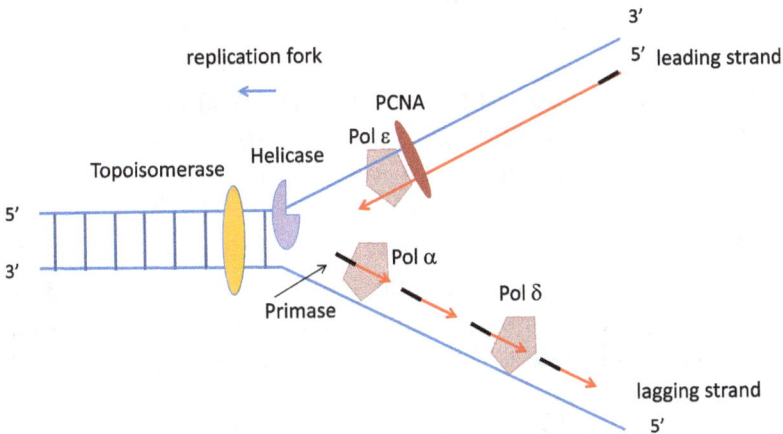

Figure 22.   DNA synthesis at replication fork. The MCM2 helicase complex unwinds the DNA, preceded by Topoisomerase to relieve superhelical stress. Synthesis begins with Primase laying down an RNA primer (short black line). Pol ε polymerase elongates the primer copying the leading strand continuously, held in place by the PCNA clamp. For the lagging strand, Primase repeatedly produces an RNA primer to initiate synthesis of Okazaki fragments by Pol α. This is then extended by Pol δ. The RNA primers are later removed and the Okazaki fragments joined.

wait until a sufficient length of template DNA is unwound to allow synthesis of at least one Okazaki fragment. The strand that can grow immediately is called the leading strand and the strand that grows discontinuously and is therefore delayed is called the lagging strand.

In replicating chromatin, we have the added complication due to the winding of the DNA in nucleosomes. For the replication machinery to access the DNA, the nucleosomes need to be disassembled just ahead of the replication fork. Early experiments showed that the overall process involved removal of the two H2A-H2B dimers, followed by the sequestration of the H3-H4 tetramer by a histone chaperone that remained bound to the replication fork and re-deposited the old H3-H4 to the newly synthesized daughter DNA molecules in an approximately symmetric fashion. Finally, H2A-H2B dimers would complete the nucleosome while entirely new nucleosomes would be deposited to restore the normal nucleosome density in the daughter chromatin molecules. Recent work has shown that the process of parental histone inheritance is intrinsically much more asymmetric and specific features are required to minimize this asymmetry.

In general, the process begins with the interaction of a nucleosome with the MCM helicase complex associated with the ASF1 histone chaperone (Figure 23). The MCM helicase is a powerful motor that uses energy from ATP hydrolysis to unwind nucleosomal DNA and displace the core histones. Two H2A-H2B dimers are released, but the $(H3-H4)_2$ tetramer remains bound to the MCM2 subunit of the helicase, which replaces the contacts it made to DNA and to H2A-H2B. At this point, the H3-H4 tetramer can be handed directly to histone-binding subunits of the DNA polymerase ε that replicates the leading strand. This would mean that the leading strand chromatin would preferentially inherit the parental H3-H4 and entirely new H3-H4 histones would need to be recruited to assemble chromatin on the lagging strand DNA molecule when it becomes available. This asymmetric outcome is not normally desirable because one daughter chromatin would retain the old H3-H4 with the pre-existing histone modifications while the other would have new H3-H4 with no histone modifications. Instead, what is normally observed is a roughly equal partitioning of the old histones between the two daughter molecules, with newly synthesized histones filling in the gaps. This equal partitioning of

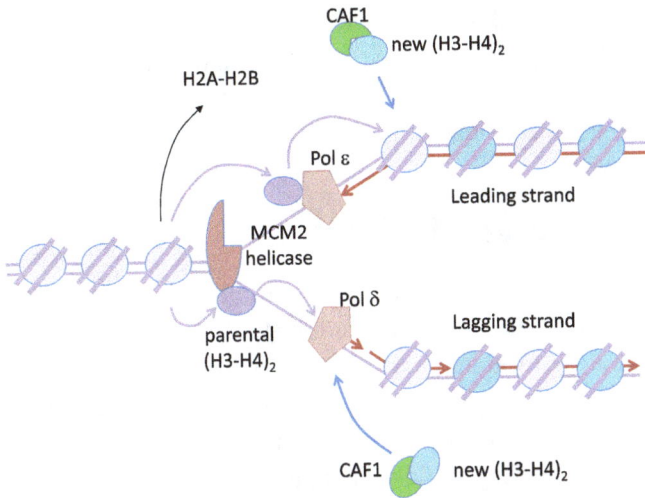

Figure 23. Nucleosome dynamics at replication fork. To replicate chromatin, nucleosomes must be dismantled at the replication fork. The H2A-H2B dimers are removed first. The (H3-H4)$_2$ tetramers bind to the MCM2 helicase complex or to the components of the Polymerase ε to form nucleosomes on the elongating leading strand. The MCM2 complex transfers the (H3-H4)$_2$ tetramers to Polymerase δ to form nucleosomes on the lagging strand. This recycling of the parental (H3-H4)$_2$ tetramers is in competition with the deposition of new (H3-H4)$_2$ tetramers (blue) by the CAF1 chaperone complex.

the old H3-H4 tetramers is due to the MCM2 subunit of the helicase hanging on sufficiently tenaciously to the H3-H4 tetramers to compete with the Pol ε polymerase. As a result, roughly half the time, the old H3-H4 tetramer is retained long enough so that the lagging strand daughter is available. If the histone-binding Pol ε subunits are deleted, the old H3-H4 tetramers go preferentially to the lagging strand. If the histone-binding domain of MCM2 is mutated, the old H3-H4 go exclusively to the leading strand. To initiate the formation of nucleosomes, the H3-H4 tetramer is handed over to another histone chaperone, the Chromatin Assembly Factor-1 (CAF-1), which deposits either the old H3-H4 histones or newly synthesized H3-H4 depending on what is first available.

This elaborate mechanism ensures that each of the two daughter chromatin molecules inherits roughly half of the old H3-H4 tetramers, bearing the histone marks that have been established during the previous cell cycle.

Two new H2A-H2B dimers are added to complete nucleosome formation. The old H3-H4 histones with their posttranscriptional marks will be important to help maintain the chromatin state, the program of gene activity, and the state of cell differentiation from one cell cycle to the next.

Histone Genes and Variants

Histones are needed in large quantities during S phase, when the genome is replicated. In *Drosophila*, the major histone genes are found in a single locus as an array of about 100 copies of a repeating unit containing the four core histones and the H1 histone (Figure 24). These are the replicative histone genes, so-called because they are specifically activated in S phase to provide very rapidly large amounts of the histone proteins in time to be incorporated in newly replicated chromatin. Histone genes in flies and mammals utilize specialized factors to regulate their expression and mRNA processing. Histone mRNAs lack 3′ poly A and have instead a characteristic stem-loop structure at the 3′ end that is cleaved by a specific endonuclease to create the mRNA 3′ end. Mammalian replicative histone genes are found in two or three smaller *HIST* clusters. Human *HIST1*, the largest cluster, contains 55 histone genes, including all the H1 genes, for a total of 10–20 copies of each histone. Unlike the *Drosophila* histone genes, the mammalian genes are not organized in tandemly repeated units but are more irregularly scattered and more variable in sequence. The single locus arrangement in *Drosophila* has provided a powerful tool to study the importance of histone sequence and modifications. In the fly, the entire locus can be genetically deleted and replaced by a transgenic set of histone genes. Fortunately, a relatively small number of copies suffices for viability. This approach has allowed the introduction

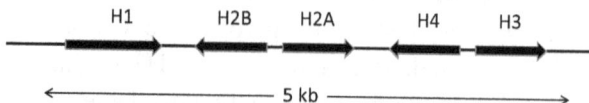

Figure 24.   *Drosophila* histone gene repeat unit. The five canonical replicative histone genes are found in a single locus. The arrangement of the genes shown is repeated in tandem about 100 times.

of any desired mutation in any one of the histones and therefore to examine the consequences for function.

In addition to the replicative histone genes, flies and mammalian genomes contain a number of histone genes that are neither clustered nor limited in expression to the S1 phase. They are transcribed throughout the cell cycle and have specific changes in the amino acid sequence they encode. These are called histone variants and are present in a few copies scattered in the genome. Unlike the replicative histones, their mRNAs are polyadenylated and, in some cases, contain introns. What are they for? This is best answered by looking at a few examples.

Centromeric H3: CENP-A

One of these variants is the H3 species that binds specifically at the centromere, called CENP-A in humans. CENP-A is a highly specialized variant and the most divergent from the replicative H3 sequence, especially in the N-terminal tail, which, although rich in basic amino acids, lacks the characteristic sites for post-translational modifications. It is also the most unusual in the way it is deposited. The centromere is the assembly site of the kinetochore, the structure to which spindle microtubules attach to guide chromosomes during cell division. In higher organisms the centromere is found usually embedded in centromeric heterochromatic repeats (the α satellite repeat in mammals) but is not sequence-determined. It depends on the incorporation of CENP-A instead of H3 in the nucleosomes. This in turn depends on the previous presence of CENP-A and high levels of H3K9me3 and H4K20me3 histone modifications (more about this in Chapter 5) . Thus the position of the centromere is epigenetically determined, although there are ways to create new centromeres if the older one is entirely lost. Since it is not expressed specifically in S-phase, when DNA is replicated, CENP-A must displace replicative H3 in pre-existing nucleosomes. A specialized histone chaperone called HJURP binds a CENP-A-H4 dimer and is apparently targeted to centromeric chromatin by proteins associated with the pre-existing centromere. The end result is a centromeric chromatin region consisting of a core of CENP-A-containing nucleosomes flanked by a region of intermixed CENP-A and H3 nucleosomes for a total of around 1 Mbp of DNA.

Histone H3 Variants

The normal histone genes, expressed during S-phase along with DNA replication, provide a large amount of histones, more than sufficient to package a full set of genomic DNA. During the rest of the cell cycle, however, there are occasions when new histone deposition might be necessary although the replicative histone genes are not active. The most common situations are the sites of strong transcriptional activity, where histones might be displaced, or regulatory sites, where nucleosome turnover occurs. It is important, therefore, to have a source of histones to provide a low level of replication-independent nucleosome assembly throughout the cell cycle. These are the variant histone genes, of which histone H3.3 is probably the best studied. In the human genome there are actually seven known sequence variants of histone H3. Most of these are minor variants of the canonical replicative histone H3 and are found in the major histone gene clusters. Histone H3.3 is the best known replication independent H3 variant. It is represented by two isolated genes transcribed throughout the cell cycle. The deposition of H3.3 occurs throughout the cell cycle, even during DNA replication, but H3.1 and minor replicative variants can only be deposited during DNA replication. This is due to the role of histone chaperones.

Replicative histone H3 and H4 tetramers are deposited by the CAF-1 chaperone at the replication fork and immediately after it. CAF-1 also recognizes H3.3-H4 tetramers during DNA replication but deposition at other stages of the cell cycle requires a different chaperone. Several alternative chaperones are known, but the most important is called Histone Regulator A (HIRA). The specificity of the replication-independent chaperones is remarkable, given that H3.3 differs from H3.1 at only four positions, one in the N-terminal tail and three in the histone fold region (Figure 25). Even more remarkably, Ahmad and Henikoff (2002) showed that changing H3.1 at any one of the three positions in the histone fold region to correspond to H3.3 allowed it to be deposited independently of replication.

H3.3 is found at genomic positions with high levels of nucleosome turnover. Typically, these are regions with high rates of transcription and some evidence indicates that the HIRA chaperone may tend to associate with the elongating RNA Pol II. More localized sites of high H3.3 content

Histone H3.3 variant amino acids

```
            10         20          30         40          50
H3.3  MARTKQTARK STGGKAPRKQ LATKAARKSA PSTGGVKKPH RYRPGTVALR
H3.1  MARTKQTARK STGGKAPRKQ LATKAARKSA PATGGVKKPH RYRPGTVALR

            60         70          80         90         100
H3.3  EIRRYQKSTE LLIRKLPFQR LVREIAQDFK TDLRFQSAAI GALQEASEAY
H3.1  EIRRYQKSTE LLIRKLPFQR LVREIAQDFK TDLRFQSSAV MALQEACEAY

           110        120         130
H3.3  LVGLFEDTNL CAIHAKRVTI MPKDIQLARR IRGERA
H3.1  LVGLFEDTNL CAIHAKRVTI MPKDIQLARR IRGERA
```

Figure 25. Comparison of histone H3.3 and H3.1. Only four positions distinguish H3.3 from H3.1. They are shown in red: one in the N-terminal tail and three in the histone fold region. Any one of the amino acid changes in the histone fold region is sufficient to permit replication-independent deposition.

are sites that recruit nucleosome remodeling complexes to mobilize nucleosomes. These are typically transcription start sites and sites that bind regulatory complexes, both activating and repressive varieties. The HIRA complex has also binding activity for naked DNA, suggesting that it can fill-in nucleosome gaps as they arise through chromatin remodeling or strong transcriptional activity.

Replication-independent histone H4 genes are similarly expressed throughout the cell cycle. In this case, the variant genes simply provide a partner for the H3.3 replication-independent variants since their sequence is identical to that of the replicative H4. In contrast, variants of H2A are not only numerous but in some cases play important roles. Variant H2A.Z is replication-independent and plays a similar role to H3.3 with respect to histone turnover. In fact, it can be introduced by nucleosome remodelers such as SWR-C or INO80 to replace canonical H2A at specific sites. Nucleosomes with the combination of H2A.Z and H3.3 have been found to be unusually unstable and prone to turnover or to give access to DNA-binding proteins. Another important H2A variant is H2AX, which normally represents a few percent of total H2A. In response to DNA damage, H2AX becomes phosphorylated at serine-139 and is commonly referred to as γH2AX.

Nucleosome Remodeling Machines

It should be clear from the preceding discussion that a nucleosome that includes a certain DNA sequence will hide that sequence from the proteins that need to read or interact with that sequence. Therefore, it will be necessary at some point to remove, displace, unwind, or in some way remodel that nucleosome to make that sequence accessible. But nucleosome assembly is energetically very favorable and nucleosomes are normally very stable structures. Therefore it will be take some work and some expenditure of energy to disassemble them even partially to carry out any remodeling. This is done by remodeling machines, multiprotein complexes that use ATP hydrolysis to provide the energy necessary. There are many different types of nucleosome remodeling machines that reorganize or even displace nucleosomes in different ways (Figure 26).

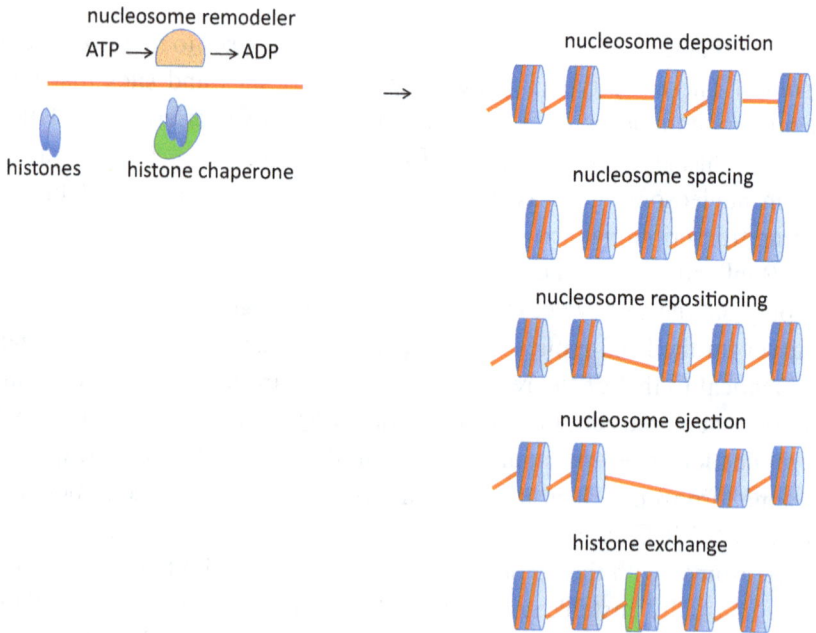

Figure 26.   Different activities of nucleosome remodeling ATPases. Remodeling complexes participate in a variety of activities, beginning with the deposition of nucleosomes. Some remodelers specialize in adjusting even spacing between nucleosomes. A major activity of many remodelers is to shift individual nucleosomes, usually to permit access to DNA. This can also partially or completely remove nucleosomes. Some remodelers specifically exchange core histones, for example replacing H2A with H2AZ.

Nucleosome remodeling was first discovered in yeast when new DNase I hypersensitive sites were found to appear within minutes of inducing new expression of genes necessary for sucrose fermentation. The functions involved were identified genetically and eventually purified biochemically. The genes and then the protein complex were named after the phenotype produced by their mutations: Sucrose Non-Fermenting or SNF. The same function was involved in switching the mating type genes (SWI), hence the current name SWI/SNF. The key component of this complex is the Swi2/Snf2 ATPase. Homologous nucleosome remodeling complexes were found in *Drosophila*, containing the Swi2/Snf2 ATPase homolog Brahma, and in mammals where two homologs are called BRG1 and hBRM. A large variety of other chromatin remodeling complexes have been isolated using assays for activities that use ATP to increase the accessibility of DNA in chromatin. Each complex contains an ATP-binding subunit that constitutes the motor of the remodeling machines. Despite the large variety of ATP-binding subunits, they are all evolutionarily derived from the same helicase superfamily. The Snf2 helicase super-family is defined by characteristic motifs within the ATPase domain. In addition, however, nucleosome remodeler subfamilies are defined by the presence of additional domains. Members of the helicase superfamily bind to double-stranded DNA and use ATP hydrolysis to move unidirectionally along one strand, generally separating the strands. The remodelers also move relative to one strand but do not separate the two strands. Beyond this level of general agreement, accounts of the mechanism of remodeling action have varied substantially in the past ten years and a number of incompatible models have been presented with equal confidence and assertiveness. A widely accepted model viewed the remodeling complex gripping tightly the nucleosome core and lifting a segment of the nucleosomal DNA loose from histone contacts, while pulling in new DNA from the entry site into the nucleosome. A translocase domain would move the detached loop along the nucleosome surface, breaking and reforming contacts with the histone core (Figure 27). This model presented problems and unsolved questions. It also predicted that DNA segments would become sensitive to nucleases as they were lifted off from the histone core. This was not observed. New biophysical studies have resulted in a new type of model in which DNA is translocated through twisting, without lifting off loops of DNA.

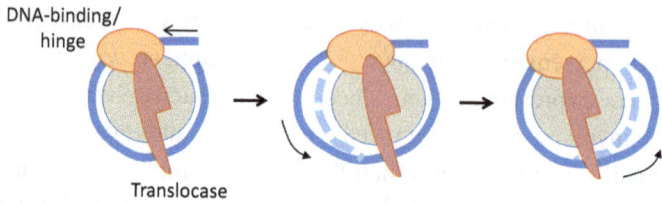

DNA-binding/
hinge

Translocase

Figure 27. Model of nucleosome remodeling. A widely accepted model viewed the remodeling machine consisting of a DNA-binding domain, which also gripped tightly the histone core and a translocase domain, which lifted a section of the nucleosomal DNA off from the histone core and moved it along, while pulling in DNA from the entry site. The DNA-binding domain would then release the DNA and bind again to the newly entered DNA to repeat the cycle.

The details and geometries of action probably vary among the large variety of remodeling machines, accounting for the different ways the nucleosome remodeling is used. However, numerous biophysical data strongly suggest that the basic action is shared by the different remodeling ATPases. The following account represents a synthesis of the latest models (Clapier *et al.*, 2017) supported by recent biophysical data for the yeast SNF2 and the yeast ISWI remodelers (Li *et al.*, 2019). The remodeling complex, which is much larger in size than the nucleosome, binds to histone octamer at a fixed position, two helical turns of the DNA from the nucleosome dyad axis (Figure 28). Both DNA and ATP are bound between two protein domains that open and close in a stroke powered by hydrolysis of the bound ATP. This ratchets the binding site on one DNA strand by one phosphate, which is pulled in toward the nucleosome midpoint. Shifting one strand causes a tilt of the base pair and a twist in the double helix. On the proximal or entry side, the DNA is undertwisted while on the distal side it is overtwisted and contains excess DNA. The twist breaks contacts of the DNA with the histone core and the excess DNA propagates on the distal side like a wave of compression, breaking contacts as it propagates and reforming them in the rear. The remodeling machine itself remains fixed on the nucleosome histone core, resulting in a sequential twisting of the DNA and displacement of the DNA relative to the histone core in steps of one nucleotide pair. The twisting strain builds up and, surprisingly, instead of immediately sliding the DNA along, the nucleosome can

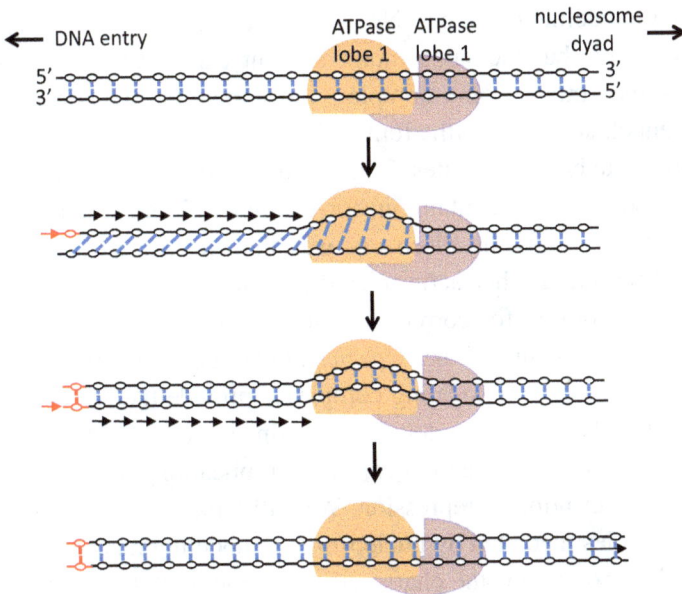

Figure 28.   Twist model for nucleosome remodeling. The remodeler ATPase binds to the nucleosomal DNA at superhelical location 2, halfway between the DNA entry site and the dyad symmetry axis of the nucleosome. The ATPase pulls the 5′ DNA strand, causing a local bulge of a few nucleotide. This causes a tilt in the base pairs corresponding to one base pair. The strain is transmitted as a twist to the DNA on the entry side, which causes the entry of one nucleotide on the 5′ strand. The ATPase shifts to a conformation that relieves the strain by shifting the 3′ strand by one nucleotide. The ATPase is re-set by hydrolyzing one ATP, restarting the cycle.

Source: Bowman (2019).

accommodate up to three additional base pairs before the accumulated twist is relieved by sliding the DNA, which moves out of the nucleosome, releasing the strain.

The details of this basic action will vary in different remodeling complexes. In some cases, the accumulation of strain may lift a loop of DNA from contact with the histone core, giving access to DNA-binding factors. In a similar way, the partial unwrapping can destabilize the histone core and, in collaboration with a histone chaperone, permit the dissociation or exchange of the H2A-H2B dimer. Different remodeling ATPases specialize in different kinds of operations, aided by associated components to form the remodeling machines. Not only is there a large variety of ATPase motor subunits, but the same motor subunit can serve in several complexes, some simple, some complex and containing a variety of other components that modulate the remodeling activity and help to target it to the appropriate chromatin sites. Some of these components are readers of histone modifications, containing, for example, chromodomains or bromodomains. A surprising discovery was that the complexes frequently contain β-actin and other actin-related proteins (Arps) that are essential components required for correct function of the remodeling complexes. The functions of actin and the Arps has not yet been identified.

These chromatin remodeling complexes provide the cell with a large panoply of tools to mold the local chromatin structure and to mediate the multitude of chromatin activities, from replication, to DNA damage repair, to transcription or repression. We will look at three general examples of activities mediated by nucleosome remodeling machines.

The first example is the characteristic action of sliding a nucleosome to create a larger gap or nucleosome-free region. This is the typical action of the SWI/SNF remodeler and its homologs in different species and accounts for the frequent presence of these remodeling complexes at transcription start sites. For a gene to be transcriptionally active, it is an essential requirement that the DNA immediately preceding the transcription site be accessible for binding of the general transcription factors and the RNA polymerase itself. This is facilitated by acetylation of the nucleosomes flanking this region. The SWI/SNF ATPase itself and often other components of the larger complex contain bromodomains that bind acetylated lysines and help recruit the remodeling complex. Regulation of the different steps in the ATPase and translocation activities determines the degree of nucleosome sliding relative to histone core ejection. The result is a typical configuration of nucleosomes around the transcription start site. A fixed reference point is the positioning of the first nucleosome immediately following the transcription start site. This is preceded by a gap usually about one nucleosome wide before less well-positioned nucleosomes in the upstream region begin again. This complex and its variants play the same role in opening the chromatin to allow binding of enhancer factors and other DNA-binding proteins.

The second situation occurs typically in the wake of the replication fork, where histones are re-deposited on the newly replicated DNA, reforming nucleosomes. The new nucleosomes are not precisely positioned: some are closer together, some a little farther apart. Two kinds of remodelers are associated with this process, ISWI subfamily and CHD subfamily remodelers. These remodelers have DNA-binding domains (SANT SLIDE or SLIDE) that bind to linker DNA and measure out the distance between nucleosomes. If sufficient linker DNA is available, the translocase activity is stimulated in proportion, drawing in linker DNA and bringing nucleosomes closer to achieve a uniform spacing until the minimum linker length is achieved. This activity is in a sense the opposite of that of the SWI/SNF type of remodeler. Overall it tends to generate chromatin that is more transcriptionally repressive while SWI/SNF tends to make chromatin more accessible and transcriptionally active. Analysis of nucleosome configurations in single cells shows that silent chromatin tends to contain uniformly spaced nucleosomes with little relationship to DNA sequence. In contrast, active chromatin tends to have precisely positioned nucleosomes but variable spacing between them.

The third case is that of the INO80 or SWR1 type of complexes. These loosen the nucleosome structure and replace histone H2A with the variant H2A.Z. This variant makes the nucleosome less stable, especially in combination with the H3.3 variant. H2A.Z is typically found in the nucleosomes flanking the gap created by the SWI/SNF type of remodeler at enhancers or promoters. The INO80 and SWR1 complexes also are recruited to DNA damage sites by the histone variant H2A.X and help displace nucleosomes to allow DNA repair.

High Mobility Group HMG Proteins

Nucleosomes are an intrinsic structural component of chromatin. They are what chromatin is made of and consequently histones, their dynamics and their modifications, play a front stage role in any discussion of chromatin. Less attention has been focused on another class of small, highly abundant proteins that are closely associated with chromatin. These are the High Mobility Group (HMG) proteins, so called because they are low molecular weight (under 30 kDa) and fast migrating in acidic gel electro-phoresis. They are all highly abundant during embryogenesis and are then progressively turned down. HMG proteins are not structural components of chromatin like the histones. They bind chromatin in a much more dynamic fashion, competing with histone H1 for binding to linker DNA but binding also to nucleosomal DNA. They control the bending and con-formation of chromatin and therefore affect the activities of chromatin in many cellular processes (Figure 29). Like histones, HMG proteins are

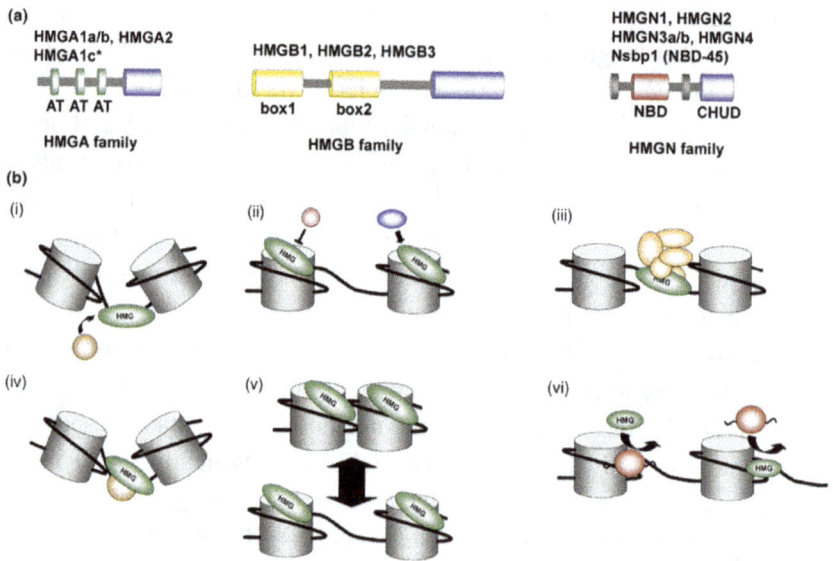

Figure 29.   Architectural functions of HMG proteins. (a) HMGAs contain two or three AT hooks that bind to AT-rich sequences, and an acidic C-terminal (blue). HMGB proteins contain two HMG boxes (yellow) and an acidic C-terminal (blue). HMGN proteins have a positively charged nucleosomal binding domain (NBD) and a negatively charged Chromatin Unfolding Domain (CHUD). (b) (i) HMGA and HMGB proteins have been shown to bend DNA. (ii) HMGN proteins have been shown to prevent or facilitate the access of chromatin factors. (iii) HMG proteins are often components of multiprotein complexes such as those that bind to enhanceosomes. (iv) They can be specifically recruited by DNA-binding factors. (v) They can promote spreading (HMGN) or compact-ing (HMGA) of nucleosomes. (vi) They can compete with binding of other proteins, for example, of linker histone H1.

Source: Hock *et al.* (2007).

subject to a wide range of post-transcriptional modifications, including acetylation, methylation of lysine and arginine, formylation, sumoylation, and phosphorylation. Unlike histone modification, little is known about the specific effects of these modifications.

The HMG proteins are subdivided into three families according to their DNA binding domains and binding specificities. All three families have a long C-terminal domain enriched in acidic amino acids The HMGA family proteins are so named because they have three AT-hooks, structural motifs that bind to the minor groove of AT-rich DNA. HMGA proteins have loose, disordered conformations that assume a defined secondary structure only when they bind to a substrate. Their best-known role is in helping to assemble enhanceosomes, DNA regions that fold in specific ways to bind multiple enhancer factors. HMGA proteins are often participants in the complex choreographies that involve histone acetylases, nucleosome remodelers, and enhancer-binding factors and result in promoter activation. Acetylation and deacetylation of the HMGA proteins themselves acts as a switch in the assembly/disassembly of enhanceosome complexes.

HMGB proteins are so named because they have two tandem HMG box domains. HMG boxes are also motifs that bind to the minor groove of DNA promoting bending at a sharp angle or binding to an already distorted DNA. HMGB proteins play a part in a variety of chromatin processes at least in part by binding to the DNA at the entry and exit from the nucleosome but, unlike histone H1, they help to recruit nucleosome remodelers that produce nucleosome sliding and favor making DNA more accessible to aid transcription, replication, and DNA repair.

The third family is called HMGN because its members contain a domain that binds directly to nucleosomes (NBD) and promote chromatin unfolding. None of the HMG proteins binds to specific sequences and all tend to compete with one another, with partially overlapping functions. In this wide variety of activities, HMG protein bind very loosely and transiently to chromatin. Their great abundance and transient interactions suggest that they participate opportunistically in any action initiated by other chromatin components, acting more as a lubricant than as a stably associated partner with either DNA or other DNA-binding proteins.

Further Reading

Ahmad K and Henikoff S (2002). The histone variant H3.3 marks active chromatin by replication-independent nucleosome assembly. *Mol Cell.* **9**, 1191–1200.

Alberts B, Bray D, Lewis J, Raff M, Roberts K and Watson JD (1989). *Molecular Biology of the Cell.* 2nd ed., Garland Publishing Inc.: New York, London.

Baldi S, Korber P and Becker PB (2020). Beads on a string — nucleosome array arrangements and folding of the chromatin fiber. *Nat Struct Mol Biol.* **27**, 109–118.

Bednar J, Horowitz RA, Grigoryev SA, Carruthers LM, Hansen JC, Koster AJ *et al.* (1998). Nucleosomes, linker DNA, and linker histone form a unique structural motif that directs the higher-order folding and compaction of chromatin. *Proc Natl Acad Sci USA.* **95**, 14173–14178.

Bianchi ME and Agresti A (2005). HMG proteins: Dynamic players in gene regulation and differentiation. *Curr Opin Genet Develop.* **15**, 496–506.

Bowman GD (2019). Uncovering a new step in sliding nucleosomes. *Trends Biochem Sci.* **44**, 643–645.

Clapier CR, Iwasa J, Cairns BR and Peterson CL (2017). Mechanisms of action and regulation of ATP-dependent chromatin-remodelling complexes. *Nat Rev Mol Cell Biol.* **18**, 407–422.

Draizen EJ, Shaytan AK, Marino-Ramirez L, Talbert PB, Landsman D and Panchenko AR (2016). HistoneDB 2.0: A histone database with variants — an integrated resource to explore histones and their variants. *Database.* PMID: 26989147.

Eltsov M, MacLellan KM, Maeshima K, Frangakis AS and Dubochet J (2008). Analysis of cryo-electron microscopy images does not support the existence of 30-nm chromatin fibers in mitotic chromosomes *in situ. Proc Natl Acad Sci USA.* **105**, 19732–19737.

Groth A, Rocha W, Verreault A and Almouzni G (2007). Chromatin challenges during DNA replication and repair. *Cell.* **128**, 721–733.

Henikoff S and Ahmad K (2019). Nucleosomes remember where they were. *Proc Natl Acad Sci USA.* **116**, 20254–2056.

Hock R, Furusawa T, Ueda T and Bustin M (2007). HMG chromosomal proteins in development and disease. *Trends Cell Biol.* **17**, 72–79.

Khorasanizadeh S (2004). The nucleosome: From genomic organization to genomic regulation. *Cell.* **116**, 259–272.

Larson DR and Misteli T (2017). The genome — seeing it clearly now. *Science.* **357**, 354–355.

Lasko P (2010). Tudor domain. *Curr Biol.* **20**, R666–R667.

Lawrence M, Daujat S and Schneider R (2016). Lateral thinking: how histone modifications regulate gene expression. *Trends Genet.* **32**, 42–56.

Li M, Xia X, Tian Y, Jia Q, Liu X, Lu Y *et al.* (2019). Mechanism of DNA translocation underlying chromatin remodelling by Snf2. *Nature.* **567**, 409–413.

Lowary PT and Widom J (1998). New DNA sequence rules for high affinity binding to histone octamer and sequence-directed nucleosome positioning. *J Mol Biol.* **276**, 19–42.

Luger K, Mäder AW, Richmond RK, Sargent DF and Richmond TJ (1997). Crystal structure of the nucleosome core particle at 2.8 A resolution. *Nature.* **389**, 251–260.

McKnight SL and Miller OL (1976). Ultrastructural patterns of RNA synthesis during early embryogenesis of *Drosophila melanogaster*. *Cell.* **8**, 305–319.

Mujtaba S, Zeng L and Zhou MM (2007). Structure and acetyl-lysine recognition of the bromodomain. *Oncogene.* **26**, 5521–5527.

Ou HD, Phan S, Deerinck TJ, Thor A, Ellisman MH and O'Shea CC (2017). ChromEMT: Visualizing 3D chromatin structure and compaction in interphase and mitotic cells. *Science.* **357**, eaag0025.

Petryk N, Dalby M, Wenger A, Stromme CB, Strandsby A, Andersson R *et al.* (2018). MCM2 promotes symmetric inheritance of modified histones during DNA replication. *Science.* **361**, 1389–1392.

Ramaswamy A and Ioshikhes I (2013). Dynamics of modeled oligonucleosomes and the role of histone variant proteins in nucleosome organization. Ch. 4 in R. Donev (ed.), *Advances in Protein Chemistry and Structural Biology*. Academic Press. Vol. **90**, pp. 119–149.

Ricci MA, Manzo C, García-Parajo MF, Lakadamyali M and Cosma MP (2015). Chromatin fibers are formed by heterogeneous groups of nucleosomes *in vivo*. *Cell.* **160**, 1145–1158.

Valouev A, Johnson SM, Boyd SD, Smith CL, Fire AZ and Sidow A (2011). Determinants of nucleosome organization in primary human cells. *Nature.* **474**, 516–520.

Wooten M, Snedeker J, Nizami ZF, Yang X, Ranjan R, Urban E *et al.* (2019). Asymmetric histone inheritance via strand-specific incorporation and biased replication fork movement. *Nat Struct Mol Biol.* **26**, 732–743.

Yu C, Gan H, Serra-Cardona A, Zhang L, Gan S, Sharma S *et al.* (2018). A mechanism for preventing asymmetric histone segregation onto replicating DNA strands. *Science.* **361**, 1386.

Zhang Q and Wang Y (2010). HMG modifications and nuclear function. *Biochim Biophys Acta.* **1799**, 28–36.

Chapter 3

DNA Methylation and Gene Silencing

Introduction

DNA methylation is an ancient DNA modification that does not change its sequence or protein-coding content but marks it in a distinct way that can be recognized by suitable proteins. Two of the nucleotide bases, adenine and cytosine, can be methylated at the 5 carbon or the 6 nitrogen to form, respectively, 5-methylcytosine (5mC) and N6-methyladenine (6mA) (Figure 1). Both kinds of DNA methylation are found in bacteria, bacteriophages, plants, and metazoans, although they have been evolutionarily lost in some species. Two well-studied model organisms, *Drosophila melanogaster* and *Caenorhabditis elegans*, have eliminated DNA methylation altogether. In bacteria, both cytosine and adenine methylation are used in restriction-modification systems to mark genomic DNA and distinguish it from infecting viral or plasmid DNA. In these systems, two different functions are involved: a DNA methyltransferase that marks specific sequence motifs and an endonuclease that cuts these sequences when they are not marked. Thus, methylated DNA is protected, but invading non-methylated DNA is cleaved and then degraded. At present, there is no indication that DNA methylation is used in a similar way in metazoans. Additional roles for DNA methylation were acquired in some bacteria such as *E. coli*, where the Dam methylase is involved in DNA replication and in the direction of DNA mismatch repair.

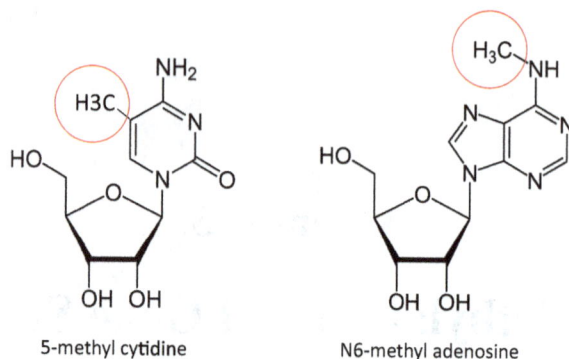

Figure 1.   5-methyl cytidine and N6-methyl adenosine.

Cytosine Methylation

In eukaryotic genomes, 5mC is much more frequent than 6mA and was found very early to be an important epigenetic modification regulating gene expression. More recently, 6mA has also been reported to have important roles to play in chromatin and gene expression that are beginning to be identified. In contrast to bacteria and plants, in vertebrates 5mC occurs primarily in the context of the self-complementary dinucleotide CpG. This has an important consequence in that the target sequence on one strand is accompanied by the same sequence on the opposite strand. Therefore, the same sequence-specific methyltransferase will target both strands producing a fully methylated CpG site. Cytosine methylation is occasionally found at other sequences that are now beginning to be thought significant.

DNA methylation serves many functions, but in vertebrates the major role is to interfere with many DNA-biding proteins and to silence transposable elements and individual genes in the course of development. It is found more abundantly in repressed parts of the genome such as the heterochromatin of many but not all metazoans. We will be primarily concerned with C-methylation because it is a critically important epigenetic repressive signal that has also played an important role in shaping the evolution of metazoan genomes.

Detection of 5mC in DNA

In a DNA sequence, cytosine residues that carry a 5-methyl group are not distinguished by standard Sanger sequencing or by massively parallel sequencing methods (also called Next Generation Sequencing. See Chapter 13). Both of these methods rely on DNA polymerase and standard base pairing with which 5mCs are simply read as Cs. Single molecule nanopore sequencing methods can distinguish them from Cs with fairly high efficiency (see Chapter 13, Nanopore Sequencing). However, the "gold standard" to detect or identify 5mC in a DNA sequence relies on a chemical treatment with bisulfite (Figure 2). 5mC residues are readily detected because they are resistant to bisulfite *in vitro*, while unmethylated cytosines are sulphonated at the 5-position. Subsequent deamination converts the cytosine to uracil, which is detected as a T in DNA sequencing. Thus, in a known DNA sequence, C residues are converted to Ts if unmethylated, while 5mC residues continue to be read as Cs. Sequencing the DNA with bisulfite treatment and comparing with the sequence

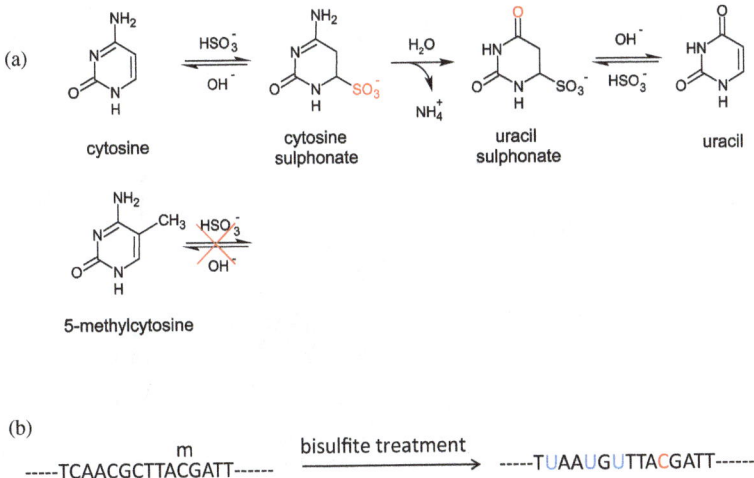

Figure 2.   Bisulfite treatment of cytosine. (a) Cytosine is converted to uracil by treatment with bisulfite. 5-methyl cytosine is resistant to bisulfite. (b) Therefore bisulfite treatment of DNA converts all Cs to Us, which are read as Ts during DNA sequencing. Only 5mCs remain unconverted and are read as Cs.

without bisulfite is therefore the most reliable method for the detection of specific methylated Cs in a sequence.

CpG Islands

Over time, cytosine can spontaneously deaminate, converting to uracil (Figure 3). This is rapidly detected by genome surveillance mechanisms in the cell and corrected. The methylation of the 5-position of cytosine corresponds to the methyl position of thymine. Therefore, deamination of 5mC converts it to thymine. This mutation is not corrected by the normal surveillance mechanisms. Since some 70% of CpGs in vertebrate genomes

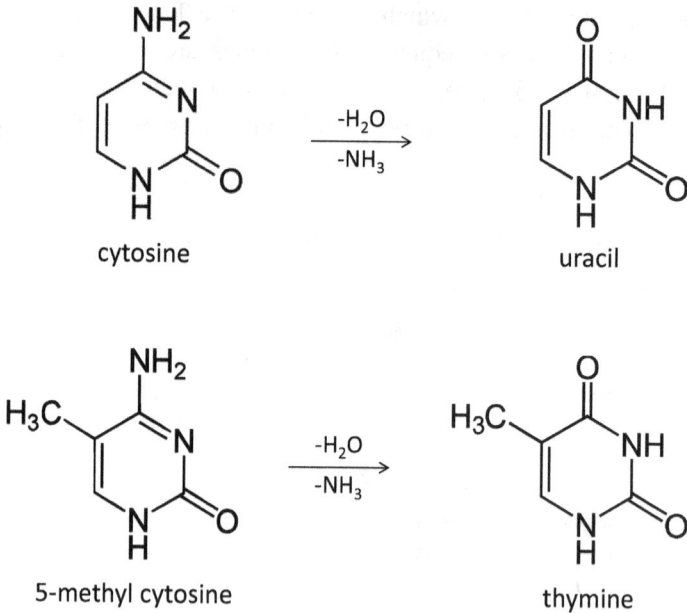

Figure 3.   Spontaneous deamination of cytosine and 5-methyl cytosine. Even under *in vivo* conditions, cytosine can spontaneously deaminate to produce uracil. This is rapidly recognized by DNA repair mechanisms that excise the mis-paired uracil and replace it with cytosine. These mechanisms do not recognize thymine as an abnormal DNA base so, although the G:T mismatch is recognized, it is corrected as A:T as likely as G:C. In evolution, therefore the occurrence of such events in the germ line lead to the loss of methylatable C:Gs.

are methylated in the germ line, as in most tissues, this results, on the evolutionary time scale, in the conversion of CpGs to TpGs. As a result, vertebrate genomes are in general depleted of CpG nucleotides. Genomic regions that tend to be protected against CpG methylation have preserved their CpGs and appear as short regions with comparatively high CpG content. These are called **CpG islands** and, in mammalian genomes, they tend to be in the range of a few hundred to a thousand bp long. The reason they are protected against DNA methylation is that they serve as promoters or regulatory sequences (see Chapter 6). Many transcription factors, including promoter factors, bind to CpG-containing sequences. The binding of a protein to a CpG protects the site from methylation. CpG island promoters are found at some 70% of mammalian genes. This is one reason CpG islands have been protected from evolutionary loss by deamination (Figure 4). The human genome contains about 25,000 CpG islands. About half of these are gene promoter regions. The rest are probably in large part enhancers or similar kinds of regulatory regions in both intergenic and

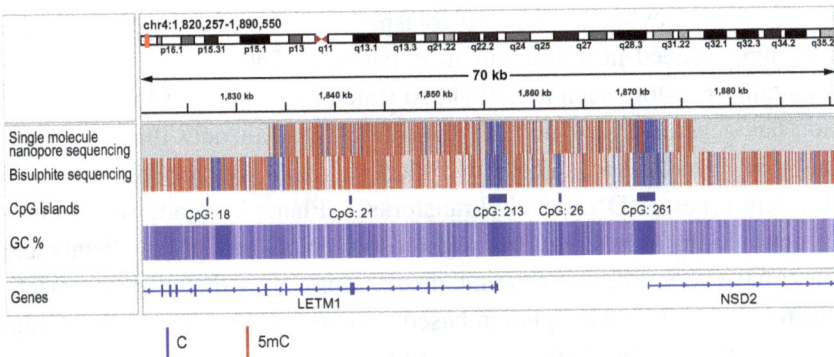

Figure 4. CpG islands in the human genome. The figure illustrates the distribution of 5mC in a region of the human genome. At the top, the genetic map of the region is shown. In the middle section, a single-molecule nanopore sequence read of about 43 kb is shown. Vertical red bars indicate 5mCs and blue bars, unmethylated Cs. The row below shows the 5mC distribution determined by bisulfite sequencing. Below this row the local %GC distribution is shown and the positions of CpG islands classified in the human genome. The lowest section maps the genes and their exon distribution in this region. Note the distinct high level of GCs corresponding to CpG islands and their low level of methylation. Sequencing data figure kindly supplied by Sofia Battaglia.

intragenic sequences. In somatic tissues, most of these CpG islands are unmethylated and methylation assumes a strongly repressive function, in most cases silencing transcription.

While in mammalian genomes promoters of developmental genes are generally undermethylated or methylated only in certain tissues or developmental stages, a large fraction of genomic CpGs are methylated, particularly in repetitive sequences, heterochromatin, and in gene bodies. Methylation of gene bodies has no effect on gene activity, methylation of promoters is generally repressive, as it prevents the binding of proteins whose binding sites contain CpG and recruits instead factors that repress transcription. Promoter methylation is carefully regulated by various mechanisms discussed as follows, including specific demethylases, to ensure that only genes whose functions are no longer needed in a differentiation pathway are silenced. In this respect, DNA methylation serves a major epigenetic role in vertebrates.

If it is to serve a reliable regulatory function in specific parts of the genome, it is evident that the methylation mechanisms need to carry out two kinds of functions: one is the specific *de novo* methylation of sites that need to be methylated to turn off transposable elements or genes that are no longer needed in a differentiation pathway. The other is to faithfully maintain or restore such a methylated state after a wave of DNA replication has generated new, unmethylated DNA in sequences that had previously been methylated. These two kinds of tasks are carried out by two different types of DNA methyltransferases. Plants have additional kinds of methyltransferases that can target also CpNpG or CpNpN. Plants and fungi have very different genomic distributions of methylation and mechanisms for *de novo* methylation based on small RNAs that are not found in vertebrates and will not be discussed here.

De novo CpG Methylation

Mammalian cells have two main *de novo* DNA methylase genes, Dnmt3A and Dnmt3B. Each of these produces multiple isoforms through alternative promoter use and splicing variants. They are assisted by a closely related protein called Dnmt3L that lacks the catalytic domain but cooperates with Dnmt3A and B to increase their DNA binding and enzymatic activity (Figure 5). An additional protein called Dnmt2 is also related but methylates some tRNAs. DNMT3A and B methylases produce the CpG methylation in vertebrate genomes. They are also responsible for the very low frequency of non-CpG methylation at CpAs or CpTs that is found in cells with very high levels of *de novo* methylases such as embryonic stem cells (see what follows). This non-CpG methylation is gradually lost because it is not maintained by the maintenance methylase, which is specific for the symmetric CpG dinucleotide.

The DNMT3 protein structure includes a catalytic domain at the C-terminal, a PWWP domain characterized by a proline-tryptophan-tryptophan-proline motif, and an inhibitory domain called ADD (ATRX-DNMT3L-DNMT3A). The PWWP domain recognizes and binds to

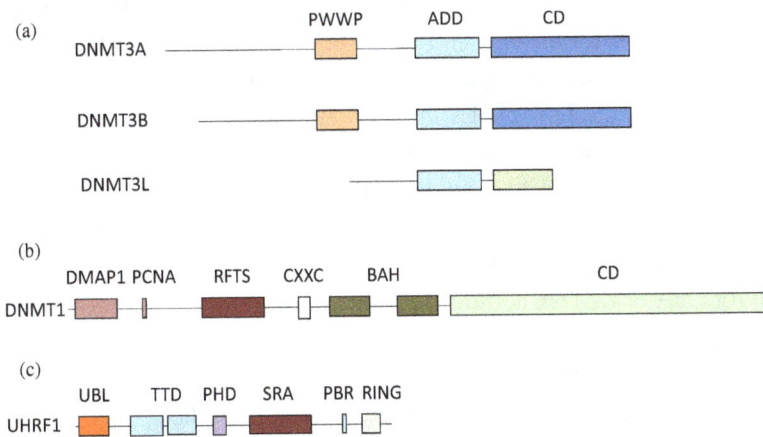

Figure 5. Mammalian cytosine DNA methyltransferases. (a) *de novo* DNMTs. The PWWP domain recognizes H3K36me3 and stimulates activity. The ADD domain recognizes H3K4 metylation and is inhibitory.The catalytic domain CD is absent in DNMT3L. Additional isoforms of the DNMT3s produced by alternative promoter use or splicing are not shown. (b) DNMT1 maintenance methylase. Binding sites for DMAP1 and PCNA are indicated. RFTS domain inhibits methylation until it binds to histone H3 ubiquitylated by UHRF1. CXXC modified zinc finger binds to CpG-rich sequences. BAH bromo-associated domains bind to replication foci. (c) UHRF1 domains. UBL targets ubiquitylation to histone H3 TTD tandem tudor domain binds to H3K9me2,3. PHD zinc finger binds unmethylated H3R2. SRA binds to hemimethylated CpGs. The RING domain ubiquitylates Histone H3K14, K18, and K23.

Source: Chen and Zhang (2020).

H3K36me3, a histone modification found in active transcription units. This ensures the DNA methylation of transcriptionally active gene bodies. The ADD domain appears to interact with the catalytic domain and decrease its binding to DNA and therefore produces an autoinhibitory effect. This autoinhibition is relieved when the ADD domain binds to unmethylated histone H3K4. At activated promoters and enhancers, which are generally marked with H3K4 methylation, the ADD domain is free to inhibit the catalytic domain, thus preventing DNA methylation of the regulatory regions of active genes.

The active DNA methylating complex is a tetramer containing two DNMT3L/DNMT3As (or DNMT3Bs) heterodimers. The DNMT3Ls have no catalytic activity and they do not themselves bind to DNA, but they still possess an ADD domain and bind to nucleosomes containing unmethylated H3K4. The fact that DNMT3A,B and DNMT3L require unmethylated H3K4 means that H3K4 methylation, associated with active enhancers and promoter regions, is a powerful inhibitor of DNA methylation. Critically, the DNMT3Ls interact with the catalytic domains of the two DNMT3B subunits and are required to maintain their active conformation. The tetramer's two catalytically active domains contact DNA at sites 10–14 base pairs apart and recognize both the C and the G of CpGs. This results in a methylation efficiency for CpG more than 20 times higher than for CpA or CpT. In addition, binding of the tetramer appears to facilitate recruitment of additional DNMT3L-DNMT3A,B heterodimers alongside. This would account for the tendency of methylation to occur preferentially in a pattern with a roughly 10 bp periodicity.

Maintenance Methylation

DNA replication of fully methylated CpG sequences separates the two strands and synthesizes a new complementary strand for each. The newly synthesized stand is entirely unmethylated. CpGs in newly replicated DNA are methylated on one strand only: they are hemimethylated. The maintenance DNA methyltransferase DNMT1 is specialized to recognize and target sites methylated on one strand only. In the absence of Dnmt1, one round of DNA replication would produce two hemimethylated daughter DNA molecules. A second round of replication would produce one hemimethylated and one fully unmethylated daughter DNA molecule. So repeated DNA replication in the absence of DNMT1 would soon result in loss of methylation (Figure 6). To ensure rapid and efficient remethylation of hemimethylated sites, the DNMT1enzyme is recruited to DNA replication foci.

DNMT1 contains a catalytic domain at the C-terminal end. The N-terminal region includes a domain that binds to DMAP1 (DNMT1-associated protein 1), a transcriptional repressor that brings along also a histone deacetylase. DNMT1 also contains a domain that binds to PCNA (proliferating nuclear antigen), the central component of the replication complex. This ensures that DNMT1 is immediately available when DNA is replicated. The N-terminal region contains also a CXXC motif, a modified zinc finger structural motif that binds preferentially to unmethylated CpG-rich regions (Figure 5). This motif will be encountered in many other proteins that associate with CpG islands, but in DNMT1 it has the key role of blocking unmethylated CpGs from the active site of the methylase and therefore preventing *de novo* methylation.

DNMT1 is recruited to replication foci by binding to PCNA but also, and critically, by interaction with UHRF1, a RING-type E3 ubiquitin

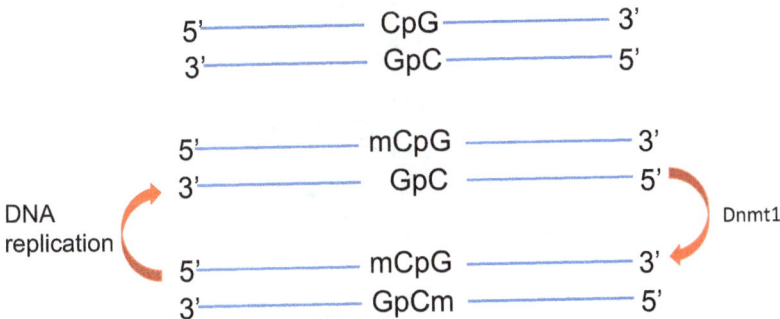

Figure 6.   The role of the maintenance methylase DNMT1. *De novo* DNA methylation methylates CpGs on both strands, but a wave of DNA replication separates the strands and synthesizes a new complementary strand along each strand. The newly synthesized strand is not methylated so the CpG sites are now methylated on the old strand only: they are hemimethylated. Hemimethylated sites need to be rapidly methylated fully. A second round of DNA replication would cause loss of methylation entirely. DNMT1 recognizes hemimethylated sites and restores full methylation.

ligase that binds to hemimethylated CpG sites through a SET and RING-Associated domain (SRA). UHRF1 also uses a tandem tudor domain (TTD) to bind to histone H3K9me2,3 and a PHD finger to bind to H3 unmethylated at arginine 2 (Figure 7). When UHRF1 is so positioned, the catalytic activity of the RING domain is stimulated to mono-ubiquitylate K14, K18, and K23 of histone H3. The ubiquitylated residues in turn provide binding sites for DNMT1. In addition, DNMT1 can also bind to a Ubiquitin-like domain of UHRF1.

Loading of DNMT1 onto the PCNA replication complex is accompanied by loading of G9a, a histone H3K9 methylase that generally produces H3K9me2. This can then be raised to H3K9me3 by other methylases such as SUV39 or SETDB1. G9a has been shown to bind directly to DNMT1 and the resulting complex stimulates both CpG methylation and H3K9 methylation. These multiple and complex interactions involved in DNMT1 recruitment mean that, while the methylase is catalytically highly active, it spares CpG islands, which normally lack hemimethylated

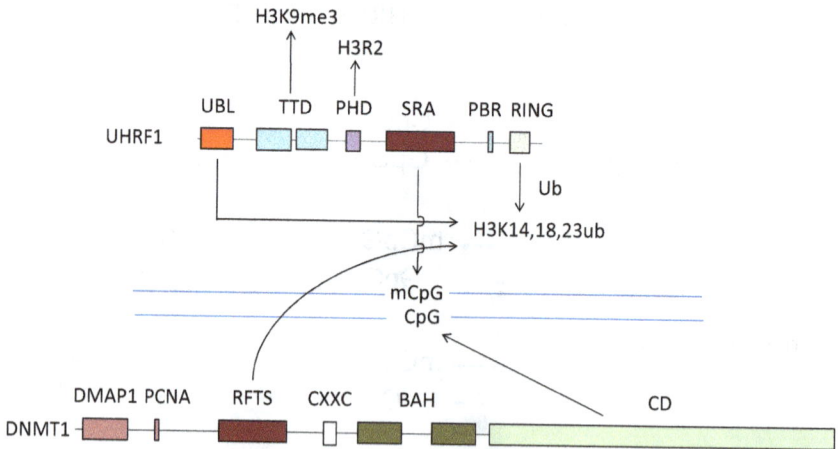

Figure 7.   Schematic summary of maintenance methylation. UHRF1 selects chromatin regions by binding to H3K9me3 and unmethylated H3R2 with its TTD and PHD domains. UHRF1 binds to hemimetylated CpG sites on DNA through its SRA domain. The SRA domain recruits ubiquitin conjugating enzymes and the RING domain ubiquitylates histone H3K14,18,23. The DNMT1 TFTS domain recognizes and binds to the ubiquitylated H3 and methylates the hemimethylated CpG site.

CpGs or H3K9 methylation. They also frequently contain symmetrically dimethylated histone H3R2, which blocks binding of UHRF1.

TET Demethylases

Before examining differentially methylated regions in more detail, we need to introduce the cytosine demethylases that counteract the DNMTs. These are the TET (Ten-Eleven Translocation) proteins, a set of closely related enzymes that act as α-ketoglutarate (also called 2-oxoglutarate)-dependent dioxygenases that target 5-methylcytosines (Figure 8). The three TET enzymes in mammals share a cysteine-rich region and catalytic domain, which binds α-ketoglutarate and iron (II) to catalyze the oxidation of 5-methylcytosine (5mC) to 5-hydroxymethylcytosine (5hmC). The TET enzymes can also, but much more slowly, further oxidize 5hmeC to 5-formylcytosine (5fC), then 5-carboxycytosine (5caC) (Figure 9). This last can be removed by decarboxylases or by the base excision DNA repair (BER) machinery, which removes the 5fC or 5caC base and restores

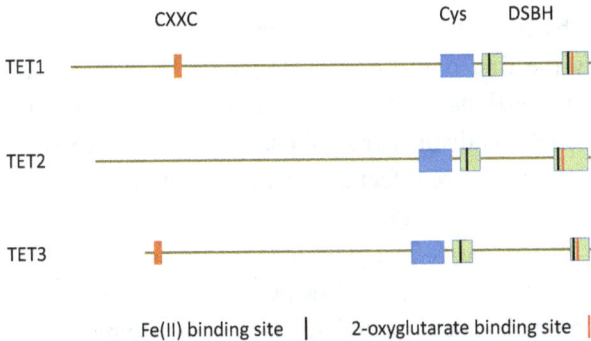

Figure 8. TET dioxygenases. All three enzymes contain a cysteine-rich region (Cys), a double-stranded beta helix region (DSBH, two Fe(II)) and one 2-oxyglutarate binding site, the latter two form part of the active site. In addition, TET1 and TET3 have a CXXC domain that targets them to CpG-rich regions. TET2 has become separated from its CXXC domain, which now is found in a separate gene upstream of TET2, called IDAX. The IDAX protein binds to TET2 and effectively also targets it to CpG islands.

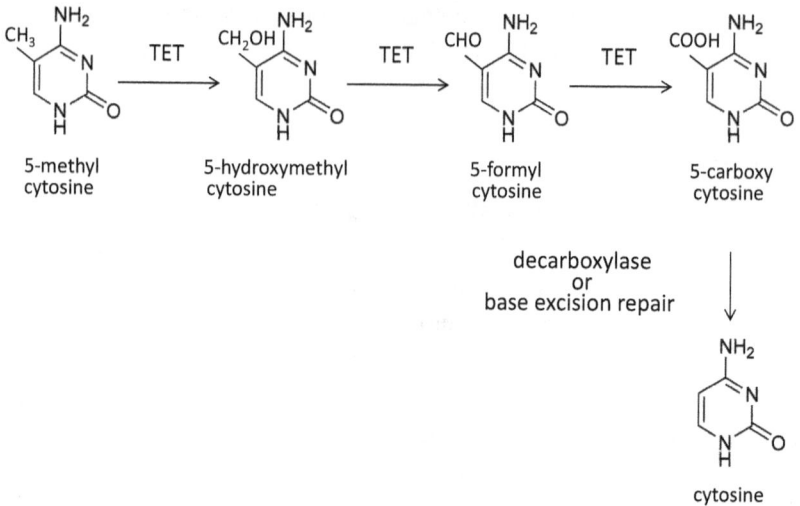

Figure 9.   Progressive oxidation of 5-methyl cytosine by TET enzymes. Repeated action by the TET enzymes on 5-methyl cytosine eventually produces 5-carboxy cytosine. The carboxyl group may be removed by a decarboxylase or the entire base can be excised by the Base Excision Repair (BER) system and the DNA repaired by resynthesis.

the cytosine by resynthesis using the other strand as template. The 5hmC produced by the first oxidation step is longer lived than the subsequent products and questions have been raised whether it might have specific epigenetic functions distinct from those of 5mC. Conversion of 5mC to 5hmC has a derepressive effect in most cases, although 5hmC still binds MeCP2, a major 5mC-binding protein involved in recruiting repressive complexes. In addition, 5-hmCpG is a very poor substrate for the DNMT1 maintenance methylase because 5mCpG/5hmCpG or CpG/5hmCpG sites are not recognized as hemimethylated targets, hence result in passive loss of methylation after DNA replication, in addition to active loss through repeated TET activity. There is little convincing evidence that 5hmC "says" something new. However, recent evidence has shown that 5hmC can accumulate and remain at stable high levels, especially in neurons and is not just a labile intermediate toward complete demethylation. In addition, it is possible that the 5hmC mark is recognized by some but not all methyl-C-binding proteins (see what follows) and thus may recruit some chromatin silencing complexes but not others. This would allow it to continue to silence in some contexts and in some cells but not in others. It should be noted that 5hmC behaves like 5mC in the standard bisulfite treatment, which therefore does not distinguish the two. A method combining TET treatment with bisulfite has been developed to distinguish 5hmC from 5mC. This method confirmed that 5hmC is enriched at gene regulatory elements such as promoters and particularly enhancers. Within these regions, 5hmC peaks around the consensus binding sites of pluripotency regulatory factors in embryonic stem cells.

Another important domain shared by TET1 and TET3 is a CXXC domain, a modified zinc finger that binds to CpG-rich sequences. TET2 lacks this domain, apparently by a rearrangement that occurred in evolution that separated the 5' end of the ancestral gene and formed a separate gene IDAX that contains the CXXC domain and interacts with TET2. This would account for the enriched presence of all three TET enzymes in regions rich in CpGs, such as CpG islands.

Targeting of DNA Methylation

In vertebrates the major DNA methylation activity takes place during the recovery from two waves of global demethylation that reset genomic programming (see Chapter 9). The first takes place in the very early embryo and the second is limited to the germ line precursor cells, as will be discussed later. Recovery from these global demethylation events is facilitated by the overexpression of the *de novo* methylases, particularly DNMT3B, which plays the major role in the first remethylation. This global remethylation is not specifically targeted and may affect cytosines in non-CpG contexts, due to the high levels of DNMT3B (see also Chapter 9, for Stem Cells). However, only CpG methylation can be maintained by the DNMT1 methylase. Global *de novo* methylation is also shaped by inhibitory and blocking effects such that, although more than 70% of all CpGs in the mammalian genome are methylated in most tissues, some regions are preferentially methylated and some are preferentially not methylated. Some of these effects are due to histone modifications that either favor or inhibit DNMTs; some are caused by blockage of CpGs by DNA binding proteins; some result from demethylation by TET demethylase enzymes; most importantly, some are produced by specific recruitment mechanisms. These are largely responsible for the differential methylation or targeting of methylation to or away from specific genomic regions as we will examine here.

Effects of Histone Modifications

We will start with the modulations resulting from the presence of histone modifications (summarized in Figure 10). As discussed above, both the *de novo* and the maintenance DNMTs are differentially affected by different histone modifications. In particular, genomic regions such as promoters or transcribed genes are associated with specific histone modifications that therefore directly affect the level of CpG methylation.

CpG islands, being particularly rich in potential methylation sites, are an important case. They also tend to be less densely occupied by nucleosomes and are therefore more accessible to methylases. However, CpG islands are also direct targets for other processes that interfere with DNA methylation. They tend to have high densities of binding sites for transcription factors, which are often rich in CpG content. These occupy DNA sequences and block the access of *de novo* DNA methyltransferases. One kind of DNA binding factor enriched at CpG islands is the family of proteins containing a CXXC type motif, which binds to regions rich in CpGs. An important CXXC factor is Cfp1, a component of SETD1A and B,

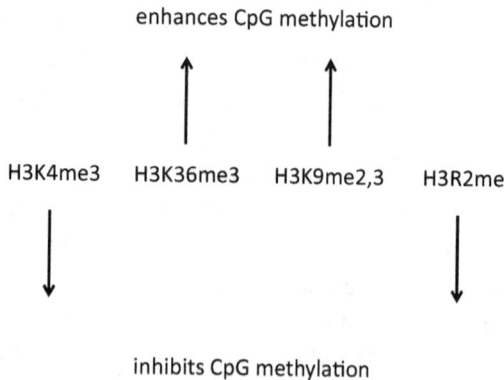

Figure 10.   Effects of histone modifications on DNA methylation.

chromatin complexes that methylate histone H3K4 at promoters. H3K4me3 is a powerful inhibitor of DNA methylation. As we have seen, TET demethylases also have CXXC motifs and tend to bind to CpG islands. As a result, CpG islands and CpG island promoters are generally protected against CpG methylation and remain potentially available as promoters.

At active genes, the advancing transcription complex includes RNA polymerase whose C-terminal domain is phosphorylated at serine2 of the C-terminal domain repeat units (see Chapter 6). This allows binding of the Set2 histone methylase, which travels with the polymerase and methylates H3K36 along the transcription unit. As we have seen, *de novo* DNMTs and associated proteins recognize and bind to histone H3K36me3. The affinity of DNMTs for H3K36me3 ensures that the bodies of actively transcribed genes are heavily methylated. This does not affect the activity of the promoter, which depends on the methylation status of the promoter and enhancer regions, nor does it affect transcription elongation. Gene body CpG methylation tends to suppress acetylation of nucleosomes and the binding of transcription factors. One possible interpretation of gene body methylation is that it prevents inappropriate transcription starts in the gene body. Transcriptional activity tends to transiently unwind nucleosomes and, in strongly transcribed genes, may decrease the nucleosome density, allowing transcription factors and RNA pol II to bind. Transcription starts in the middle of a gene would lead to the synthesis of partial proteins that in many cases would interfere or even antagonize with the functioning of the gene product.

Related to this is the role of another CXXC protein called FBXL10, also known as KDM2B, a H3K36 demethylase. This protein is characteristically associated with most CpG islands and contributes to keeping them free of DNA methylation both by blocking CpG sites and by removing H3K36 methylation that might stimulate DNA methylation. KDM2B is not entirely favorable to transcriptional activity, however, it can help to recruit another repressive mechanism independent of DNA methylation or H3K9 methylation: this is the Polycomb repressive mechanism as we shall see later (see Chapter 7).

H3K9 methylation has a close but more indirect relationship to CpG methylation. In regions containing H3K9 di- or tri-methylation, CpG methylation is preferentially maintained by the DNMT1-UHRF1 complex, as we have seen. In addition, *de novo* DNMTs have been found to be associated with complexes that deposit H3K9 methylation. Knockout experiments show that, although there are several histone H3K9 methylases, knocking each out individually causes loss of DNA methylation in some particular context. SUV39H1 can be found in the same complex with the *de novo* DNA methyltransferase, DNMT3B, while SETDB1, a methyltransferase that produces H3K9me3, has been detected in complex with DNMT3A. As a result, satellite clusters and heterochromatin in general tend to be strongly DNA methylated.

To summarize, H3K9 methylation promotes DNMT1, but H3R2 methylation inhibits it; H3K4 methylation inhibits DNMT3s, but H3K36me3 promotes it. And, in fact, CpG methylation is well correlated with heterochromatin and with genomic regions rich in H3K9 methylation. CpG methylation is high in the gene bodies of actively transcribed genes, low at promoters of active genes, which are instead generally enriched for H3K4 methylation and symmetric H3R2 methylation. In the long run, CpGs that are not associated with H3K4me3 or with histone acetylation tend to acquire both H3K9 methylation and CpG methylation and become transcriptionally silenced.

Recruitment of DNMTs to Transposable Elements

Silencing repetitive elements is probably the most conserved function of DNA methylation, preserved also in plants and lower eukaryotes. In mammals, transposable elements, either intact or partially deleted, constitute about 40% of the genome and consist of three major types: Long terminal repeat (LTR) elements such as endogenous retroviruses, long interspersed nuclear elements (LINEs), and short interspersed nuclear elements (SINEs). LTR elements and LINES contain promoters, which in intact elements drive reverse transcriptases and transposition-related functions. These need to be silenced to prevent transposition activity and genomic instability. SINEs generally utilize functions expressed by the other types of transposons.

Different mechanisms have developed to silence different types of transposable elements in embryonic stem cells. Many endogenous retroviruses are targeted by a zinc finger DNA-binding protein ZFP809 that binds to a sequence in the LTR promoter that is conserved in many retroviruses because it is the binding site of a cellular tRNA that serves as primer for reverse transcriptase. ZFP809 in turn recruits a silencing complex containing TRIM28 and SETDB1, which methylates H3K9, silencing the retroviral promoter. This is accompanied by the recruitment of DNMT3A, which establishes long-lasting CpG methylation-based silencing.

Genome integrity is particularly important in the germ line. In mammalian germ line progenitors, the genome undergoes a wave of global DNA demethylation to reset the methylation status to that of gametes. DNA methylation of transposable elements must quickly be silenced again to prevent the propagation of retroviruses as well as non-LTR repetitive elements such as LINEs. In male gametogenesis, the PIWI mechanism (see description in Chapter 5) is activated when transcription of transposable elements begins to be derepressed. The RNAs are processed by the PIWI proteins. In mouse germ line cells, these are the MILI and MIWI2 proteins. The RNA transcripts are reduced to 26 nucleotide primary piRNAs. These serve as guides to bind MILI to antisense transcripts produced by the PIWI clusters. These are in turn processed to produce secondary piRNAs, which bind to MIWI2 and target it to the sense transposable element transcripts in the cytoplasm. This is the so-called ping-pong amplification in which transposable element transcripts are consumed while at the same time increasing the supply of primary piRNAs. Simultaneously, secondary piRNAs complexes analogous to the *Drosophila* piRISC complexes enter the nucleus, target nascent transposable element transcripts, and recruit silencing complexes containing H3K9 methylases and HP1. These complexes also involve DNMT3L and DNMT3A, which carry out *de novo* CpG methylation of transposable elements. The details of DNMT recruitment are not fully elucidated, but it is clear that loss of MILI in the male germ line results in loss of transposable element CpG methylation, massive expression of transposable element transcripts, and meiotic arrest. DNA methylation continues in sperms until the genome is almost completely methylated. This is important to prevent unregulated gene expression in the fertilized egg, when the sperm genome is not yet assembled into chromatin (see Chapter 9).

In contrast to sperms, the oocyte genome has a more specific DNA methylation pattern. While millions of sperms are produced in male gametogenesis, oocytes are produced only one or a few at a time. Oocytes are active cells that need to prepare for fertilization and for the initial steps of embryogenesis, which means that many genes need to remain active. Although the full story of *de novo* CpG methylation in the female germ line is complex, it appears that much of the genomic methylation is the consequence of H3K36me3 produced by transcriptional activity. Loss of function of the SETD2 histone methylase responsible for H3K36me3 results in loss of DNA methylation in oocytes. Whether and to what extent the PIWI pathway is active in the female germ line or in somatic tissues is not yet clear. There is evidence of somatic PIWI activity in *Drosophila*. In mammals, the machinery required for repetitive element silencing is not present in somatic tissues other than the early embryo. In general, transposable elements remain silenced in somatic tissues, DNA methylation is maintained by the DNMT1 maintenance pathway and there is little transcriptional activity of repetitive elements.

Developmental Gene Silencing by *de novo* Methylation

During development some genes need to be turned off, for example: when a cell enters a differentiation pathway (as we shall see later), genes controlling other pathways must be turned off for the long term. DNA methylation cannot turn off active genes: active epigenetic marks at CpG island promoters inhibit DNMTs. These genes must be first turned off by repressive transcription factors. Generally this involves histone deacetylases and H3K9 methylases. Subsequently, DNMTs promoted by H3K9 methylation are recruited to render the repression stable and long-term. A common feature of promoters that are turned off during development is the recruitment of the H3K9 methylase G9a by DNA-binding transcriptional regulators. This produces H3K9me1,2. This is followed by DNA methylation and transcriptional shutdown. Knockout mutation of G9a prevents CpG methylation at these genes, but knockout of DNMT3b does not interfere with H3K9 methylation. This implies that G9a acts first and then recruits CpG methylation. Detailed analysis at these genes shows in fact that H3K9 methylation and HP1 binding usually occurs first, followed by recruitment of DNMT3B and DNA methylation. *In vitro* experiments show that G9a binds directly to DNMT3B through its ANK domain and recruits it to its chromatin targets. Consistent with this structural role, DNA methylation at some target genes was found to be dependent on G9a but not on its catalytic activity.

Methyl-binding Proteins

How does DNA methylation silence transcription? Silencing is generally initiated by H3K9 methylation. DNA methylation takes over a chromatin that has already been silenced. This prevents binding of many transcription factors.

A broader repressive effect results from the involvement of repressive complexes associated with the establishment of repressive chromatin by recruiting histone deacetylases and chromatin remodeling machines that make chromatin more compact. Such repressive complexes are recruited to DNA enriched in 5mC by proteins that bind preferentially to this modification. Two classes of methyl-binding proteins are known: MBD proteins and KAISO proteins (Figure 11). The MBD group contains a conserved Methyl Binding Domain (MBD). MBD proteins generally bind to symmetrically methylated CpG sites and recruit repressive complexes. The KAISO group is characterized by a POZ/BTB domain, a powerful protein–protein interaction motif that forms homodimers or heterodimers with other POZ/BTB proteins. KAISO proteins bind to 5mC through some of the multiple zinc finger motifs they contain.

MBD is a structural domain of about 70 amino acids that binds to DNA that contains one or more symmetrically methylated CpGs. MECP2, MBD1,2,3,4 are known human MBD proteins, although each has alternative splicing variants that produce protein isoforms. Each has also special features that modulate whether and how they bind to CpGs. In addition, MBD proteins often contain additional structural motifs that interact with chromatin, such as bromodomains, SET domains, PHD fingers that help to recruit other chromatin proteins such as histone deacetylases, histone methylases SETDB1 and SUV39, and chromatin remodeling complexes. MBD proteins accumulate at genomic regions depending on the local

(a)

(b)

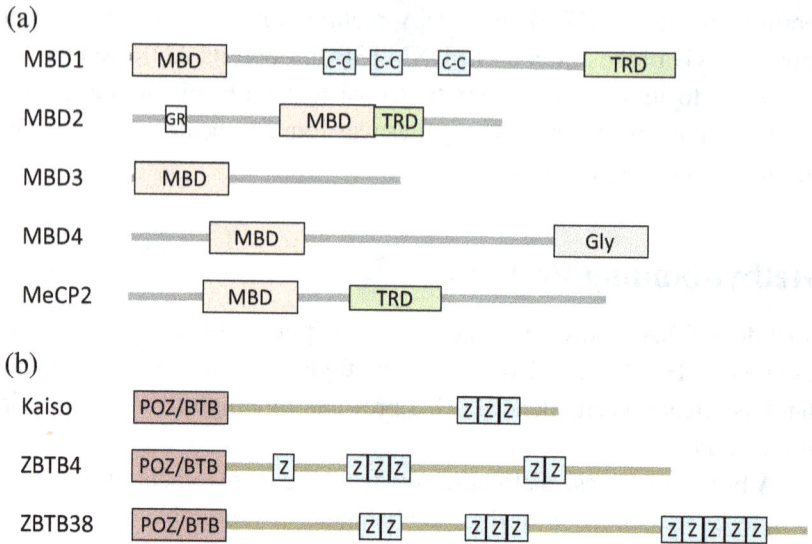

Figure 11.   5-methyl cytosine-binding proteins. (a) MBD proteins share the MBD domain. Transcriptional Repression Domains (TRD) identified in MeCP2, MBD1, and MBD2 are non-homologous. CXXC (C-C) domains in MBD1 permit binding also to unmethylated CpG-rich regions. The glycine- and arginine-rich GR domain may serve as a low complexity intrinsically disordered region (IDR). MBD3 has a mutated MBD domain that does not bind 5mCpGs. MBD4 has a glycosylase domain that can excise a DNA base from its pentose, prior to DNA repair. (b) The KAISO family of proteins uses triple zinc fingers to bind to 5mCpG. The POZ/BTB domain is a powerful protein/protein interaction domain.

density of methylated CpG sites, and lead to chromatin compaction and transcriptional repression.

Individual MBD proteins have particular distinguishing features. For example, some splicing variants of MBD1 contain three CXXC domains. As a result, they can, potentially, bind to CpG-rich regions whether or not they are methylated.

MBD3 is somewhat unusual among the MDB proteins. Unlike the others, MBD3 has a modified MBD domain that does not bind to methylated CpG. There have been some claims that it binds to 5hmC, but the significance of this finding, if correct, has not been established. MBD3 is a subunit of the NuRD, a multisubunit complex containing nucleosome remodeling and histone deacetylase activities, that is involved in the repression of many genes. MBD3 also contains a coiled-coil domain that helps to recruit Polycomb Repressive Complex 2 (PRC2) to a subset of genes, thus establishing a transition between DNA methylation-mediated gene silencing and the more flexible and dynamic Polycomb repression (see Chapter 7). MBD4 binds preferentially to fully methylated CpG sites but also to their deamination derivative G:U and G:T sites. MBD4 is in fact a glycosylase that catalyzes an initial step of base excision repair, removing T and U paired with G in CpG sites. If unrepaired, G:T or G:U pairs are the most frequent cause of mutations in human cancer.

Perhaps the best-studied MBD protein is MeCP2, an abundant chromatin protein found in all tissues but particularly enriched in neurons. MeCP2 binds to symmetrically methylated CpGs but with additional specificity. *In vitro* selection showed that MeCP2 prefers sites containing multiple A/T nucleotides adjacent to the methylated CpG and such sequences are generally found *in vivo* at sites known to bind MeCP2. MeCP2 recruits histone deacetylase proteins and effectively represses transcription. Together with HP1, MeCP2 is a major constituent of heterochromatin. Both form liquid phase condensates (see Genome Architecture chapter), particularly when bound to chromatin. MeCP2 mutations in mammals result in severe neurological and behavioral defects. In the human genome the gene encoding MeCP2 is on the X chromosome and males bearing loss of function mutations die shortly after birth. Heterozygous females survive and display devastating symptoms, referred to as Rett Syndrome. These are due to mosaic tissue patches in which the X chromosome bearing the normal gene copy has become inactivated (see Chapter 11). MeCP2 has a highly flexible and disordered structure that forms many weak interactions, as is typical of proteins containing intrinsically disordered regions (IDRs). Such proteins interact with themselves and other IDR proteins to form liquid phase condensates, physical domains that exclude water and tend to concentrate certain other IDR proteins. In the case of MeCP2, this includes heterochromatin protein HP1 and a number of other heterochromatin proteins such as histone H3K9 methyltransferases, histone deacetylases, and other repressive proteins and complexes. By generating a condensed, non-aqueous phase, MeCP2 induces the coalescence of MeCP2-binding heterochromatic domains, which further concentrates heterochromatin proteins and stabilizes the condensed, silenced chromatin domains. In general, MeCP2 has repressive effects on transcription and this has been confirmed by targeting it to a specific reporter gene. In some cases, however, positive transcriptional effects have been reported, suggesting that the effect of MeCP2 on transcription may be context-dependent.

Very recently, an important other target for the binding of MeCP2 was found to be 5mC in contexts other than CpG. The protein also binds 5mCpN, where N is A, C, or T. Such methylated dinucleotides are relatively abundant in nerve cells and the ability of MeCP2 to bind to such sites has turned out to be necessary to avoid neurological symptoms similar to those of Rett Syndrome. Non-CpG methylation is produced by DNMT3A, B, particularly in the early embryo, when they are very abundant. Non-CpG methylation is normally lost in dividing cells because the methylation maintenance mechanism of DNMT1 requires hemimethylated CpGs. DNMT3A persists in the early post-natal brain and binds to regions that are poorly transcribed, leaving a trail of 5mCpN, most frequently 5mCpApC. Neurons are differentiated, post-mitotic cells: they have stopped dividing and therefore no longer lose methylation through replicating their DNA. Neurons therefore retain their 5mCpApC throughout their life. They also contain levels of MeCP2 much higher than those in any other cell type, allowing this protein to saturate the binding to 5mC. Adrian Bird and co-workers found that these non-CpG sites are key binding sites for MeCP2 (Klose *et al.* 2005). They showed that failure to recognize and bind 5mCpApC results in symptoms as severe as those due to the complete loss of MeCP2.

Adenine Methylation

Adenine methylation at the N6 position is widespread in bacteria. Recent work has confirmed its presence in eukaryotes, including the model organisms *Caenorhabditis elegans, Drosophila melanogaster,* and mouse, though at a level much lower than that of 5mC. Methyltransferases responsible for this methylation have been identified, as have corresponding oxidative demethylases. The effects of 6mA deposition appear to be to enhance transcription in the cases studied in *C. elegans* and *Drosophila,* but in mammals 6mA is associated with transcriptional repression. In mouse, the adenine methyltransferase is Mettl4 and the demethylase is Alkbh4, both orthologous to enzymes found in *C. elegans* and *Drosophila*. Homozygous *Mettl4* knockout mice are viable and fertile but die early with hematopoietic deficiencies. They produce small litters with a frequency of anatomical and hematopoietic defects. Biochemical analyses suggest that the 6mA enhances Polycomb repression (see Chapter 7) by promoting the degradation of deubiquitinases that would otherwise remove the Polycomb-induced ubiquitylation of histone H3K119. Target sequences for adenine methylation have a consensus motif A*GAAGA*GGA where the asterisk indicates the methylated As. The sequence is not symmetric, meaning that the methylation is only on one strand of the DNA and lacks therefore the self-maintaining feature of CpG methylation. After every round of DNA replication, adenine methylation is lost in one of the two daughter DNA molecules unless new methylation is targeted. Unlike CpG methylation, therefore, adenine methylation is not as suitable as a long-term epigenetic mark.

Further Reading

Agarwal N, Hardt T, Brero A, Nowak D, Rohlbauer U, Becker A *et al.* (2007). MeCP2 interacts with HP1 and modulates its heterochromatin association during myogenic differentiation. *Nucleic Acids Res.* **35**, 5402–5408.

Bogdanović O and Veenstra GJC (2009). DNA methylation and methyl-CpG binding proteins: Developmental requirements and function. *Chromosoma.* **118**, 549–565.

Chen Z and Zhang Y (2020). Role of mammalian DNA methyltransferases in development. *Annu Rev Biochem.* **89**, 135–158.

Deniz Ö, Frost JM and Branco MR (2019). Regulation of transposable elements by DNA modifications. *Nat Rev Genet.* **20**, 417–431.

Dennis K, Fan T, Geiman T, Yan Q and Muegge K (2001). Lsh, a member of the SNF2 family, is required for genome-wide methylation. *Genes Dev.* **15**, 2940–2944.

Esteve PO, Chin HG, Smallwood A, Feehery GR, Gangisetty O, Karpf AR *et al.* (2006). Direct interaction between DNMT1 and G9a coordinates DNA and histone methylation during replication. *Genes Dev.* **20**, 3089–3103.

Greenberg MVC and Bourc'his D (2019). The diverse roles of DNA methylation in mammalian development and disease. *Nat Rev Mol Cell Biol.* **20**, 590–607.

Jones PA (2012). Functions of DNA methylation: Islands, start sites, gene bodies and beyond. *Nat Rev Genet.* **13**, 484–492.

Klose RJ, Sarraf SA, Schmiedeberg L, McDermott SM, Stancheva I and Bird AP (2005). DNA binding selectivity due to a requirement for A/T sequences adjacent to methyl-CpG. *Mol Cell.* **19**, 667–678.

Lande-Diner L, Zhang J, Ben-Porath I, Amariglio N, Keshet I, Hecht M *et al.* (2007). Role of DNA methylation in stable gene repression. *J Biol Chem.* **282**, 12194–12200.

Lyko F (2017). The DNA methyltransferase family: A versatile toolkit for epigenetic regulation. *Nat Rev Genet.* **19**, 81.

Myant K, Termanis A, Sundaram AYM, Boe T, Merusi C *et al.* (2011). LSH and G9a/GLP complex are required for developmentally programmed DNA methylation. *Genome Res.* **21**, 83–94.

Rasmussen KD and Helin K (2016). Role of TET enzymes in DNA methylation, development, and cancer. *Genes Dev.* **30**, 733–750.

Smith ZD and Meissner A (2013). DNA methylation: roles in mammalian development. *Nat Rev Genet.* **14**, 204–220.

Spruijt CG and Vermeulen M (2014). DNA methylation: old dog, new tricks? *Nat Struct Mol Biol.* **21**, 949–954.

Tao Y, Xi S, Shan J, Maunakea A, Che A, Briones V *et al.* (2011). Lsh, chromatin remodeling family member, modulates genome-wide cytosine methylation patterns at nonrepeat sequences. *Proc Natl Acad Sci USA.* **108**, 5626–5631.

Weinberg DN, Papillon-Cavanagh S, Chen H, Yue Y, Chen X, Rajagopalan KN *et al.* (2019). The histone mark H3K36me2 recruits DNMT3A and shapes the intergenic DNA methylation landscape. *Nature.* **573**, 281–286.

Chapter 4

Genome Organization

Introduction

The genome is clearly visible during cell division when the genomic chromatin becomes tightly packaged and condensed into the familiar mitotic chromosomes: well-defined dense bodies that can be pulled apart and segregated into the daughter cells (Figure 1). The tight condensation is essential for this process: the DNA in each of the 46 chromosomes that make up the diploid complement in a human cell is a thread roughly 5 cm long and all 46 chromosomes are contained in a cell nucleus about 6 microns in diameter. It would be impossible to untangle and sort out the chromatin threads into the daughter cells. After mitosis, most of the chromatin is unpackaged and at least partly decondensed. This is the normal chromatin state in interphase cells and it is called **euchromatin**. When stained with dyes (such as ethidium bromide) that bind to DNA, this appears as a diffuse mass. A smaller fraction of the chromatin does not decondense and remains as strongly staining areas of the nucleus (Figure 2). This was called **heterochromatin** by Emil Heitz, who first observed it in 1929 (see Chapter 5).

If we look through the microscope at the nucleus of an interphase cell to try to visualize euchromatin, there is not much structure to be seen. The nucleolus stands out. This is the site of very strong transcriptional activity in all cells. The nucleolus stains weakly with DNA-staining dyes but is rich in RNA. The nucleolus is the site of the ribosomal RNA genes, usually present in 100 or more copies most of which are very actively transcribed. Their RNA products accumulate in the nucleolus as they are

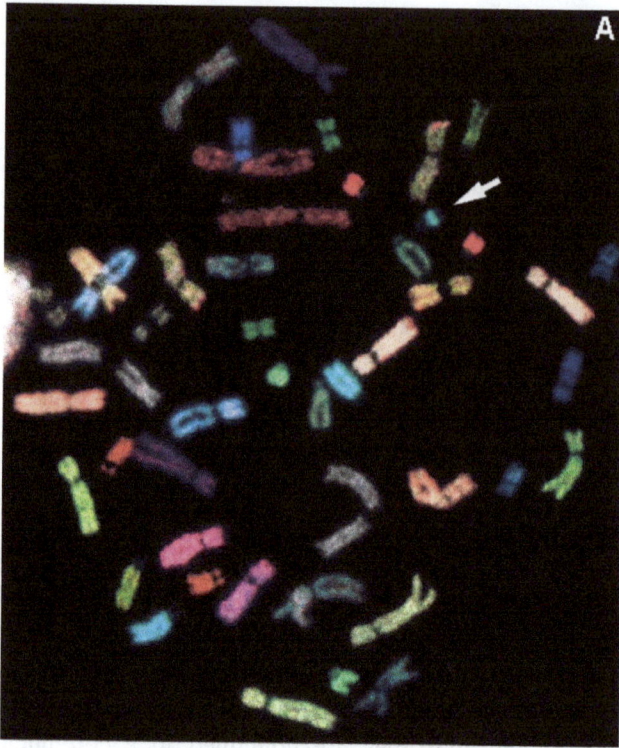

Figure 1.   Mitotic chromosomes. A mitotic cell at the metaphase stage is made to lyse and spread the condensed mitotic chromosomes on a glass slide. The chromosomes are hybridized with a multiplex fluorescent probe that labels each of the 22 autosomes, X and Y chromosomes with a different color. Each chromosome appears double, having replicated in preparation for mitosis. The two copies are still held together by their centromeric regions, which appear as constrictions. The tips of the chromosomes contain the telomere, chromatin regions designed to ensure that the chromosome ends are appropriately replicated and protected against degradation or fusion with other chromosome regions.

Source: Uhrig *et al.* (1999).

simultaneously transcribed, folded, and associated with the appropriate proteins that will lead to the assembly of ribosomes in the cytoplasm. The nucleolus is the largest and most noticeable of a class of nuclear bodies that appear as distinct nuclear compartments but are not separated from the rest of the nuclear space by any membrane. These structures are

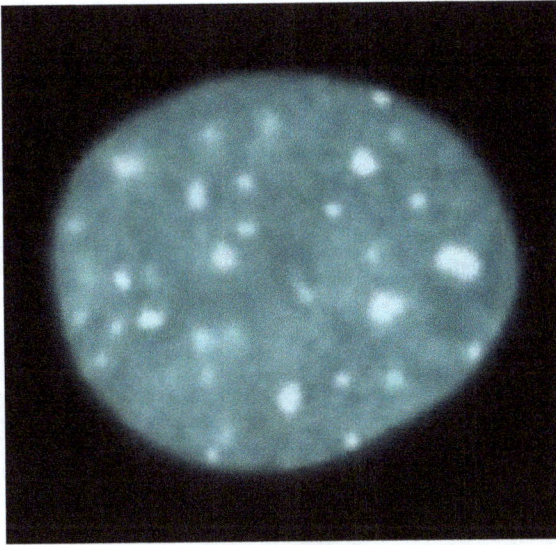

Figure 2. Brightly staining heterochromatin. This mouse nucleus was stained with ethidium bromide, a chemical dye that fluoresces brightly when bound to DNA. The brighter foci are chromatin regions that remain condensed during interphase, when the rest of the chromatin is decondensed. These are heterochromatin regions.

Source: Maison *et al.* (2002).

produced by the assembly of proteins through multiple, dynamic, weak interactions that condense to form a separate liquid phase.

Nucleoli are liquid droplets that themselves contain phase-separated subcompartments. In mammals, these are the fibrillar centers within the dense fibrillar components, embedded within a granular component (Figure 3). The fibrillar centers correspond to sites of ribosomal RNA gene transcription, the dense fibrillar components surrounding them are sites of initial processing of the rRNA transcripts, which are matured to ribosomal subunits in the granular component. Distinct proteins and distinct condensation properties separate these compartments into immiscible liquid phases, droplets within droplets.

In the rest of the nucleus some regions look darker than others. If we stain cells with dyes that bind to DNA, we can see that the darker regions are more densely packed with DNA: this is heterochromatin. It remains condensed during interphase. In the electron microscope we can see that

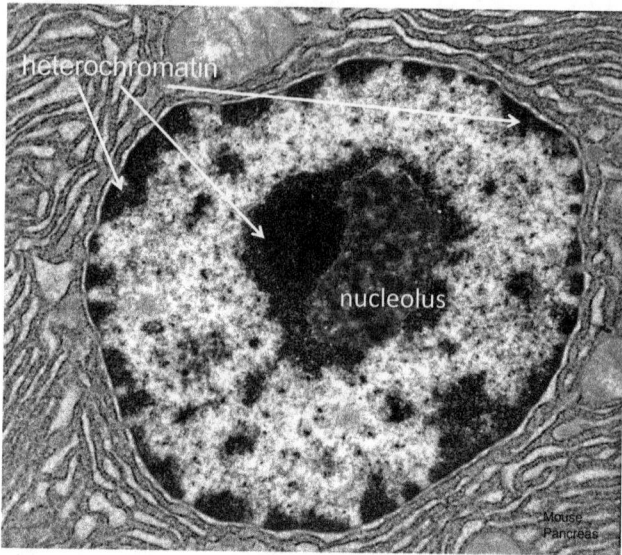

Figure 3.   Electron micrograph of a cell nucleus. Denser heterochromatic regions are frequently associated with the nuclear envelope or the surface of the nucleolus. Image by Kenneth M. Barth, Hamilton College.

the heterochromatin is often associated with the nuclear periphery and with the nucleolus (Figure 4). We cannot visualize what most of the genomic euchromatin looks like: it is too diffuse.

In recent years, it has been possible to develop a package of oligonucleotide probes with sequences specific for each of the human chromosomes. If these oligonucleotides are tagged with a particular colored dye and then hybridized *in situ* to a human cell, we can visualize the space occupied by that particular chromosome during interphase. This is called chromosome painting. A virtuoso extreme of this kind of experiment was done by using 23 sets of such packages each specific for one of the 23 human chromosomes and each tagged with a different color dye (Figure 5). The result shows that each chromosome appears to keep much to itself in its own chromosome territory with little mingling with the sequences of neighboring chromosomes, at least at this scale. This is still a vastly larger scale than a chromatin fiber. But what happens to individual genes?

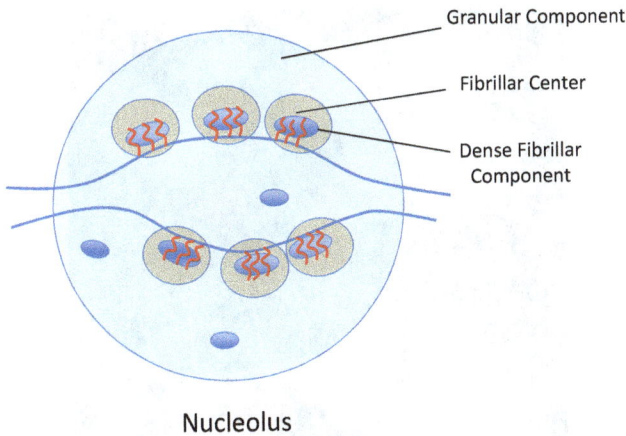

Nucleolus

Figure 4. Nucleolar organization. The nucleolus is a membraneless organelle held together by the formation of a separate liquid phase, within which other, non-miscible phases are assembled by dense association of proteins. The nucleolus assembles around genomic sites of ribosomal RNA gene transcription. The Fibrillar Centers represent the sites of transcription of the ribosomal RNA genes by RNA Pol I. The Dense Fibrillar Components are sites of initial processing of the transcripts, which are assembled into ribosomal subunits in the Granular Component.

We can get some more information by using as hybridization probes DNA sequences that we know are found in heterochromatin. This confirms the impression that heterochromatin tends to be associated with the nuclear periphery. Some chromosomes are densely packed with genes while others are relatively gene-poor. If we do chromosome painting for specific chromosomes, we see that gene-poor chromosomes tend to lie next to the nuclear periphery while gene-rich chromosomes are more centrally located. In another experiment, hybridization was done with a chromosome painting set of probes in one color and with another set of sequences corresponding to the RNA transcribed from active genes in that chromosome labeled with a different color. The results show that the regions that are being transcribed form a cloud spreading beyond the chromosome territory and toward the interior of the nucleus (Figure 6).

This tendency agrees with the electron microscopy observation that the more condensed, heterochromatic parts of the genome appear to concentrate near the periphery of the nucleus and around the nucleolus. This was

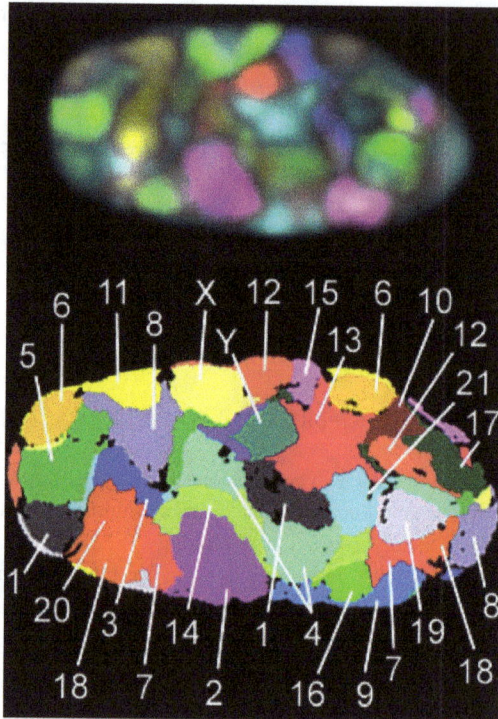

Figure 5.   Chromosome territories. This nucleus was hybridized with 23 different chromosome-specific oligonucleotide probes, each tagged with a different color dye. Each chromosome tends to occupy its own specific volume in the interphase nucleus, rather than mingling and tangling with other chromosomes.

Source: Bolzer *et al*. (2005).

confirmed by a direct experiment. Using a technique called DamID (see Chapter 13), a nuclear envelope protein such as lamin was fused to a bacterial adenine methyltransferase (Dam). DNA regions that reside very close to the nuclear envelope are labeled *in vivo* by DNA methylation. When the methylated regions are sequenced and identified, they generally corresponded to untranscribed, repressed, or heterochromatic regions. More dramatically, when the labeled sequences were used as a hybridization probe on cultured cells, they mapped to parts of the nucleus immediately underlying the nuclear envelope (Figure 7). Overall then transcriptionally active sequences reach out toward the interior of the nucleus while silent

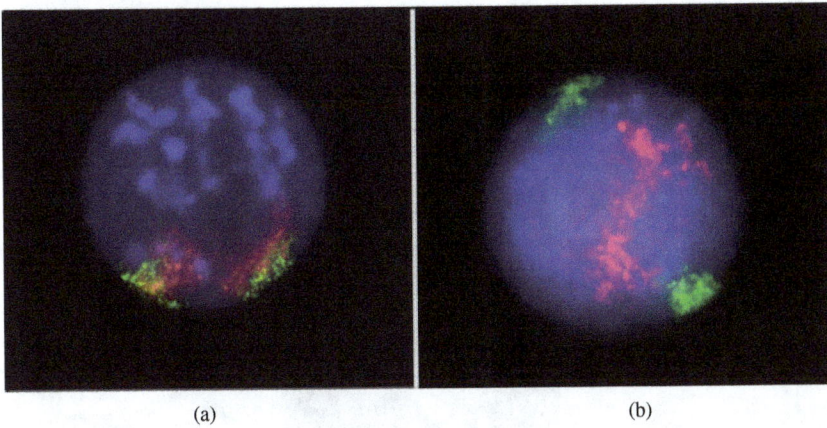

(a)   (b)

Figure 6.   Positioning of transcriptionally active regions in the nucleus. These nuclei were hybridized with oligonucleotide probes specific for individual chromosomes. On the left, a probe specific for chromosome 2 (green) and a probe specific for chromosome 2 RNA (red), showing that the transcriptionally active regions of the two copies of chromosome 2 tend to be more interiorly located. On the right, gene-poor chromosome 18 (green) lies close to the nuclear envelope while gene-rich chromosome 19 (red) is in the nuclear interior.

Source: Bickmore and van Steensel (2013).

sequences are often attached to the nuclear envelope. In fact, certain chromosomal regions that are transcriptionally inactive in a given cell tend to associate with the nuclear lamina: these are Lamin Associated Domains or LADs. Heterochromatin is then the part of the genome that is poorly transcribed either because it contains few genes or because it is prevented from being transcribed by specific mechanisms that tend to maintain it in a silent and condensed state (see Chapters 5 and 7). Heterochromatin and transcriptionally inactive chromatin tend to be associated with the nuclear lamina or with the periphery of the nucleolus.

Structure of the Nucleus

The nucleus is enclosed by two lipid bilayer plasma membranes (Figure 8). The outer membrane is continuous with the endoplasmic reticulum (ER) so that proteins transported through this structure can enter directly the space between the inner and outer nuclear membrane.

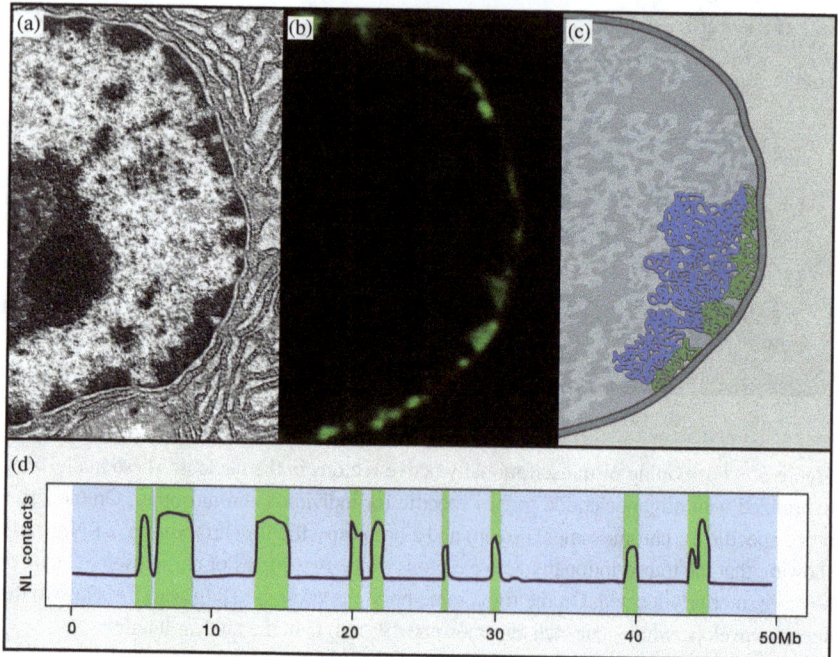

Figure 7.   Lamin-associated domains (LADs). DNA sequences that lie close to the nuclear lamina were labeled with the DamID technique. They were then hybridized *in situ* to a nucleus (green in the middle image). (c) These sequences represent untranscribed or condensed chromatin as shown schematically. (d) When mapped in a genome browser, these sequences corresponded to genomic domains (shaded in green).

Source: van Steensel and Belmont (2017).

Both membranes are traversed by nuclear pores, multiprotein structures responsible for diffusion and active transport of macromolecules in and out of the nucleus. Nuclear pore traffic is essential for growth and the higher the growth rate of a cell, the higher the number of nuclear pores in the nuclear envelope. The inner membrane is lined by the nuclear lamina, a fibrous meshwork composed of intermediate filament proteins called lamins (Figure 9). Intermediate filaments are cytoskeletal fibers of a thickness intermediate between that of actin fibers and myosin fibers or tubulin fibers. Like other intermediate filaments, such as keratin fibers, lamin filaments are composed of monomers that have an amino-terminal head domain, a long helical coiled-coil central rod domain ending in a C-terminal globular domain.

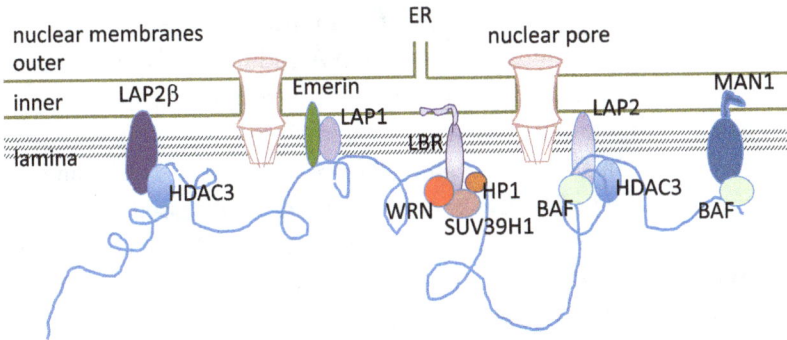

Figure 8. Nuclear envelope. The nucleus is enclosed by two nuclear membranes. The outer membrane is continuous with the endoplasmic reticulum ER. The nuclear lamina, composed of lamin Bs and lamin A/C, forms a stiff inner layer anchored to the nuclear membrane by proteins such as MAN1, Lamin Associated Proteins 1, 2, 2beta, Emerin. Emerin and Nesprin proteins traverse the nuclear envelope and link it to the cytoskeleton. Nuclear pores are complex assemblies that mediate both active and passive transport of proteins and nucleic acids into and out of the nucleus. Numerous proteins connect the lamins with chromatin regions and bind chromatin proteins such as HDACs, HP1, SUV39H.

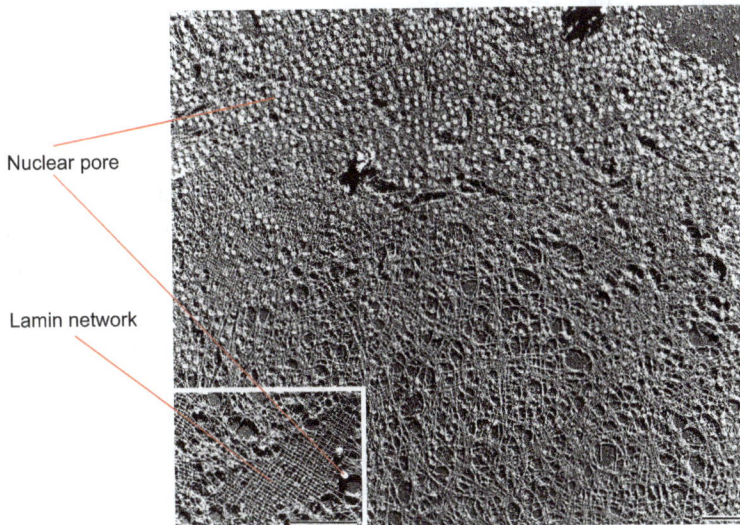

Figure 9. Nuclear lamina. Electron micrograph of a remarkable spread of the nuclear lamina from a Xenopus oocyte, freeze-dried and metal shadowed. The numerous round white objects are the nuclear pores. The meshwork pattern of the lamin filaments is visible, particularly well preserved in the inset picture, a sample in which the nuclear pores have been mechanically removed. The nuclear lamina is a meshwork of intermediate-type filaments.

Source: Aebi *et al.* (1986).

In animals the lamins are of two main types, lamin A/C and lamin B that play somewhat different roles. Lamin A and lamin C are the product of alternative splicing of the same genes. Humans have two lamin B genes (B1 and B2). Structurally, B-type lamins, lamin B1 and lamin B2, are the most important. In fact, embryonic stem cells lack lamin A/C and their lamina is composed of B lamins only. Lamin A is expressed and required only when embryonic stem cells start to differentiate. At the C-terminal of lamin proteins, a CAAX domain (where A is an aliphatic amino acid) is the site of farnesylation, the attachment of a farnesyl hydrocarbon group that is necessary for the interaction of the lamin with the nuclear membrane and its positioning to assemble the lamin meshwork. To assemble this, the lamin coiled-coil domains first form dimers in which two lamin monomers associate in parallel with the helical regions forming a coiled coil. These dimers further associate head to tail, forming long polar polymers. Two such polymers pair in inverted orientation forming a protofilament. Finally, three or four protofilaments cohere to form a thicker filament about 10 nm in diameter (Figure 10). How the crosslinks that form the mesh-like structures are made is not clear but may require the participation of lamin A and C. Lamin C lacks the CAAX domain and is therefore not farnesylated, while lamin A is farnesylated but the C-ter domain is then cleaved off by a peptidase to allow the proper assembly with the lamin B network. This structure is remarkably elastic and the nuclear lamina confers rigidity to the nuclear envelope and retains its shape, which can be deformed, squashed, dented, but then springs back.

Lamins bind to proteins such as Nesprin and Emerin that form part of a network connecting the nuclear envelope to the actin cytoskeleton, intermediate filaments, and microtubules on the cytoplasmic side and anchor the lamin meshwork on the nuclear side. These structures are important to position and shape the nucleus within the cytoplasm of the cell. Lamins attach to chromatin through numerous proteins that bind to both, but they also can bind directly to chromatin. The lamina anchors specific chromatin regions, both important for the proper architecture and functioning of the genome. A number of lamin associated proteins (LAPs) link the lamina to the inner nuclear membrane. They include lamina-associated proteins 1 and 2 (LAP1,2), lamin B receptor (LBR), MAN1. They also bind to chromatin-interacting proteins that bind to specific features of

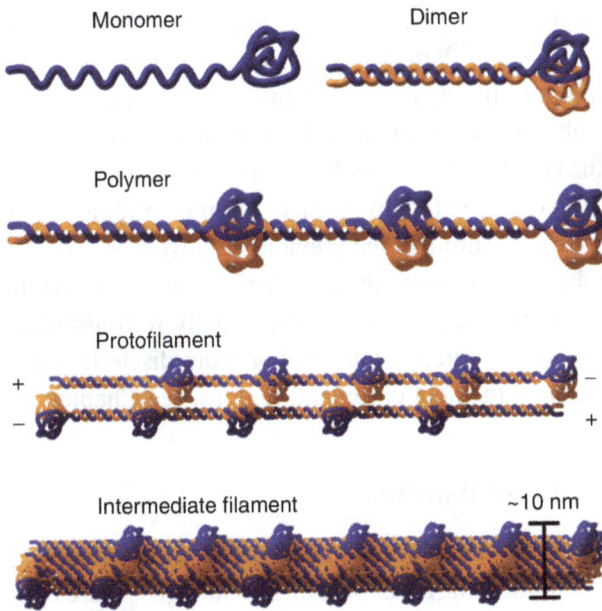

Figure 10.   Assembly of intermediate filaments. The helical regions of two lamin mono-mers intertwine by a coiled coil pairing to form a dimer with the two globular heads paired. Dimers further assemble by a head to tail interaction that embeds the coiled coil end of one dimer in the paired globular head of another. Two such polymers can now further pair in inverted orientation to form a protofilament. Note that because of the inverted orientation of the two polymers, the protofilament has no polarity, unlike actin fibers or tubulin fila-ments. Three or four protofilaments assemble to give the intermediate filament about 10 nm thickness.

Source: Dittmer and Misteli (2011).

chromatin and therefore recruit these chromatin regions to the nuclear envelope. Most of these proteins, such as HP1, BAF, histone methylases, histone deacetylases, are associated with heterochromatin and create a concentration of heterochromatin-promoting factors in the periphery of the nucleus. As a result, the sub-lamina region is specifically enriched for and promotes formation of heterochromatin and other transcriptionally silent chromatin (see Chapter 5).

In higher eukaryotes, the nuclear envelope disassembles when the cell undergoes mitosis although in lower eukaryotes, such as fungi, nuclei can remain bound by the nuclear envelope. In animals the lamina depolymerizes upon a phosphorylation signal. Lamin B remains associated with nuclear membrane fragments and forms small vesicles while lamin A/C remains soluble or associated with chromatin. The nuclear envelope reforms at the end of mitosis and the lamins reassemble to form the lamina meshwork. Importantly, the appropriate chromatin regions that had been associated with the lamina in the previous cell cycle are again recruited to the re-assembled lamina or to the periphery of the nucleolus. It appears in fact that some chromatin regions can be equally well associated with the nucleolus or with the nuclear lamina. For more discussion of lamins and their association with silent chromatin regions, see Chapters 8 and 12.

Polytene Chromosomes

To get a picture of what chromatin looks like in interphase, the polytene chromosomes of the fruit fly *Drosophila melanogaster* are extremely useful. This type of chromosome is found in most of the larval tissues of dipteran insects. Polytenic tissues are post-mitotic but still growing: the cells no longer divide but the genomic DNA continues to replicate for about 10 more rounds without cell division and without separating the products of replication. This failure to separate the DNA copies results in giant chromosomes where each chromosome is a bundle of some $2 \times 2^{10} = 2048$ DNA molecules all aligned in register (Figure 11). As a consequence, the chromosome is much more linearly organized and is made visible even during interphase because a region that is condensed in one copy of the DNA molecule or chromatid is associated with 2000 corresponding condensed regions from the 2000 other chromatids. This gives rise to the characteristic appearance of polytene chromosomes with alternating dark and light bands.

Another characteristic of polytene chromosomes is that the chromosome arms radiate from a common chromocenter composed of the pericentric heterochromatin and centromeric regions of all the chromosomes (Figure 12). In *Drosophila*, as in many other organisms, including mammals, the chromosomal regions surrounding the centromere form heterochromatin. In polytene chromosomes, pericentric heterochromatin from each chromosome assembles together forming the chromocenter from

Polytenic chromosomes

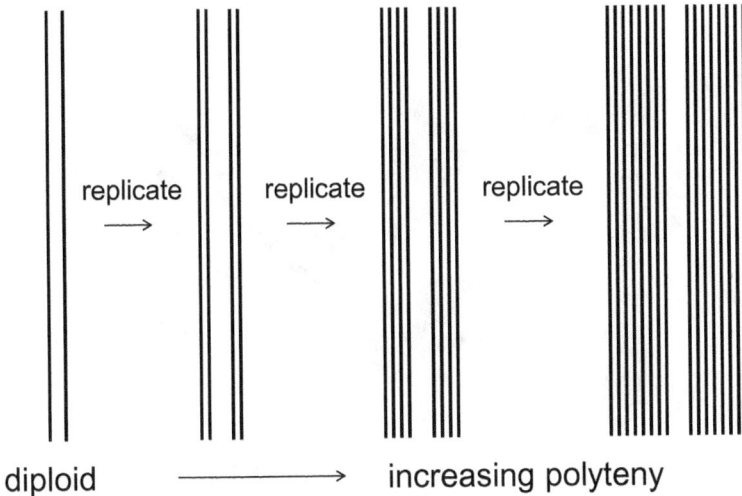

Figure 11. Polytenization in dipteran insects. In most larval tissues, chromosomes replicate without cell division and the copies remain associated together in perfect alignment. In *Drosophila* salivary gland cells, the diploid genome replicates about 10 times reaching a total of 2048 copies of the genome.

which all the chromosome arms spread out. This is an illustration of a general property of heterochromatin: heterochromatic regions tend to associate with one another. This is true both at the large scale and at the finer scale and is an important principle of chromatin architecture, as we will see later.

Late Replicating Regions

Genomic regions that have little or no transcriptional activity and are therefore more condensed are also harder to replicate because the DNA has to be unpacked before it can be replicated. Therefore, they tend to be late-replicating during interphase. In general, heterochromatin and poorly transcribed regions are late-replicating. This was first discovered by looking at polytene chromosomes. In polytenic tissues some parts of the genome may be so delayed that they do not get replicated in time before

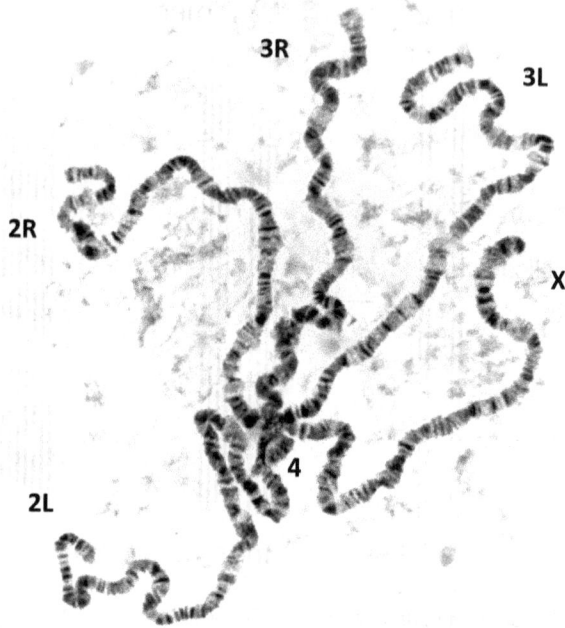

Figure 12.   *Drosophila melanogaster* polytene chromosome squash. Chromosomes 2 and 3 have a right and a left arm; the X chromosome has a single arm, as does the very small chromosome 4. The heterochromatic centromeric regions of all four chromosomes become attached in polytenic cells, forming the chromocenter. The characteristic band–interband pattern is highly reproducible and can be mapped genetically.

Source: image by B.P. Kaufmann, from John W. Kimball, https://bio.libretexts.org/Bookshelves/ Introductory_and_General_Biology/Book%3A_Biology_(Kimball)/07%3A_Cell_Division/7.05% 3A_Endoreplication.

the end of a cell cycle and remain under-replicated: they are present in fewer copies than the rest of the genome. Therefore, in the *Drosophila* polytene chromosomes, certain sites on the chromosome arms look highly condensed (dark) and pinched and may look like splits or breaks in the chromosome. These are regions that are under-replicated. We now know that these regions are highly repressed by chromatin silencing mechanisms. Pericentric heterochromatin comprising about one-third of the *Drosophila* genome is so under-replicated in polytene chromosomes that it appears as a relatively small undifferentiated mass, the chromocenter.

Although pericentric heterochromatin makes up about 40% of each chromosome, it is so underreplicated in polytene chromosomes that it looks very small compared with the banded chromosome arms.

The most characteristic feature of polytene chromosomes is the pattern of dark bands alternating with light interband regions (Figures 12 and 13). These bands and interbands physically correspond to more condensed and less condensed chromatin and it can be estimated that the thicker bands contain as much as 300 Kb of chromatin length while interbands range from a few kb to 30 kb. It is evident therefore that band chromatin is 10–20 times more condensed than interband chromatin. When these band patterns were first noticed, they were interpreted as physical evidence that chromosomes were strings of genes: one band, one gene. The position of many genes was mapped on the polytene chromosomes using the cytological breakpoints of genetically mapped deletions or inversions so that a gene can usually be fairly precisely localized to a given band or interband or portion of one. It soon became clear, however, that there were many more genes than bands. We now know that interbands are chromosome regions that are decondensed and transcriptionally active. Interbands

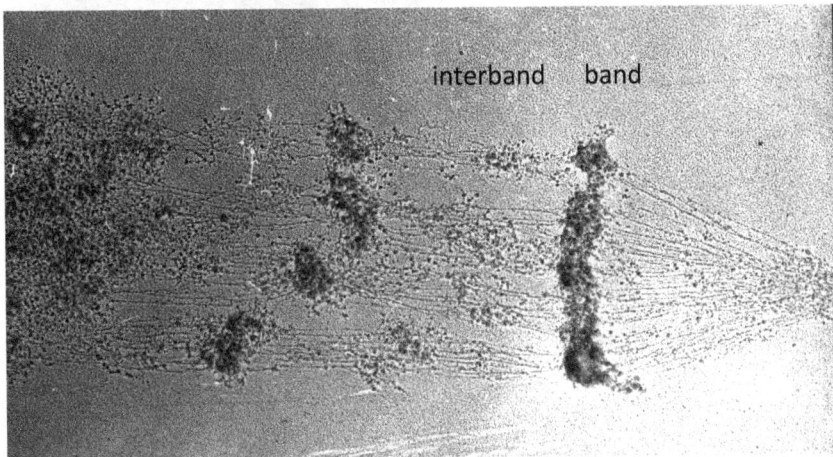

Figure 13.   Electron micrograph of a short segment of a *Drosophila* polytene chromosome at the 32 copy stage. The individual strands can be visualized in interband regions but become clumped together and tangled in band regions.

Source: Ananiev and Barsky (1985).

and not bands are where RNA polymerase is found and where nascent RNA is produced. This can be shown by staining polytene chromosomes with antibodies against RNA polymerase. If the antibody is tagged with a fluorescent dye visible under ultraviolet light, the result is a pattern of fluorescent bands that is a faithful inverted image of the band pattern seen with visible light (Figure 14). Labeling nascent RNA confirms that inter-bands are not just a repository of RNA polymerase: this is where transcription occurs.

Accidental exposure to higher temperature (37°C) showed that a few sites in the polytene chromosomes became greatly enlarged, blown up (Figure 15). These are the sites of heat shock genes, genes that are massively induced by a shift to higher temperature. Similarly, at certain stages in development, some chromosome regions become massively activated by the hormone ecdysone. These regions swell up, become decondensed and look like blown up balloons (Figure 16). These expanded and decondensed regions are in fact called puffs. Staining these chromosomes with

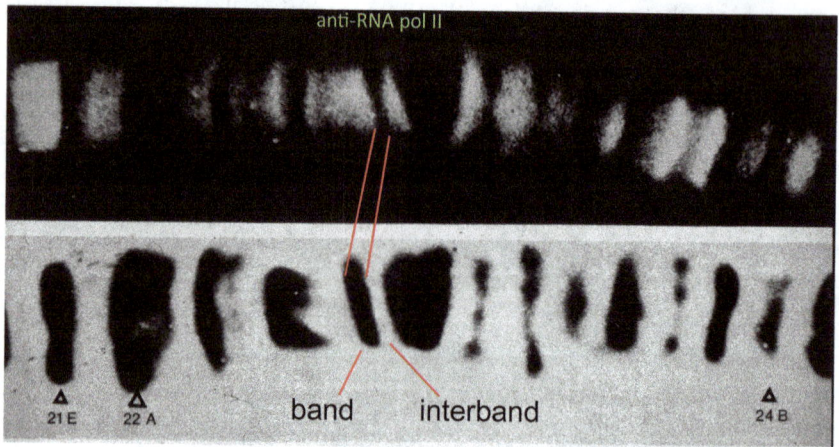

Jamrich, Greenleaf & Bautz, 1977

Figure 14.   RNA Pol II is found in interbands. The lower image shows a section of a polytene chromosome showing the pattern of bands and interbands viewed under phase contrast microscopy. The upper image shows the same section stained with a fluorescent antibody against RNA Pol II, viewed by immunofluorescence. A comparison of the two images shows that the polymerase is found in all the interband regions.

Source: Jamrich *et al.* (1977).

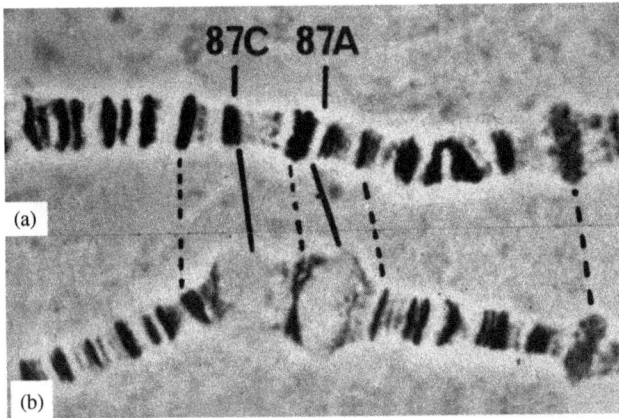

Figure 15. Heat shock puffs in *Drosophila* polytene chromosomes. The upper image shows a section of chromosome 3R at fixed room temperature. The lower image shows the same chromosome region in a preparation that had been briefly exposed to 37°C before fixing. The puffed regions correspond to 87C and 87A, the sites of two sets of hsp70 heat shock genes.

Source: Ashburner and Bonner (1979).

an antibody that detects RNA polymerase shows that puffs are sites that suddenly recruit massive amounts of RNA polymerase, are transcribed at a great rate, and accumulate nascent RNA. We can consider interbands as a sort of low grade puff and the nucleolus as the mother of all puffs. In contrast, bands are regions that either contain few genes or contain genes that are transcriptionally inactive. The chromatin of a gene that is transcriptionally inactive tends to pack in a more condensed form. For more discussion of the organization of active and inactive genomic domains, see Chapter 8.

Genomic DNA Sequences

In the 1990s, a massive DNA sequencing effort was undertaken worldwide but particularly through the US National Institutes of Health and by Celera Genomics, a private company. These efforts utilized for the most part DNA sequencing technologies derived from the Sanger chain termination method (see Chapter 13, for DNA Sequencing). By the time the

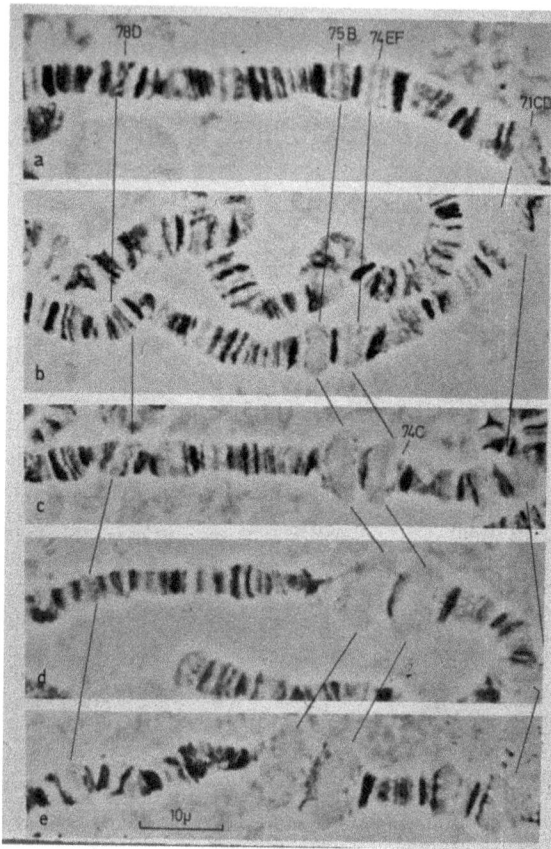

Figure 16.   Ecdysone puffs developing in *Drosophila* larvae approaching pupation. As larvae approach pupation, the levels of the steroid hormone ecdysone rise and induce the dramatic formation of puffs at specific chromosome sites, the location of genes strongly activated by the hormone.

Source: Ashburner (1972).

human genome sequence was declared accomplished, drastically new, massively parallel sequencing technologies began to be available (see Chapter 13, for DNA Sequencing). These methods vastly increased sequencing speed and cut the costs of sequencing by one hundred thousand-fold. As a result of both DNA and RNA sequencing efforts, we are now in possession of the sequence of the genome of not only *Homo sapiens* and a few model organisms but literally tens of thousands of animal and plant species and even of thousands of individual humans. Combined with the sequencing of mRNA (through the synthesis of cDNA), this has allowed the construction of annotated genome sequence maps that include the precise positions of genes, transcripts, splice sites. In many cases these maps are regularly updated to include regulatory elements, transposon insertions, mutations, and other sequence features as they become available in the scientific literature. These sequences and associated information are stored in data base repositories and are available online. To visualize such a wealth and extent of sequence information, many invaluable computational and display tools have been developed, among which the fundamental instrument is the genome browser. This computer display tool represents the genome, usually one chromosome at a time on a scale that can be modified continuously from the chromosome scale to the nucleotide sequence scale. The genes and transcripts and other sequence features are displayed so that transcription units on one strand are mapped above the sequence bar (usually 5′ on the left to 3′ on the right) and those on the other strand are shown below the sequence bar (5′ on the right to 3′ on the left). The genome browser displays in addition alternative transcripts coming from the same sequence (Figure 17). Additional data files

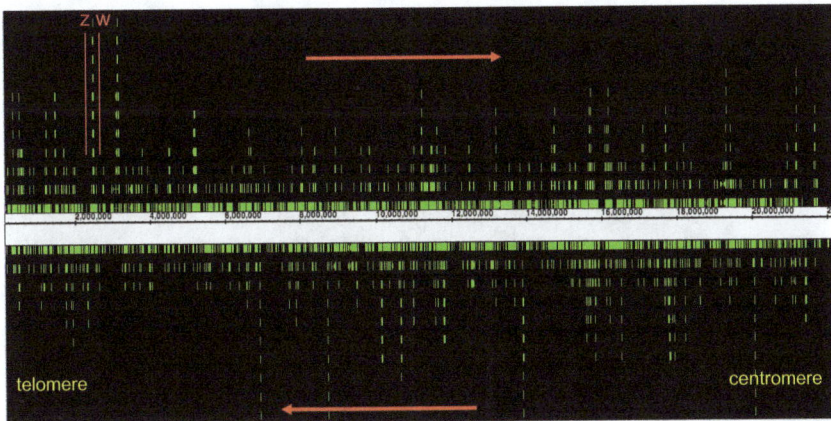

Figure 17. The *Drosophila* X chromosome viewed on a genome browser. Genes are shown in green. Genes above the line are transcribed toward the right. Genes below the line are transcribed to the right. Alternative transcripts from the same sequence are shown on additional rows. The interval containing the *zeste* and *white* genes, expanded in Figure 18, is indicated.

can be loaded on to the browser to display, for example, the results of histone modification data or of specific protein binding sites, obtained from chromatin immunoprecipitation and sequencing (ChIP-seq) experiments.

Genome browsers are extremely useful to gain both overviews and detailed views of how genes are distributed, how they are put together, how they function. From even a cursory inspection of a low resolution view of a genome, it is evident that gene distribution is very variable. Some chromosome regions, or even whole chromosomes, are very sparsely populated while other regions have high densities of genes and transcripts. It is instructive to compare the view of the genome provided by the *Drosophila* polytene chromosomes with that given by the genome browser view. Figure 18 gives an example. In general, dense bands correspond to genomic regions that contain few genes, but genes that are known to be transcriptionally inactive in the larval salivary glands (the

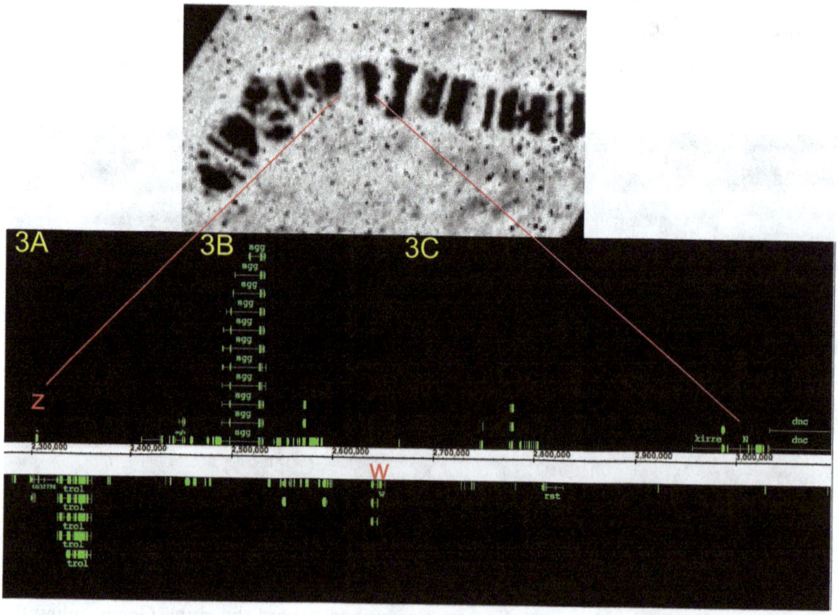

Figure 18.   The zeste-white region of the X chromosome. This region was once used to show genetically that there were many more genes than bands. It shows in fact that bands are gene-poor. Interband regions contain most of the genes.

tissue most commonly used to make polytene chromosome spreads) may also be located in a band region. In interband regions, genes are closely spaced. Surprisingly, overlapping genes are not uncommon both in the same orientation and in opposite orientation. Some very long genes can be shown to contain one or more other genes in their entirety, usually within introns. Adjacent, divergently transcribed genes are common but mapping of regulatory elements shows that some genes have very extensive regulatory regions that may be over 100 kb distant from the promoter. In mammals, extensive regulatory regions are very common and may lie more than one megabase from the promoter they regulate. Some of the features seen in the *Drosophila* genome may be due to its generally smaller and more compact nature, compared to mammalian genomes, but gene overlap can also be found on occasion in mammals. Overall, the number of genes in higher organisms ranging from nematodes to man varies from ~15,000 to 25,000. The value of these numbers is difficult to estimate since it is unclear how to enumerate genes. Alternative splicing patterns can produce a remarkable number of different proteins, often with different functions, from the same basic genome sequence. In addition, increasingly complex regulatory regions can result in the acquisition of new functions depending on the timing, stage, tissue, and signals controlling the activity of promoters. Therefore, the complexity of the repertory of functions available to an organism is not necessarily limited by the size of its genome.

Genome Composition

Genome size and composition varies enormously among living organisms from a few thousand nucleotides to more than 100 giga base pairs (10^{11} bp). Only part of the genome actually encodes protein sequences. While a bacterium like *E. coli* contains some 4,000 genes making up a genome of 4.6 Mb, the budding yeast *Saccharomyces cerevisiae* contains about 6,000 genes that constitute 85% of the 14Mb genome. Of the remainder, half represents regulatory sequences and half are repetitive sequences and transposable elements (Figure 19). A higher eukaryote such as *Drosophila melanogaster* contains some 15,000 genes but their coding regions constitutes only 30% of the genome. Regulatory and

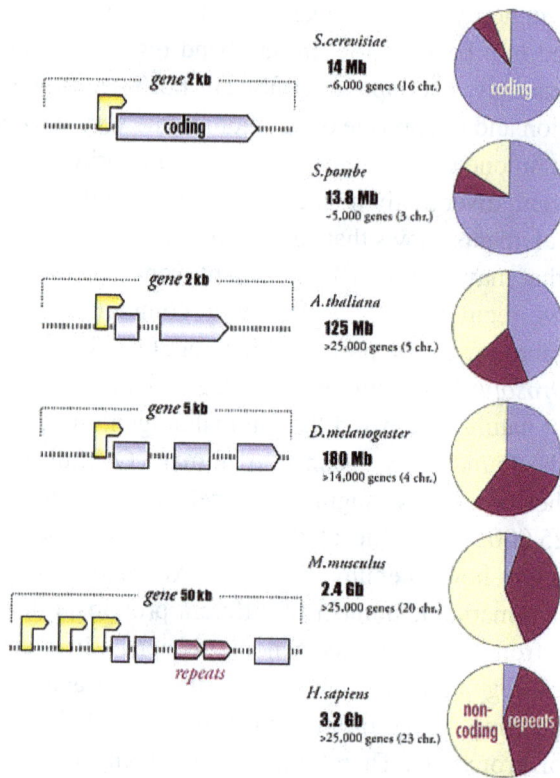

Figure 19.   Comparison of genomic contents. The figure illustrates the expansion of the genome in higher eukaryotes. From microorganisms like yeast to mammals, the total genome has expanded some 200-fold, but the gene content has increased only four-fold. The diagrams on the left illustrate that much of the expansion has gone into non-coding gene regulatory elements, including introns and transcriptional regulatory sequences. Equally increased are repetitive sequences: satellite sequences and transposable elements of different types.

Source: Kosi Gramatikoff (Creative Commons, https://en.wikipedia.org/wiki/File:Genomic Organization_140_percent.jpg).

non-coding sequences now account for close to 40% and repetitive sequences for 30% of the 180 Mb genome. When we come to mammals, the human genome is fairly typical in containing some 25,000 genes accounting for little more than 5% of the 3.6 Gb genome. Non-coding regions make up more than 50% and repetitive sequences about 45% of the genome. So, while genome size increased 50-fold from yeast to man, the number of protein-coding genes increased only five-fold. The great increases have occurred in the regulatory and intronic sequences and in the repetitive sequences. Introns, non-coding sequences that are transcribed as part of a gene but must be excised from the functional messenger RNA, were discovered in 1977. Introns are rare in yeast genes but frequent in higher eukaryotes. They can be very short (30–50 bp) or extremely long (up to 3 Mbp) and are generally more numerous in mammalian genes than in genes of organisms with smaller genomes such as *Drosophila*. Some extremely long genes such as the human dystrophin gene (2.4 Mbp) may take one or two days to transcribe. The increase in length and complexity of regulatory regions corresponds to the increased complexity in the structure of tissues, the variety of cells, and the developmental usage of coding regions. While in yeast regulatory regions are at most a few kilobases in length or distance from the gene they regulate, they can be up to 100 kb away in *Drosophila* and megabases in distance in mammals. The regulatory complexity of genes in higher eukaryotes is such that patterns of expression and alternative splicing regimes in different tissues mean that a single coding region can act as the equivalent of many different genes in terms of usage. Many regions that are not protein-coding are nevertheless transcribed, producing non-coding RNAs. In fact, it now appears that most of the genome may be transcribed, though at very different levels. Much of this transcription may be noise but many such ncRNAs have been found to have important functions in regulating other genes at the transcriptional or translational level.

Repetitive Sequences

It is evident that a striking expansion has occurred in the amount of repetitive sequence contained in the genomes of higher eukaryotes. There are two basic types of repetitive regions: (1) simple, highly repetitive tandem sequences, also called satellite sequences make up about 20% of the *Drosophila* genome, and (2) middle repetitive sequences that tend to be more scattered, making up about 15% of the *Drosophila* genome. Satellite sequences consist of short sequence motifs, usually 5–12 nucleotides long, tandemly repeated tens of thousands of times (Figure 20). They were

Drosophila Satellite Sequences

Sequence	CsCl density	% genome
ATAAT	1.672	3.1
AATAG	1.693	0.23
AAGAC	1.689	2.4
AAGAGAG	-	1.5
AATAACATAG	1.686	2.1
359 bp	1.688	5.1

Figure 20. *Drosophila* satellite sequences. *Satellite sequences* are short, tandem, highly repetitive sequences. In *Drosophila* they make up about 20% of the genome. Most are found in centric heterochromatin, but some blocks are also scattered in the chromosome arms.

so called because their highly repeated sequences produced satellite bands of different buoyant density than the main band of heterogeneous genomic DNA, when purified by density gradient centrifugation. Satellite sequence regions are generally found surrounding centromeres and are in fact important in helping the centromeric regions of chromosomes stick together, facilitating the lining up and sorting of chromosomes at mitosis. The human α-satellite repeat has a unit length of 171 bp, is found in all chromosomes, and is the preferred site for the formation of centromeres.

Middle repetitive sequences are longer, from a few hundred to a few thousand base pairs and are present in the *Drosophila* genome in up to a few hundred copies. These are scattered throughout the genome and generally correspond to transposable elements or fragments of what were once transposable elements. These are mobile genetic elements that either invaded the genome in the form of a virus or derive from endogenous sequences that acquired the ability to become mobile, that is to replicate and insert copies at new genomic sites. Virtually all eukaryotic genomes contain transposable elements and in many cases they constitute a large fraction of the genome. In humans, they make up about 40% of the total genomic DNA. In maize, where they were first discovered by Barbara McClintock through genetic experiments, they add up to 80% of the genome.

There are many different kinds of transposable elements (Figure 21). The main distinction is that between elements that exist exclusively as DNA (Class II transposable elements) and those that go through an RNA stage from which they are copied back into DNA for insertion into new sites (Class I transposable element). The latter are known as retrotransposons and include a large class of retroviruses. Most class II elements transpose by cutting out the original and inserting it in a new location by a "cut and paste" mechanism. Class I elements are transcribed into many RNA copies which are then copied back into DNA by a reverse transcriptase, often encoded by the element itself. The DNA copy can then be inserted into the genome potentially at many new sites without loss of the original insert by a "copy and paste" mechanism. Retrotransposons contain long terminal repeats (LTRs) several hundred nucleotides long, which include a promoter from which the RNA copy is transcribed. Non-LTR retroposons are another type of Class I elements that uses an internal

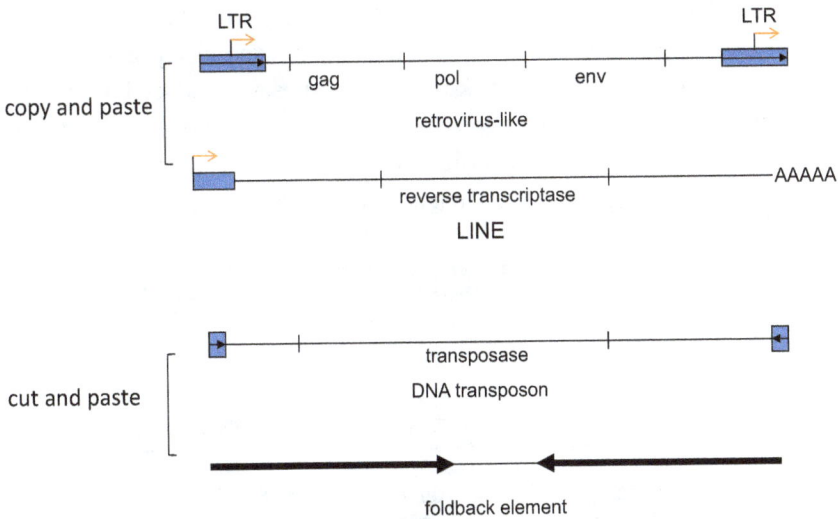

Figure 21. Transposable elements. Some of the main types of transposable elements are shown. The top two are retrotransposons. Some encode a transposase enzyme. Others exploit the transposase made by other transposons. A typical retrovirus type of element encodes proteins that form the viral particle, in addition to the transposase enzyme. The bottom two are cut-and-paste DNA transposons that move by excising from one site and inserting in a new site.

promoter very close to the 5′ end that directs RNA polymerase to initiate transcription including the promoter sequences. Long Interspersed Nuclear Elements (LINEs) are an abundant type of non-LTR retroposons in mammalian genomes. Short Interspersed Nuclear Elements (SINEs) are usually just a few hundred nucleotides long and are transcribed by RNA polymerase III. They do not encode a reverse transcriptase but generally utilize the reverse transcriptase produced by LINEs. A particular kind of SINE that is specific for primates is the Alu element, originally derived from the cytoplasmic 7SL RNA, a small RNA that is an essential component of the signal recognition complex necessary to insert membrane proteins into the membrane of the endoplasmic reticulum. In the evolution of primates, this 300 nt long RNA was hijacked by a reverse transcriptase and its DNA copy was re-inserted into the genome and greatly expanded. In human genome, Alu elements corresponding to a modified dimer of the 7SL sequence (Figure 22) have invaded the genome to the extent of more than a million copies, including some 7,000 copies that have been inserted since the divergence of *homo sapiens* from other primates.

Class II transposable elements tend to have inverted repeats and may contain a transposase gene or make use of transposase produced by another element. The transposase recognizes sequences in the inverted repeats and catalyzes a cut-and-paste transposition mechanism in which the transposon sequence is excised and inserted in a new site, usually by making staggered

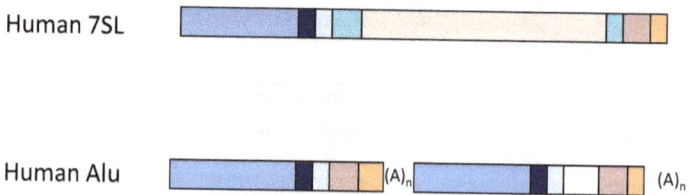

Figure 22.   The human Alu element. Alu elements are SINEs (Short INterspersed Elements) evolutionarily derived from 7SL RNA, a component of the signal peptide recognition complex. Alu elements have fused parts of two 7SL sequence. They do not code for any protein but use the transposase made by LINE elements. They arose in a primate ancestor 65 million years ago and now are present in ~1 million copies in the human genome. Most are now altered and no longer active, most are ancient but some have inserted into gene introns or even coding sequences.

Source: Ullu and Tschudi (1984).

cuts in the target DNA. As a result, the insertion is accompanied by the duplication of a short sequence (corresponding to the interval between the staggered cuts) at the two ends of the newly inserted transposon.

Most transposon sequences found in the genome are fragmentary, or mutated and no longer functional. The human genome, for example, contains some 500,000 copies of the LINE1 element, or 17% of the genome, but only about one hundred of these are still intact and only 10 or so per individual are likely to transpose. This is due to the fact that reverse transcription frequently terminates before reaching the 5′ end, where the promoter is located, resulting in a new insertion unable to transcribe. In the human genome, LINE1 transposition events still occur both in the germ line and in somatic cells with the potential to insert in genes and cause disease. It is estimated that about one new insertion occurs in the germ line of one in 150 births. Clearly the activity of transposons needs to be controlled and the genome has in fact developed mechanisms to silence transposon transcription and inhibit transposition. Nevertheless, transposons have also been a source of innovation in genomes, contributing to the creation of new genes and regulatory elements. An important example is a transposable element that is thought to have given rise to the RAG1 protein, one of the proteins involved in the recombination of V(D)J immunoglobulin sequences in vertebrates.

Silencing mechanisms are essential to prevent the transcription not only of transposons but also of many genes at inappropriate stages of development or in different tissues of higher organisms. They are also important in generating condensed chromatin that provides structural support for chromosomal regions such as telomeres and centromeres that have roles to play in the mechanics of chromosome behavior. These structural elements are in fact flanked by blocks of repetitive sequences that are constitutively silenced and are sometimes referred to as constitutive heterochromatin. Transposable elements whether functional or degraded need to be silenced in all cells but particularly so in germ line cells, to prevent transmission of new transpositions to new generations. Special mechanisms are devoted to ensure their transcriptional silencing (see Chapters 3 and 5). Other specialized mechanisms and, in particular, Polycomb silencing mechanisms are used to regulate silencing of specific genes at particular stages of specific tissues (see Chapter 7).

Non-coding Sequences

Equally dramatic is the expansion of non-repetitive non-coding sequences. These are diverse kinds of sequences. They include introns within genes: sequences that are transcribed but are spliced out of the coding mRNA. They are often somewhat less complex in sequence content than protein-coding regions and often include degraded transposable element sequences. It may seem paradoxical and counter-productive to have coding regions within genes interrupted by extraneous sequences that need to be removed and much debate has taken place and is still occurring about their source in evolution. One school of thought has argued that they are ancient relics of the process of gene evolution. An alternative view is that they have accumulated in evolution through the invasion of genes by foreign sequences. Genomic sequences show that introns were present very early in eukaryotes, but they are completely absent in present day bacteria and archaea. It is also clear that evolution has resulted in extensive creation as well as loss of introns. Introns have at least two important useful features. One is the process of alternative splicing, which allows a single gene to produce several different proteins with different selections of functional domains. Another valuable consequence of introns that are rapidly spliced during transcription is that, by removing newly transcribed sequences, they reduce the danger of R-loop formation. This is the tendency of newly transcribed RNA to form RNA–DNA hybrid regions, displacing the non-template DNA strand. R-loops are a hazard for DNA damage, are a drag on transcription elongation, and may create problems in DNA replication. It has been proposed that these features may explain the retention or introduction of introns. A typical mammalian gene has numerous introns that have often evolved to be very large, generally several kb. These in turn have collected during evolution large numbers of transposon sequences, usually inactive. In contrast, mammalian exons tend to be small, probably under selective pressure, so that in mammals internal exons (excluding the 5′ and 3′ exons) have an average length of 140–150 nucleotides, about the size of the DNA wrapped around the histone core in a nucleosome.

This is not just a coincidence. Exon sequences tend to favor nucleosome formation and nucleosome occupancy in exons is distinctly higher than in introns, the more so, the more frequently the exon tends to be spliced. Furthermore, splice sites occur preferentially at the edges of nucleosomes. Exons tend to be more GC-rich than introns and more likely to contain sequences favoring nucleosome assembly. Stronger pyrimidine tracts at the 3′ end of introns are correlated to a more pronounced difference in nucleosome occupancy between the end of the intron and the beginning of the exon. A similar discontinuity in nucleosome occupancy was found at the 3′ exon /5′ intron border. This is probably largely driven by the GC richness of exons. Similar discontinuities occur for the level of some histone modifications, particularly H3K36me3. This is at least in part due to the higher nucleosome occupancy at exons rather than a specific preference of exons for H3K36 methylation. Nevertheless, the presence of H3K36me3 may favor the recruitment of splicing factors. The presence of RNA Pol II is distinctly higher in exons compared to introns, independently of the level of expression of the gene. This implies that the polymerase slows down when it reaches an intron, probably because of the higher nucleosome occupancy. This slow-down of transcription is correlated with splicing efficiency. Thus, alternatively spliced exons with poorer splicing consensus sequences are more likely to be included when transcription rate is lower. These observations strongly suggest that the intron–exon structure of genes and the splicing architecture itself is encoded in the DNA sequence (Figure 23).

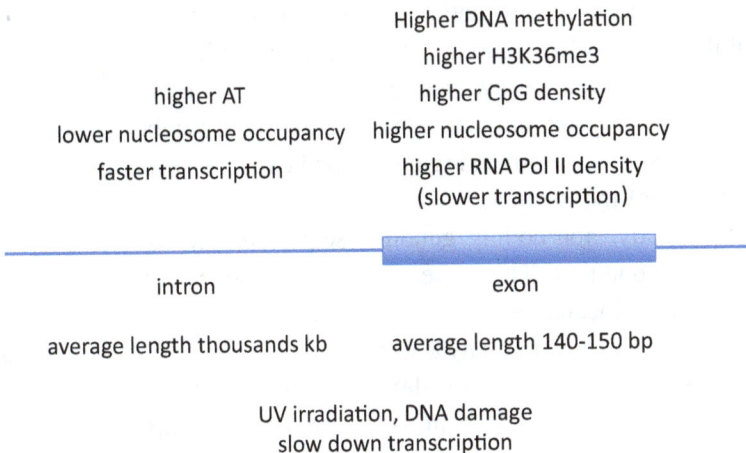

Higher DNA methylation
higher H3K36me3

higher AT
higher CpG density

lower nucleosome occupancy
higher nucleosome occupancy

faster transcription
higher RNA Pol II density
(slower transcription)

intron

exon

average length thousands kb

average length 140-150 bp

UV irradiation, DNA damage
slow down transcription

Figure 23.   A summary of features distinguishing mammalian exons from introns.

Splicing involves a large number of factors associated with many small RNAs to form a large splicing machine called the spliceosome. Splicing factors select splice donor and acceptor sites according to certain sequence requirements. The 5′ end of the intron is the donor site with a consensus sequence 5′ exon GG (cut) GURGU-intron. At the 3′ end of the intron, the acceptor site consists of a few pyrimidine-rich nucleotides followed by CAG (cut) G-intron. These sequence requirements are fairly loose and there are better and less good splicing donor and acceptor sites, which usually affect the order in which they are utilized. The splicing reaction goes through an intermediate step in which the spliceosome selects a branchpoint nucleotide with consensus pyUpuAC some 20–50 nucleotides upstream of the splicing acceptor site. This site attacks the 5′ donor site, forming a lariat and releasing the GG at the 3′ end of the exon to attack in turn the splice acceptor site ligating donor to acceptor and releasing the lariat. The process requires the hydrolysis of one ATP for each bond formed, thus two ATPs for a simple splicing reaction (Figure 24). Splicing generally occurs during transcription and various devices are used to slow down the RNA polymerase to allow splicing without accumulating too much unspliced transcript (see Chapter 12). In the case of very long introns, instead of waiting for the whole intron to be transcribed, intermediate splice sites are used, progressively removing the intron piecemeal. Regulatory mechanisms and suboptimal splicing consensus sequences may sometimes allow a range of alternative splicing possibilities (see also Chapter 12). Alternative splicing is infrequent in lower metazoans but has evolved to become an important resource in vertebrates. In many mammalian genes it allows a number of alternative proteins to be made from a single gene and expands several fold the coding capacity of the genome.

Importantly, non-coding genomic sequences include transcriptional regulatory sequences. These are greatly expanded in higher eukaryotes and are usually located between genes, sometimes as far as one Mb distant from their target gene, but may also be found within introns. A single gene may have multiple regulatory elements at different distances from the promoter. The vast increase in gene regulatory complexity in higher organisms accounts for the expansion of this type of sequence. In the following chapters much space is devoted to the mechanisms by which

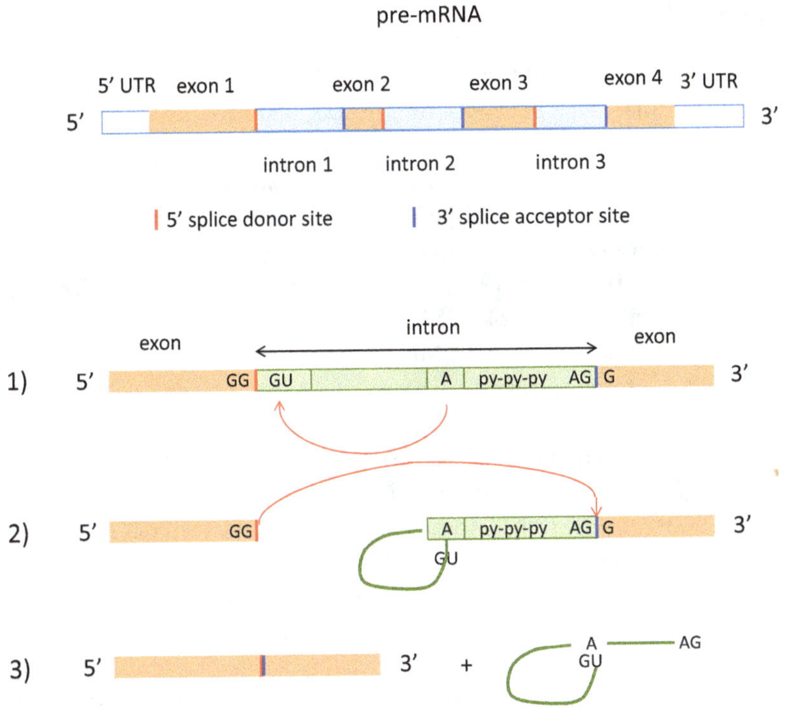

Figure 24. Pre-mRNA splicing. The diagram above represents a pre-mRNA with four exons and 3 introns. The three diagrams below show a sequence of steps in the splicing of an intron. (1) The splicing factors assembled in a spliceosome select a site A in the intron that will be the branchpoint. The 2′ OH of that nucleotide attacks the GU at the 5′ donor site forming the lariat intermediate with hydrolysis of one ATP. (2) The 3′ OH at the splice donor site now attacks the splice acceptor site, which is a G, preceded by a pyrimidine-rich sequence ending in AG, hydrolyzing one ATP. This joins the two exons and releases the lariat for later degradation.

regulatory sequences of different kinds operate to produce the patterns of gene expression that are necessary for the growth, differentiation, and function of the different tissues that make up a higher organism. Finally, some non-coding regulatory sequences are necessary for the mechanics that make possible and regulate the replication and partitioning of the genome during the cell cycle and cell division. These are exemplified by the chromosomal telomeres and centromeres (see Chapter 1).

Further Reading

Aebi U, Cohn J, Buhle and Gerace L (1986). The nuclear lamina is a meshwork of intermediate-type filaments. *Nature.* **323**, 560–564.

Ananiev EV and Barsky VE (1985). Elementary structures in polytene chromosomes of *Drosophila melanogaster. Chromosoma.* **93**, 104–115.

Ashburner M (1972). Patterns of puffing activity in the salivary gland chromosomes of *Drosophila. Chromosoma.* **38**, 255–281.

Ashburner M and Bonner JJ (1979). The induction of gene activity in *Drosophila* by heat shock. *Cell.* **17**, 241–254.

Beck CR, Collier P, Macfarlane C, Malig M, Kidd JM, Eichler EE *et al.* (2010). LINE-1 retrotransposition activity in human genomes. *Cell.* **141**, 1159–1170.

Bickmore WA and van Steensel B (2013). Genome architecture: Domain organization of interphase chromosomes. *Cell.* **152**, 1270–1284.

Bolzer A, Kreth G, Solovei I, Koehler D, Saracoglu K, Fauth C *et al.* (2005). Three-dimensional maps of all chromosomes in human male fibroblast nuclei and prometaphase rosettes. *PLoS Biol.* **3**, e157.

Dittmer TA and Misteli T (2011). The lamin protein family. *Genome Biol.* **12**, 222.

Goodier JL (2016). Restricting retrotransposons: A review. *Mobile DNA.* **7**, 16.

Gruenbaum Y and Foisner R (2015). Lamins: Nuclear intermediate filament proteins with fundamental functions in nuclear mechanics and genome regulation. *Annu Rev Biochem.* **84**, 131–164.

Jamrich M, Greenleaf AL and Bautz EKF (1977). Localization of RNA polymerase in polytene chromosomes of *Drosophila melanogatser. Proc Natl Acad Sci USA.* **74**, 2079–2083.

Lafontaine DLJ, Riback JA, Bascetin R and Brangwynne CP (2021). The nucleolus as a multiphase liquid condensate. *Nat Rev Mol Cell Biol.* **22**, 165–182.

Luco RF, Allo M, Schor IE, Kornbliht AR and Misteli T (2011). Epigenetics in alternative pre-mRNA splicing. *Cell.* **144**, 16–26.

Maison C, Bailly D, Peters AHFM, Quivy J-P, Roche D, Taddei A *et al.* (2002). Higher-order structure in pericentric heterochromatin involves a distinct pattern of histone modification and an RNA component. *Nat Genet.* **30**, 329–334.

Matera AG and Wang Z (2014). A day in the life of the spliceosome. *Nat Rev Mol Cell Biol.* **15**. 108–121.

Padeken J, Zeller P and Gasser SM (2015). Repeat DNA in genome organization and stability. *Curr Opin Genet Develop.* **31**, 12–19.

Ullu E and Tschudi C (1984). Alu sequences are processed 7SL RNA genes. *Nature.* **312**, 171–172.

Uhrig S, Schuffenhauer S, Fauth C, Wirtz A, Daumer-Haas, C, Apacol C *et al.* (1999). Multiplex-FISH for pre- and postnatal diagnostic applications. *Am J Hum Genet.* **65**, 448–462.

Van Bortle K and Corces VG (2012). Nuclear organization and genome function. *Annu Rev Cell Develop Biol.* **28**, 163–187.

van Steensel B and Belmont AS (2017). Lamina-associated domains: Links with chromosome architecture, heterochromatin, and gene repression. *Cell.* **169**, 780–791.

Wells JN and Feschotte C (2020). A field guide to eukaryotic transposable elements. *Annu Rev Genet.* **54**, 539–561.

Chapter 5

Heterochromatin

Introduction

Heterochromatin, the part of the genome that remains condensed and largely transcriptionally inactive, is a distinct genomic region in terms of sequence composition, chromatin structure, histone modifications, and associated proteins. Among other things, it contains most of the highly repeated, satellite-type sequence component of the genome and a large fraction of the interspersed repeat sequences: transposable elements or remnants of former transposable elements. Most of the heterochromatic material comes from the pericentric region, the part of the chromosome surrounding the centromere, but islands of heterochromatin can also be found in other parts of the chromosome and in the subtelomeric region. Pericentric heterochromatin can be roughly visualized even in mitotic chromosomes because it is hypercondensed and forms the constricted chromosomal region surrounding centromeres (Figure 1). Heterochromatic elements are also associated with subtelomeric regions and can occasionally be found scattered amidst euchromatin. Not surprisingly, heterochromatin is low in those histone modifications that are usually found in transcriptionally active regions, such as histone acetylation of all sorts, H3K4me3 and H3K36me3. Instead, heterochromatin is highly enriched in H3K9me2, H3K9me3, H4K20me3, as well as 5mC DNA methylation (see Chapter 3).

In general, we can distinguish between centric heterochromatin, the part of the genome immediately surrounding the centromeric region, and

145

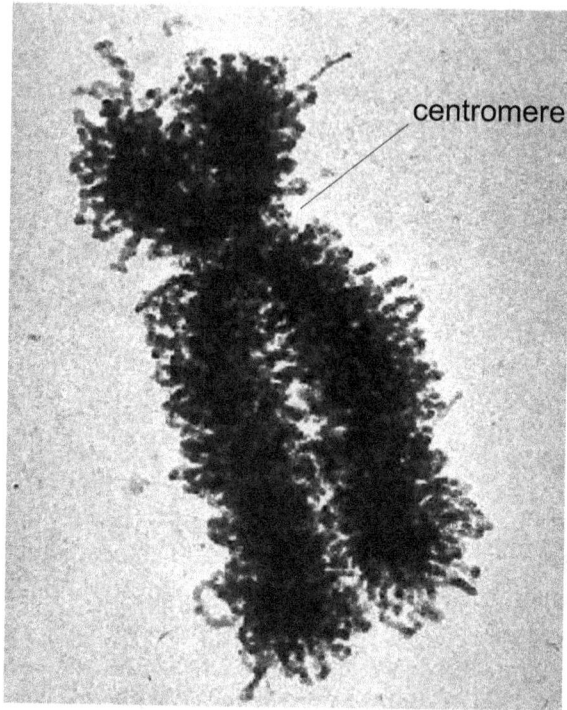

Figure 1.   Mitotic chromosome. This typical mitotic chromosome shows the two sister chromatids held together at the centromere. Even when the chromosome is tightly condensed in preparation for mitosis, the heterochromatic pericentromeric region is even more condensed and forms a constriction in the chromosome.

Source: DuPraw (1968).

pericentric heterochromatin, more distal and bordering with euchromatic regions. While centric heterochromatin consists largely of satellite-type repeats, pericentric heterochromatin includes many transposable elements or decayed transposable elements. Although heterochromatin is poor in gene content, it is not entirely lacking in functional genes. These are in some way protected from heterochromatic silencing. The high content of repetitive sequence has made it difficult to map and sequence in detail much of the heterochromatin of higher eukaryotes but much progress has been made in recent years to complete the sequencing of this part of the genome in selected organisms. For example, we now know that of 24 Mb of *Drosophila* pericentromeric heterochromatin more than 74% consist of transposable element and other repeated sequences, often fragmented and nested one inside another. Islands of unique sequences within this repetitive material contain a small number of functional genes, often with large introns containing repetitive sequences. Repetitive sequences are also found in subtelomeric regions where they are thought to play a role similar to that of pericentromeric heterochromatin in helping to arrange these chromosome regions relative to one another and to the nuclear architecture (see Chapter 8).

In *Drosophila* polytene chromosomes, the onset of pericentric heterochromatin can be readily identified by the loss of band morphology, followed by the constriction reflecting DNA underreplication. Staining the polytene chromosomes with antibodies against heterochromatin proteins such as HP1 or histone modifications such as histone H3K9 di- or trimethylation also allows the mapping of the pericentromeric heterochromatin boundary. At the sequence level, the onset of high levels of H3K9 methylation characteristic of pericentric heterochromatin can be visualized by chromatin immunoprecipitation and sequencing. Figure 2 shows the border region where the sudden rise in H3K9me2 creates a fairly well-defined boundary. H3K9 methylation is high on the centromeric side of this boundary while H3K4me3, characteristic of active promoters, is low. However, scattered individual spikes of H3K4me3 can still be seen on the heterochromatin side and correspond to the promoters of known genes that continue to be functional even though surrounded by heterochromatin.

Properties of Heterochromatin

Heterochromatin has a number of characteristic properties that we will summarize here. The subsequent discussion will clarify the molecular bases for many of these properties. The first characteristic, which is part of the definition of heterochromatin, is that it remains highly condensed throughout the cell cycle and is condensed not only in appearance but also in its DNA content, its nucleosome organization, and its consequent resistance to nucleases and to other factors and enzymes that require access to the underlying DNA. For many years, it was assumed that in heterochromatin, nucleosomes stack in the regular way they do *in vitro* under optimal

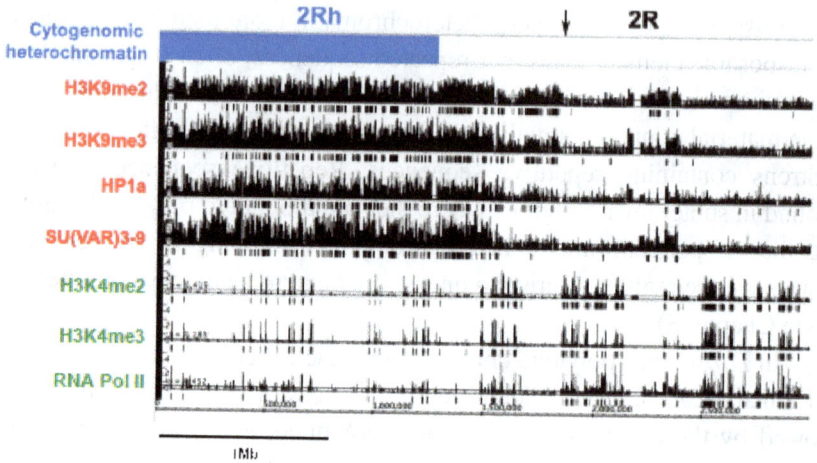

Figure 2.   Boundary region between euchromatin and heterochromatin. Chromatin immunoprecipitation mapping of active transcription marks and heterochromatin marks at the border region of chromosome 2R in *Drosophila* cultured cells. The region marked in blue as cytogenomic heterochromatin is what appears heterochromatic in polytene chromosomes. In this cultured cell line, the heterochromatin boundary appears to be almost 1 Mb to the right, as indicated by the black arrow. Although less frequent, both H3K4 methylation marks and RNA Pol II, indicative of active transcription, are found also in pericentric heterochromatin.

Source: Riddle *et al.* (2011).

conditions to form a 30 nm fiber (see Chapter 2). This regular stacking is stabilized by the regular interactions between nucleosomes and prevents the access of proteins to the underlying DNA. Recent optical and electron microscopy studies have shown that, even in heterochromatin, the nucleosome chain does not assume an ordered stacking. Instead, it remains disordered though more densely packed than in euchromatic regions and with closer nucleosome interactions that hinder the access of nucleases or DNA-binding proteins. According to these studies, no higher-order, regular organization of nucleosomes was seen even in mitotic chromosomes, only a higher concentration of the same lumpy nucleosome string.

The denser packing of heterochromatic nucleosomes results in large part from the proteins and protein complexes that are recruited to bind to heterochromatin. Locally, these proteins are responsible for the denser interactions among nucleosomes, and on a nuclear scale, they are also responsible for the physical association among different heterochromatic regions in the genome. An extreme example of this is visible in the nuclei of *Drosophila* salivary glands, where all four polytene chromosomes come together at their centric heterochromatin to form a single chromocenter. Heterochromatin also tends to be associated with the nucleolus and, in particular, with the nuclear envelope, where it binds to a stiff network of fibers formed by the lamin proteins (see Chapters 4 and 8).

Heterochromatin is highly deficient in genetic recombination. This is not only consistent with its dense packing and the consequent loss of access to the DNA but also essential to protect the integrity of this part of the genome. Given the high content of repetitive sequences, genetic recombination would frequently involve pairing and recombination between two sequences at different sites and therefore result in genetic rearrangements, duplications, and deletions of chromosome regions.

The dense nature of heterochromatin and the difficult access to its DNA content also suggest that it would be difficult to replicate and also to transcribe. Replication timing is a complex matter and regulated for different chromosome regions in ways that are not fully understood. Nevertheless, in general, heterochromatic regions of the genome tend to replicate late in the cell cycle. Similarly, dense packing and difficulty in accessing the DNA would lead us to expect that heterochromatin would be deficient in transcriptional activity. This is largely the case although a few functional genes do reside in heterochromatin and therefore must have ways to overcome these difficulties. Although transcriptional activity is very low in heterochromatin, it is not entirely absent and may in fact be necessary for the maintenance of the heterochromatic state (see the following sections).

A characteristic of heterochromatin and the transcriptional repression that results from heterochromatin formation is its ability to spread along the chromosome. This is observed when genes normally residing in euchromatin are placed next to heterochromatin either by a chromosomal rearrangement or by insertion of a transgene. In such cases, there is a tendency for heterochromatin to invade the gene and silence its expression entirely or in part. The silencing is stochastic and cell-autonomous. That is, it occurs at random with a certain frequency in each cell during early development. As these cells divide and produce progeny cells, the adult tissue contains patches of cells in which the gene has been silenced and patches in which it remains active. This haphazard but cell-autonomous process reveals another key feature of heterochromatic silencing: once established, the heterochromatic state of the gene is transmitted to the cellular progeny from one cell cycle to the next. This was one of the key properties that led to the understanding of the epigenetic features of many chromatin modifications.

Position-effect Variegation: PEV

Heterochromatin spreading into new regions can cause striking effects when it affects the expression of a gene with a readily visible phenotype. Many of the properties and constituents of heterochromatin were first discovered by geneticists studying these effects in *Drosophila melanogaster*. A typical example and a model used for fundamental work in the study of heterochromatin is that of the *Drosophila white* gene. This is a small gene normally located near one end of the X chromosome and required for the brilliant red pigmentation of the large compound *Drosophila* eyes. Mutations or loss of function of the *white* gene results in loss of eye pigmentation and in the totally white eye phenotype for which the gene is named (Figure 3). A surprising recessive mutation of *white*

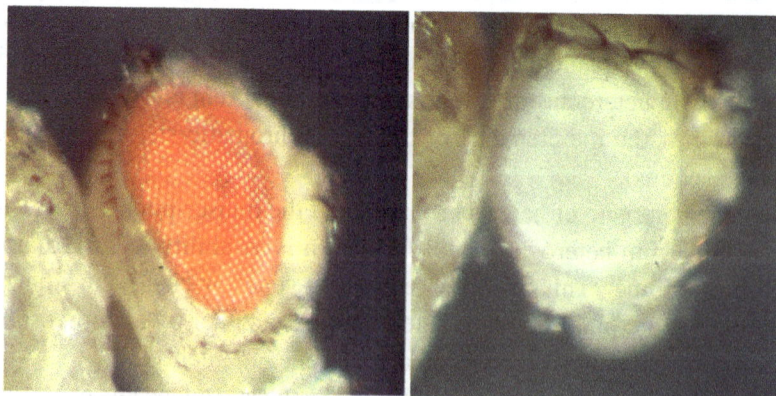

Figure 3.   The *Drosophila white* gene phenotype. On the left is the wild-type eye. On the right is the eye of a null mutant of the *white* gene.

Source: V. Pirrotta.

resulted, however, in a variegated eye color: the compound eye contains patches of red and patches of unpigmented tissue. The w^{m4} mutation is due to a chromosomal rearrangement in which a chromosomal region comprising most of the X chromosome has become inverted, with one break next to the *white* gene and the other in the middle of centric heterochromatin (Figure 4). The variegation dependent on the chromosomal position of the gene is called position-effect variegation (PEV). The rearrangement places the *white* gene in immediate contact with tandemly repeated sequences deep in heterochromatin. As a result, heterochromatic silencing can spread into the *white* gene, making it heterochromatic and transcriptionally silenced. This generally happens in the early stages of embryonic development, when heterochromatin first becomes established. Each cell

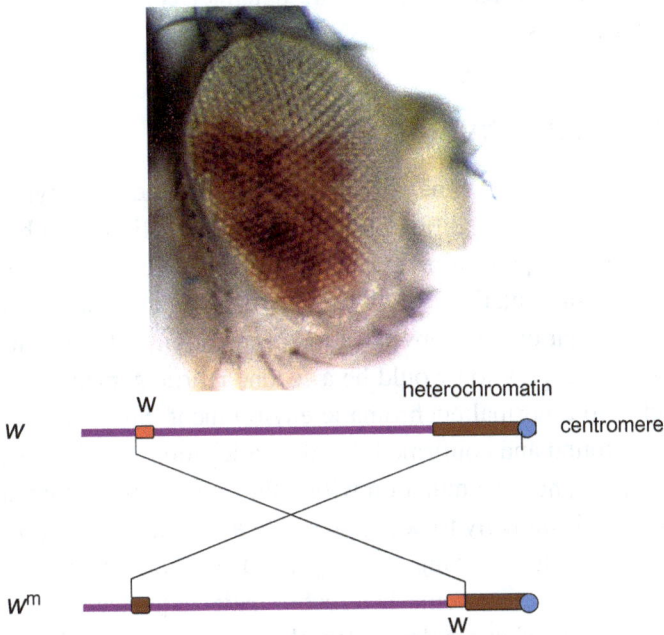

Figure 4. The w^{m4} chromosome inversion. An inversion called *white*^{mottled4} (w^{m4}) places the *white* gene *w* next to most of the centric heterochromatin. Heterochromatin spreads in a variable, stochastic manner into the *white* gene causing silencing in a variable, mosaic pattern called variegation.

Source: V. Pirrotta.

at this stage "decides" independently whether heterochromatin spreads into the *white* gene or not, but once the gene is silenced, it remains silenced in all the progeny cells. This random or stochastic silencing results in a mosaic eye in which clones of cells have a silenced *white* gene and other clones have an active *white* gene. An alternative view of the variegated expression is that silencing occurs early in development and is indeed inherited by daughter cells for several generations but stochastically lost at some point. It is also possible that both mechanisms can operate and that their relative importance depends on the characteristics of the heterochromatin that causes the silencing. In any case, these observations illustrate two important points: (1) heterochromatic silencing can spread from sequences that originate it to sequences that normally are not heterochromatic; (2) the heterochromatic state is established at one point in development and is maintained in the daughter cells produced through many cell divisions.

Mutations Affecting PEV

Variegation of the *white* gene not only is a very visible phenotype but also allows the distinction of different degrees of variegation from barely different from wild type to nearly completely white eyes. It was easy therefore to look for mutations elsewhere in the genome that affected the degree of variegation. One obvious kind of mutation that will cause reversion to normal expression would be a second rearrangement that puts the gene back into a normal euchromatic environment. Such mutations have in fact been found and confirmed that the variegation was due to the position of the gene, not to a mutation within the gene. Furthermore, a second rearrangement is unlikely to occur precisely at the same breakpoint as the first and, in fact, the reverting rearrangements generally have breakpoints near the first but retain some heterochromatic sequence near the *white* gene. Variegation of eye color is largely but not completely abolished. This illustrates another important point: the more heterochromatic sequence, the more likely and stronger the degree of silencing.

Much more frequent than second rearrangements are mutations in other genes that can either enhance or suppress variegation (Figure 5). Such mutations have been found in more than 150 genes in the *Drosophila*

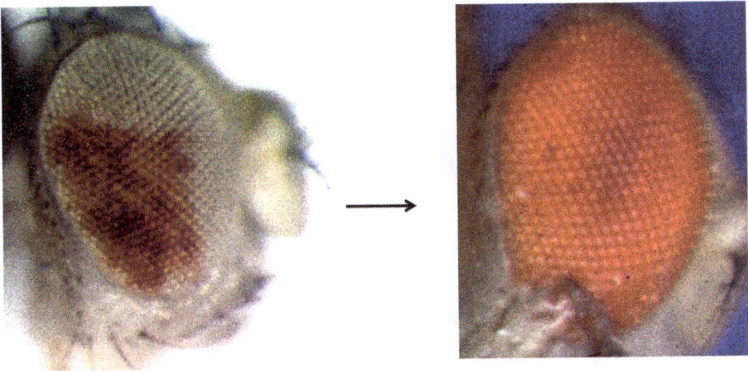

Figure 5. Suppressors of variegation. Mutations in many other genes called *Su(var)* genes suppress partially or totally the effects of Position-Effect Variegation (PEV), showing that their gene products are needed for heterochromatic silencing.

Source: Wallrath and Elgin (1995).

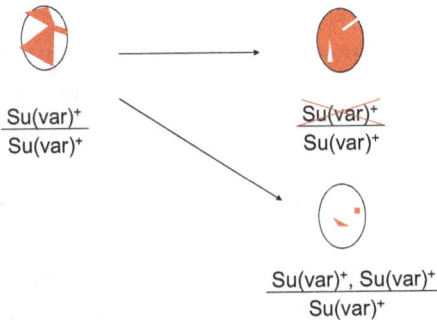

Figure 6. Suppressors of variegation have quantitative effects. Knocking out one copy of a *Su(var)* gene suppresses variegation: the less Su(var) product, the less silencing. Similarly, adding an extra copy of a *Su(var)* gene increases the degree of silencing.

genome. Of particular interest are those genes whose function is necessary for variegation since they would be candidates for functions necessary for heterochromatic silencing or its spread. Mutations in such genes will suppress variegation and are called therefore *Su(var)* genes (Figure 6). These mutations have generally dominant phenotypes, with effects detectable even when only one copy of the gene is mutated, implying that a decreased amount of gene product has a visible effect on the degree of heterochromatic silencing or spreading. This suggested that the more the *Su(var)* gene product, the more the repression would result. In fact, adding an extra copy of a *Su(var)* gene (three copies instead of two) increased the degree of silencing or variegation.

The *white* gene is not the only gene subject to PEV. The genes that lie next to *white* and are also placed near heterochromatin by the same chromosomal inversion can be shown to acquire variegated expression. Many other genes can become silenced or acquire variegated expression when placed next to heterochromatin. Similar effects were seen using transgenes: they too can be silenced or variegated when inserted in heterochromatin. The same spreading and silencing mechanism is responsible in most of these cases and, in fact, is suppressed by the same *Su(var)* mutations.

Su(var) Gene Products are Heterochromatin Proteins

The first Su(var) gene product to be identified was a protein highly abundant in extracts from a *Drosophila* chromatin fraction enriched in heterochromatin. This was called Heterochromatin Protein 1 or HP1. When the distribution of HP1 protein in chromosomes was examined using an antibody that binds to HP1, it was found that this protein binds to all the heterochromatic regions of the genome, in particular pericentric heterochromatin and telomeric regions (Figure 7). Another *Su(var)* gene is *Su(var)*3-9. Its protein is also preferentially associated with heterochromatin and with the HP1 protein itself. Although these genes were first discovered in *Drosophila*, it was soon found that most eukaryotes have similar genes, closely related to the *Drosophila Su(var)* genes. These discoveries supported the idea that heterochromatin was kept in a repressed and condensed state by the binding of the Su(var) proteins. A common idea at the time was that Su(var) proteins packaged heterochromatin into a tight, highly condensed form that was inaccessible to transcription factors or RNA polymerase and thus transcriptionally disabled. But the epigenetic nature of heterochromatic silencing remained to be explained. How is the silenced or active state maintained in the progeny of the cell in which it had been established? The epigenetic nature of heterochromatic silencing strongly suggested that the silenced chromatin becomes marked

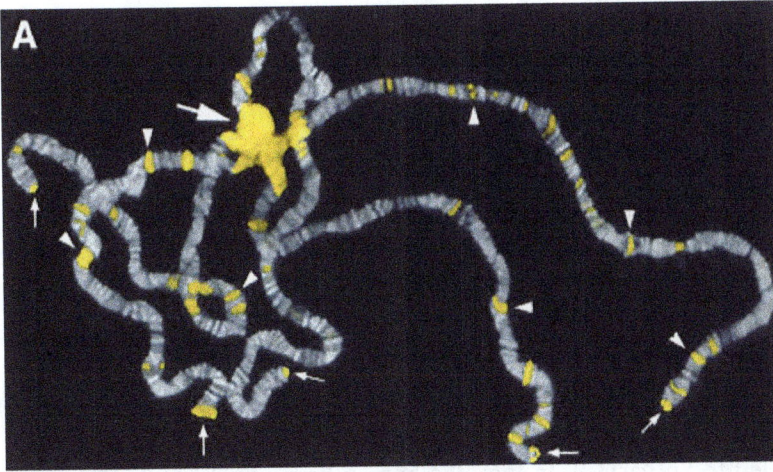

Figure 7.   HP1, the product of *Su(var)205*, is a heterochromatin protein. Heterochromatin Protein 1 (HP1) was identified as a heterochromatin-binding protein, here shown using an anti-HP1 antibody on *Drosophila* polytene chromosomes. By far, the greatest binding of HP1 is at the heterochromatic chromocenter (arrow) but distinct binding sites occur also on the euchromatic chromosome arms (arrowheads) and telomeres (small arrows). HP1 was subsequently found to be the product of the *Su(var)205* gene.

Source: Fanti *et al.* (1998).

with a relatively stable mark so that it "knows" that it had been silenced in the previous cell cycle and becomes silenced again in the daughter cells. The only well-understood mechanism for this kind of "marking" at that time was DNA methylation. This is because DNA methylation in vertebrates occurs primarily at the C of CpG sequences. A CpG on one strand will have a CpG on the complementary strand, therefore both strands are targets of DNA methylation. If both strands of DNA are methylated at a given site, when the two strands separate for the semiconservative replication of DNA, each strand retains a methyl mark. The DNA methyltransferase 1 (Dnmt1) enzyme recognizes hemimethylated DNA as a target and fully methylates it again (see Chapter 3). DNA methylation is in fact abundant in vertebrate heterochromatin but it is also widespread in non-heterochromatic regions of the genome. There must be other ways to maintain a chromatin mark because *Drosophila* contains very little, if any, DNA methylation and many other organisms lack DNA methylation but have typical heterochromatin and heterochromatic silencing whose epigenetic states are maintained through many cell divisions.

The Heterochromatic Histone Methylation Mark

A major breakthrough came in the year 2000 when the laboratory of Thomas Jenuwein discovered that the mammalian *Su(var)3-9* homolog encoded a protein with enzymatic activity that could methylate the N-terminal tail of histone H3 at lysine 9 (Figure 8). It was immediately recognized that H3K9 methylation might be the epigenetic "mark" of heterochromatin. We now know that heterochromatin in most higher eukaryotes contains methylated H3K9 and one or more proteins closely related to Su(var)3-9. In fact, the human homolog, SUV39H1, can completely substitute for the *Drosophila* enzyme. The catalytic activity of Su(var)3-9 resides in the SET domain, a highly recognizable structure so called because it was first discovered as a shared domain found in the three histone methyltransferases: Su(var)3-9, Enhancer of zeste, and

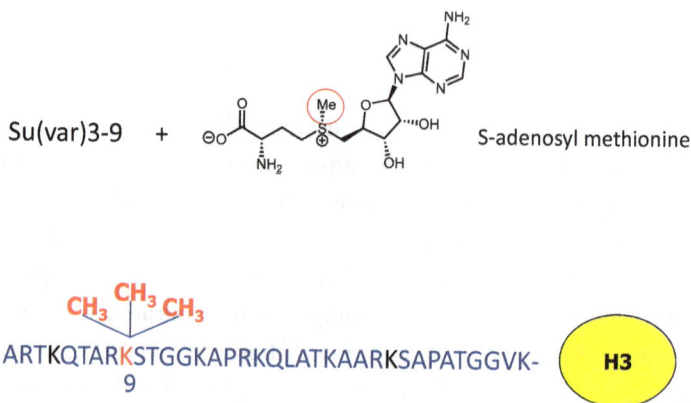

Figure 8.   Histone H3K9 methylation. In 2000, Thomas Jenuwein and co-workers discovered that Su(var)3-9 or its human homolog is an enzyme that methylates the N-terminal tail of histone H3 at lysine 9 using S-adenosyl methionine as the methyl donor. The enzyme progressively adds one, two, and three methyl groups to lysine 9. Heterochromatin contains predominantly H3K9me2 and H3K9me3.

Source: S-adenosyl methionine illustration from https://commons.wikimedia.org/wiki/File:S-adenosyl_methionine.png.

Trithorax. The SET domain is in fact characteristically found in almost all histone methyltransferases. Like all other methyltransferases, Su(var)3-9 uses S-adenosyl methionine as the methyl donor. An abundant supply of S-adenosyl methionine is therefore essential to maintain heterochromatin and, not surprisingly, the enzyme that synthesizes S-adenosyl methionine, S-adenosyl synthase, is the product of another *Su(var)* gene, *Su(var)5* in *Drosophila*.

Histone H3 K9 di- or tri-methylation is highly enriched in heterochromatin and provides a mark for chromatin regions that are to be made into heterochromatin but this immediately raises the question of what identifies or reads this mark. *In vitro* binding studies showed that a particular structural domain of HP1 bound specifically a peptide containing the N-terminal tail of histone H3 trimethylated at lysine 9. This HP1 domain, called the chromodomain, includes a hydrophobic pocket that at the same time includes two negatively charged residues, providing a good fit for the positively charged trimethylated amine of lysine 9 (Figure 9). A suitably

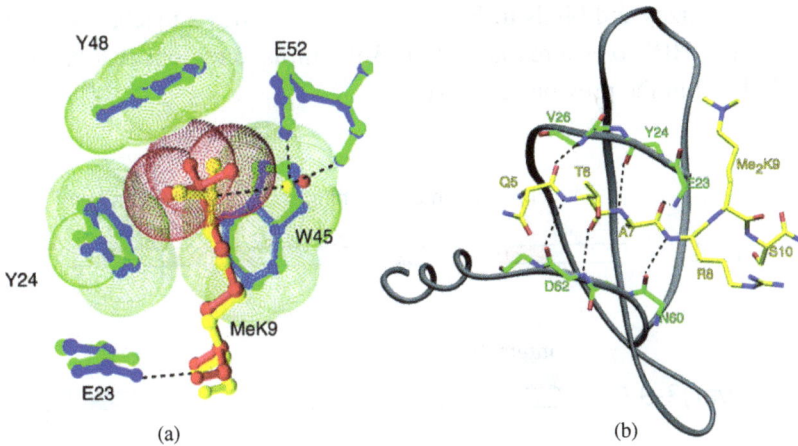

Figure 9. The HP1 chromodomain. The chromodomain is shown in (b) interacting with the N-terminal tail of histone H3 dimethylated at lysine 9. The tail fits in a long groove that is positioned by specific contacts. (a) shows the K9me2 (yellow) fitting in the aromatic pocket (green) and the K9me3 (red) fitting in the aromatic pocket (blue). The red clouds in (a) indicate the van der Waals field around the three methyl groups of K9me3.

Source: Jacobs and Khorasanizadeh (2002).

positioned groove provides additional interactions with the amino acids preceding lysine 9 and renders the binding specific for this particular tri-methyl lysine rather than, for example, lysine 4 or lysine 27 of histone H3.

The chromodomain at the N-terminal of HP1 is connected by a hinge region to a C-terminal domain that is distantly related to the chromodo-main and has been called the chromoshadow domain (Figure 10). Both the chromodomain and the chromoshadow domain can mediate dimerization of HP1. As a result, when HP1 binds to chromatin containing H3K9 meth-ylation, it can, in principle, form chains or spread along from one methyl-ated nucleosome to the next. In addition, the chromoshadow domain mediates the dimerization of HP1 and the interaction with a number of other chromatin proteins and, in particular, with Su(var)3-9, which recog-nizes a surface formed by the dimerization of two HP1 chromoshadow domains. This set of interactions provide a mechanism for the spreading of a heterochromatic domain. Binding of one HP1-Su(var)3-9 complex to a nucleosome mediates both the binding of another copy of the complex to a neighboring nucleosome and its methylation (Figure 11). Su(var)3-9 also contains a chromodomain near its N-terminal. This chromodomain also recognizes and binds to H3K9me3 and provides a mechanism inde-pendent of HP1 to ensure that Su(var)3-9 returns to regions that had been methylated in the previous cell cycle.

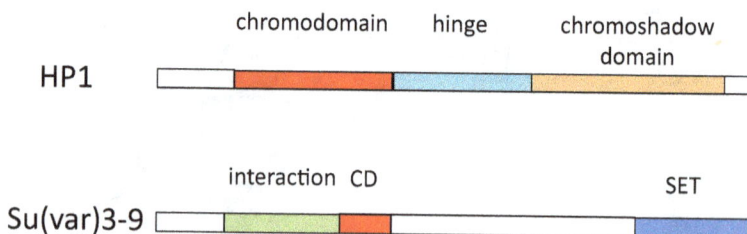

Figure 10.   Domain structure of HP1 and Su(var)3-9. (a) The HP1chromodomain binds to histone H3K9me2,3. The chromoshadow domain is distantly related to the chromodo-main. It interacts with itself, forming HP1 dimers. The interaction surface binds to Su(var)3-9. The hinge region binds to RNA. (b) Su(var)3-9 is not drawn on the same scale as HP1. The interaction domain binds to HP1 and to another Su(var) protein, Su(var)3-7. The chromodomain, CD, binds to H3K9me2,3. SET is the catalytic methyltransferase domain.

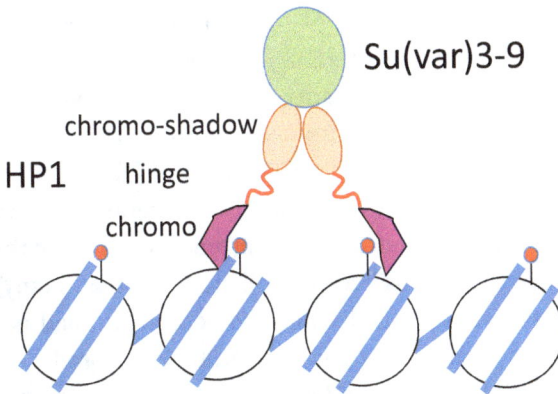

Figure 11. HP1 binding to nucleosomes. HP1 dimerizes through the chromoshadow domain. The HP1 chromodomain binds to the di- or tri-methylated H3K9, thus linking two nucleosomes together. The chromodomain can also dimerize, potentially allowing interactions to spread to additional nucleosomes. The interaction of two chromoshadow domains generates a surface to which Su(var)3-9 binds.

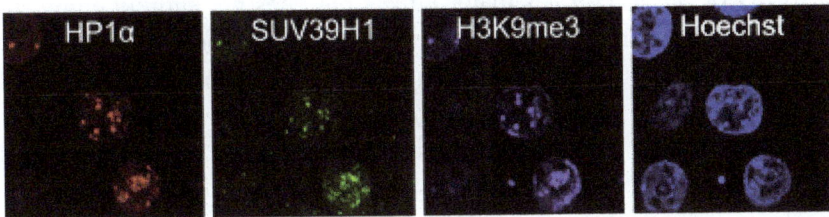

Figure 12. DNA concentration and heterochromatin marks. Staining nuclei with antibodies specific for three heterochromatin marks: HP1a, SUV39H1 and histone H3K9me3 show that they co-localize with one another and with foci of DNA density, shown by the DNA dye Hoechst.

Source: Wang *et al.* (2019).

HP1 and Su(var)3-9 are in fact heavily concentrated in parts of the genome known to be heterochromatically condensed and their enrichment coincides with that of H3K9 methylation (Figure 12). They also spread to the *white* gene in genomic rearrangements that place *white* next to heterochromatin and cause PEV of *white*. The spread of these proteins is accompanied by the spread of H3K9me2,3, the chromatin mark they produce. Mutations in Su(var)3-9 cause a massive loss of H3K9me2,3 and also a loss of binding of HP1 to heterochromatin. Mutations that abolish HP1 result in loss of effective targeting of Su(var)3-9, which now frequently associates with euchromatic regions. This is consistent with the association of HP1 and Su(var)3-9. Loss of HP1 does not cause loss of H3K9 methylation, however, because the methyltransferase can also function independently and its own chromodomain helps maintain the methylated state once it has been established. Another methylation mark, H4K20me3, is also associated with heterochromatin and is required for effective heterochromatic silencing. H4K20me3 is produced by the histone methylase SUV4-20, encoded by the *Suv4-20* gene, now known as *Hmt4-20*. Loss of HP1 or of Su(var)3-9 causes a strong reduction of H4K20me3 and mutations in the *Hmt4-20* gene suppress PEV and heterochromatic silencing. Loss of SUV4-20 reduces H3K9 methylation and HP1 binding to heterochromatin. SUV4-20, HP1, and Su(var)3-9 are in fact components of a heterochromatic complex that requires all three for function.

Loss of Su(var)3-9 has major effects but does not entirely eliminate visible heterochromatin. In polytene chromosomes, the heterochromatic chromocenter is still visible although partially decondensed and condensed chromatin is still visible in diploid cells. Furthermore, cellular H3K9 methylation is not entirely lost. Clearly, Su(var)3-9 is not the only H3K9 methyltransferase. Mammals have at least four others, in addition to the two SUV39H1/SUV39H2: SETDB1/SETDB2 and G9A/GLP. SUV39H1,2 is responsible for most of the H3K9me3 in the nucleus. While SETDB1,2 contributes only a fraction of the total H3K9me3, it is known to be important for repression of transposable elements and knockout of both these enzymes results in deformation of the nuclear envelope and a tendency to fragment, forming multiple small nuclei. G9A and GLP produce H3K9me1,2 and are important for the regulation of gene expression during development. *Drosophila* has also dSetdb1, shown to be responsible for chromosome 4 and some centric heterochromatin. A G9a homolog is also present in *Drosophila*. Recent work shows that if all six mammalian H3K9 methylases are inactivated by mutations in mouse, all three degrees of H3K9 methylation are lost. The result is the derepression of nearly all types of repetitive elements and the total loss of condensed heterochromatin. This indicates clearly that there are different kinds of heterochromatin, produced in different ways. We will return to some of these mechanisms further down.

Heterochromatin Genes

The phenomenon of PEV shows that heterochromatin can spread and invade genes that are normally euchromatic. In the *Drosophila w*^{m4} chromosomal inversion and other similar inversions that place euchromatic regions next to heterochromatin, the spreading of heterochromatic marks can extend up to 175 kb and include multiple genes. Yet, the spreading of HP1 binding and H3K9 methylation varies considerably and the effects on gene expression vary even more, showing that some genes are more sensitive to the repressive effects than others. These examples make it clear that spreading of heterochromatin is highly sensitive to the chromatin state of the region to be invaded. It is not surprising therefore that a large number of gene functions and the specific features of the genes involved can affect the tendency of heterochromatin to spread into euchromatic territory. What prevents heterochromatin from spreading beyond the normal pericentromeric regions in which it is normally found? The boundary between constitutive heterochromatin and euchromatin is generally a fairly sharp one, as shown by the distribution of H3K9me2 and HP1 binding at this boundary region in a *Drosophila* chromosome, as shown by chromatin immunoprecipitation (Figure 2). The gene browser display shows a sudden increase in parallel of H3K9 methylation and of HP1 binding occurring over a region of 100 kb or less. At the same time, marks of gene activity such as H3K4me3 become more sparse. Note, however, that they do not disappear entirely. There are in fact genes that normally reside within pericentromeric heterochromatin and that are active and are in some cases essential genes. Most of these genes are larger than the typical *Drosophila* gene because they have large introns containing repetitive sequences, usually inactive fragments of transposable elements. The heterochromatic genes have high levels of H3K9 methylation and bind HP1 in their gene bodies but not in their promoter region. The promoter is poorly defined and transcription initiates at multiple positions. In these and other ways, *Drosophila* heterochromatic genes come to resemble a typical mammalian gene (Figure 13) and it could be argued that mammalian euchromatin, with its abundance and broad distribution of repetitive sequences and high level of DNA methylation, is in fact a more repressive environment than typical *Drosophila* euchromatin. Interestingly, the homologs of a few *D. melanogaster* heterochromatin-resident genes have been examined in several other *Drosophila* species. Perhaps not surprisingly, the homologs do not always reside in heterochromatin in other species. When they are found in a euchromatic environment, they shed the very large introns and the repetitive sequences they contain and resemble normal euchromatic genes.

How do heterochromatin genes successfully fight off heterochromatic silencing? There are clearly mechanisms that protect these genes or at least their promoters from the effects of surrounding heterochromatin. One relevant feature is that, although heterochromatin genes reside in chromatin that is enriched in H3K9me2, the 5′ end of these genes is specifically depleted of H3K9 methylation. Evidently, the promoter region can either prevent methylation or recruit a demethylase to remove it.

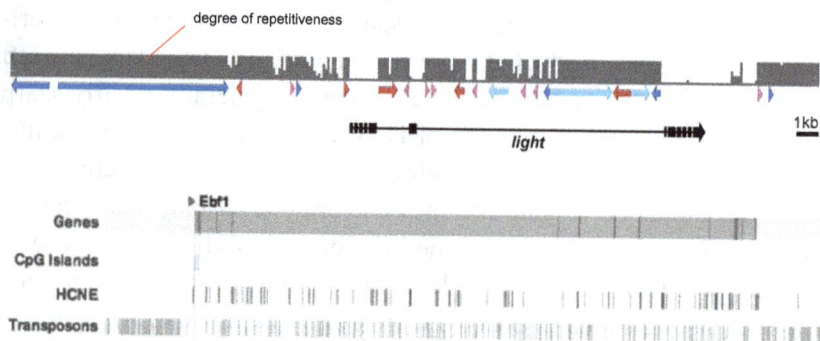

Figure 13. Comparison of a *Drosophila* heterochromatin gene and a typical mammalian gene. The upper figure shows the region containing the *light* gene, a *Drosophila* gene essential for viability that resides deep in heterochromatin. Note the unusually large intron and the high content of repetitive sequences. Source: Yasuhara and Wakimoto (2008). The lower figure shows a typical mammalian gene, *Ebf1*. Note the large introns and the high content of transponson-derived repetitive sequences. HCNE denotes highly conserved non-coding elements.

Source: Bernstein *et al.* (2006).

Perhaps more surprising is that in *Drosophila* many of these heterochromatin-resident genes actually function best when they are in a heterochromatic environment and lose activity if they are transposed to a euchromatic chromosome region. This is the opposite of the normal PEV and suggests that heterochromatin genes have come to require the chromatin folding produced by HP1 and other heterochromatin proteins. The role of heterochromatin proteins in facilitating the expression of heterochromatin-residing genes has not been determined but some mechanisms are known that might help neutralize the repressive effects of the heterochromatin environment.

Histone Deacetylation and Phosphorylation

Transcriptional activity produces chromatin marks and chromatin states that are antagonistic to heterochromatic silencing. In order to spread heterochromatin, the Su(var) complexes must inhibit these euchromatic marks. The most important of these is histone acetylation. Acetylation of histone H3 and H4 at several lysines accompanies gene activity but lysine methylation is incompatible with lysine acetylation. It is not unexpected, therefore, that a histone deacetylase is associated with a complex that includes HP1 and Su(var)3-9. This enzyme, called HDAC1 and encoded by the *rpd3* gene in *Drosophila*, is required to allow the establishment of domains of H3K9 methylation, and mutations in *rpd3* are strong suppressors of variegation. Consistently, inhibitors of histone deacetylases, such as butyric acid, Trichostatin A (TSA), or various more specific inhibitors that have been developed for cancer treatment, prevent heterochromatin spreading and reactivate genes that had been silenced by H3K9 methylation. Conversely, genome studies have shown that certain gene regulatory elements recruit histone acetylases. The specific binding of a histone acetylase to a promoter region can successfully hold heterochromatin at bay and prevent its spreading to silence the promoter.

Another histone modification produced in the course of transcriptional activation is the phosphorylation of H3S10 (see Chapter 2). This places a strong negatively charged phosphate next to the lysine whose methylation is recognized by the HP1 chromodomain. Not surprisingly, phosphorylation of H3S10 prevents the binding of HP1 to H3K9me2,3 and produces dissociation of HP1 previously bound to methylated H3K9. In fact, phosphorylation of H3S10 by specific enzymes causes the massive eviction of HP1 from chromatin at the onset of mitosis. Clearly, this phosphorylation mark must be removed or prevented in order to establish heterochromatin. Like H3K9 acetylation, H3S10 phosphorylation is a very effective way to antagonize the spread of heterochromatin. Also associated with transcription is H3K4 methylation, where H3K4me3 is typically found at activated promoters and H3K4me1 is a signature of activated enhancers. Since transcriptional activity produces histone acetylation and phosphorylation, which are antagonistic to heterochromatin spreading, H3K4 methylation would also be expected to be a suppressor of variegation. Mutations in the *Lsd-1* gene, encoding a H3K4me1,2 demethylase, were in fact discovered as suppressors of variegation *Su(var)3-3* mutations in *Drosophila*.

Liquid Phase Condensation

The hinge region of HP1 proteins is an Intrinsically Disordered Region (IDR), a domain that lacks a stable three-dimensional organization but can form a multiplicity of weak interactions with other IDRs, assuming flexible, dynamically variable condensed structures that tend to exclude water. At a certain concentration, IDR proteins undergo a sharp transition and form a separate phase from the aqueous environment. Globules of condensed IDR proteins behave like liquid droplets that can fuse with other similar droplets and, by excluding water, concentrate the protein components in a separate phase (Figure 14). Many chromatin proteins and transcription factors contain IDRs and can form liquid phase condensates, often aided by interactions with RNA. These condensates, each with a specific ability to meld with certain other condensates, are now thought to play important roles in the organization of chromatin in the nucleus. Such condensates can be surprisingly stable even while the IDR-containing proteins within them can diffuse rapidly. This high mobility means that modification of the IDR proteins, for example, by phosphorylation, acetylation or methylation, or interaction with other proteins affecting IDR properties, can have very rapid effects causing condensates to form or to

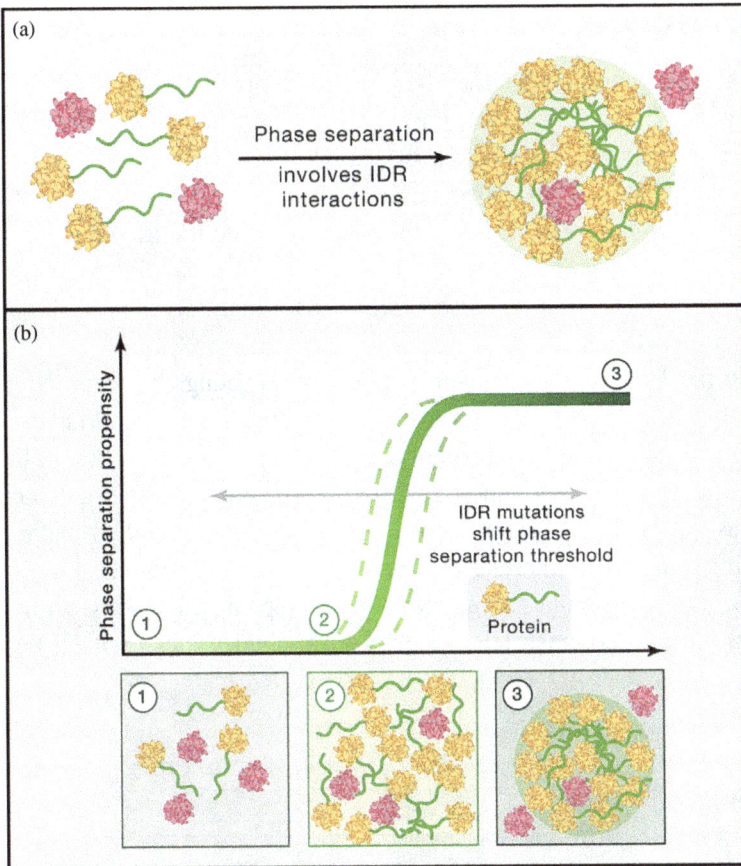

Figure 14. Intrinsically disordered proteins. (a) Proteins containing an intrinsically disordered region (IDR), indicated by the wiggly green line, associate through multiple weak interactions. At a certain concentration, such proteins can undergo a phase transition. (b) At a critical concentration, IDR proteins are thought to transit to a separate liquid phase, forming droplets that do not mix with the aqueous environment. IDR proteins can enter freely such droplets but other proteins are less favored.

Source: Tsang *et al.* (2020).

dissolve. In general, the formation of condensates provides a rapid way to separate certain proteins, or the chromatin regions to which they bind, from the nuclear environment, while allowing access to factors that interact with the condensing proteins themselves.

HP1 Paralogs

The human genome, like the fly genome, contains three closely related HP1 genes (paralogs), HP1α, HP1β, and HP1γ (*Drosophila* HP1a, HP1b, and HP1c), that differ slightly in sequence but have distinct functions (Figure 15). HP1b, HP1β and HP1c, HP1γ can also have transcriptional activating effects. The small differences in amino acid sequence have important consequences for the multiplicity of weak interactions that result in condensation of these proteins with themselves or with certain other proteins.

In the HP1 protein, the hinge region connecting the chromodomain with the chromoshadow domain is the IDR and is sufficient to cause formation of condensates. Phosphorylation tends to increase the ability of HP1 dimers to interact and to form phase-separated condensates and, in the case of HP1α, is required for the formation of heterochromatic foci. Binding to RNA or to certain peptides can have similar effects. The human HP1α, like Drosophila HP1a, forms phase-separated condensates *in vivo* and *in vitro*. In contrast, HP1β cannot form condensates by itself but can

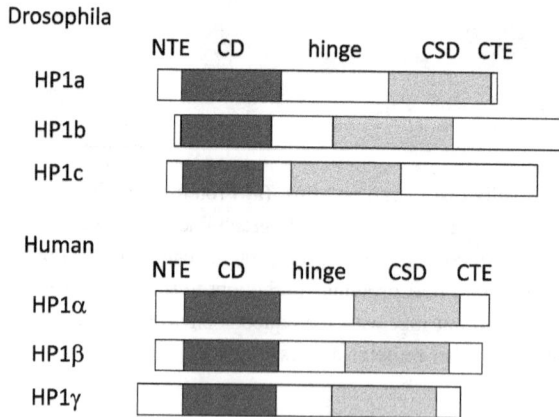

Figure 15.   Structure of HP1 family proteins. The protein domains, N-terminal end, chromodomain, hinge, chromoshadow domain, and C-terminal end are shown with the chromodomains aligned. HP1a and HP1α are mostly nuclear but HP1b, HP1β and HP1c, HP1γ are partially nuclear and partially cytoplasmic. Note the smaller hinge regions of HP1b, HP1β and HP1c, HP1γ, which reduces their ability to form liquid condensates.

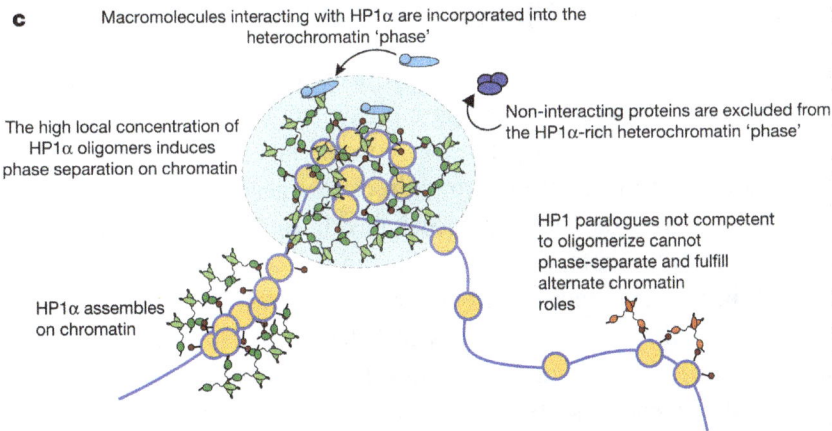

c

Macromolecules interacting with HP1α are incorporated into the heterochromatin 'phase'

The high local concentration of HP1α oligomers induces phase separation on chromatin

Non-interacting proteins are excluded from the HP1α-rich heterochromatin 'phase'

HP1 paralogues not competent to oligomerize cannot phase-separate and fulfill alternate chromatin roles

HP1α assembles on chromatin

Figure 16. Formation of liquid phase condensates by HP1α bound to chromatin. HP1α, with the CD and CSD shown in green and connected by the hinge region, binds to nucleosomes containing H3K9me3. At a critical concentration, HP1α forms a separate liquid phase. This allows interacting proteins to enter the HP1 phase but excludes other, non-interacting proteins in the aqueous phase.

Source: Larson *et al.* (2017).

associate with previously formed, chromatin-containing condensates. Adding HP1β to a HP1α condensate results in invasion of the condensate by HP1β and eventual decondensation due to the replacement of HP1α (Figure 16). However, HP1β can initiate condensates when interacting with chromatin containing H3K9 methylation. This behavior suggests that HP1β could be important in establishing heterochromatin boundaries.

While HP1α is preferentially associated with silenced heterochromatin, HP1β and HP1γ can both silence and stimulate transcription. It is thought that the different properties of the HP1 paralogs are most likely due to the differences in the less structured regions, hinge, N-, and C-terminals. While the three different paralogs have different localization and different primary roles, it is clear that each one can also play more than one role. HP1 α, for example, can still be recruited by DNA methylation to transcribed regions where it can help recruit RNA splicing factors or histone heacetylases. All three HP1 isoforms are recruited to sites of DNA damage and contribute to DNA repair.

Heterochromatic Silencing and RNAi

We have talked about the properties of heterochromatin and the mechanisms of heterochromatic silencing but have not confronted the question of what determines which sequences become heterochromatic and why. There is evidence that heterochromatin can be generated by a variety of processes. Some satellite sequences may intrinsically generate hetero chromatin. For example, if a protein that binds to a specific DNA sequence can recruit key heterochromatin factors such as HP1 or Su(var)3-9, such a sequence will clearly be a focus of heterochromatin initiation. Some satellite sequences have such properties. In general, however, there are no conserved sequence motifs that characterize heterochromatin. Although repetitive sequences both of the short satellite type and the long interspersed repeats or transposable elements are typically found in heterochromatin, non-repetitive sequences can also be heterochromatic. The fact that heterochromatic silencing can spread into sequences that are normally euchromatic argues that the sequence itself is not, in principle, necessary to specify heterochromatin.

Satellite repeats, repetitive sequences, and transposable elements are known foci that initiate heterochromatin formation. But what is it about these sequences that singles them out for this role? Before we look into this question, we have to consider a surprising set of mechanisms that depend on RNA and were first revealed by studies in plants, fungi, and nematodes. To understand the multiple roles of RNA, we need to recapitulate the discovery of RNA interference or RNAi. In the 1990s, it was thought that one way to inhibit viral infections in plants and animals might be to introduce RNA molecules with antisense sequences relative to the viral RNA. The antisense RNA was expected to hybridize to the sense viral RNA and prevent its translation by ribosomes. In other words, the effect of the antisense RNA would be post-transcriptional. It was surprising therefore that, in some cases, plant biologists found that the transcription of the gene in question was also inhibited. The interfering RNA effect worked well also in animals, particularly in the nematode *Caenorhabditis elegans*. In 1998, Andrew Fire and Craig Mello (both Nobel laureates, 2006) independently made surprising discoveries showing that, in fact, antisense RNA alone had only feeble effects but double-stranded RNA induced a powerful inhibition of the expression of the corresponding endogenous gene. Only a few molecules of the double-stranded RNA per cell were sufficient to produce the inhibition, arguing against a simple competitive mechanism. Double-stranded RNA or RNA containing significant double-stranded or fold-back regions is in fact the effective inactivating agent in what were collectively called RNA interference phenomena or RNAi and the range of targets involves not just mRNA but also chromatin and transcription.

The trigger that initiates RNAi processes is in general the presence of double-stranded RNA. *In vivo*, this can be generated in various ways, some of which we will examine in more detail. One possible mechanism, particularly relevant for repetitive sequences results from low-level random transcription or read-through from flanking regions. Such RNAs can be produced from either strand and, particularly for repeated sequences, provide a pool of complementary RNAs that can yield double-stranded structures (Figure 17). However, even stem-loop structures from fold-back of inverted repeats in RNA molecules can initiate some RNAi processes. These can be divided into three principal types, all three involving the

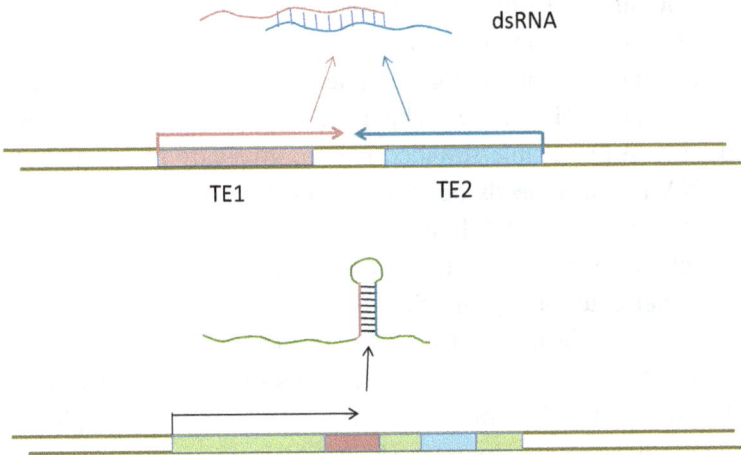

Figure 17. Sources of double-stranded RNA. Heterochromatin can give rise to overlapping transcripts in opposite directions, due to frequent presence of transposable elements that can insert randomly, sometimes even one inside another. Double-stranded RNA can arise from stem-loop structures in transcripts with palindromic or base-pairing sequences.

production of small RNAs but using somewhat different pathways and different targets. They are pathways involving microRNAs (miRNAs), small interfering RNAs (siRNAs), and PIWI-interacting RNAs (piRNAs). miRNAs are cytoplasmic and regulate in a variety of ways the utilization of mRNAs containing appropriate sequences, affecting translation, adenylation, capping, and more. The function of many genes is regulated post-transcriptionally by corresponding miRNAs. siRNAs direct the endonucleolytic cleavage of mRNAs containing complementary sequences. The most important activity of piRNAs is to associate with nascent transcripts as they are being transcribed and target chromatin silencing machinery to the chromatin itself. All three classes of small RNAs are handled by Argonaute proteins, a family of RNA-binding proteins that constitute the core of RNA-Induced Silencing Complexes (RISCs). A branch of this family contains the PIWI proteins that bind to piRNAs.

The miRNA pathway utilizes the transcripts of endogenous genes that have evolved to provide the source material for specific miRNAs. In some cases, the RNA comes from introns or from 3′ UTRs. In other cases, it is produced by specific miRNA genes that are usually developmentally regulated and target and in turn regulate developmental genes. In the miRNA and siRNA pathways, the double-stranded RNA material, after some preliminary trimming by an exonuclease, is escorted out of the nucleus and then cut into double-stranded fragments by an endonuclease of the Dicer family (Figure 18). The miRNA formation requires imperfect base pairing in the double-stranded region, involving some mismatches. The siRNA pathway needs perfect pairing. Dicers contain two tandem RNase III domains. A PAZ domain that binds to a 3′ end overhang positions the cleavages and the distance between PAZ and the RNase domains acts as a ruler determining the size of the fragment produced. The fragment sizes are characteristic for each specific Dicer involved and range from 21 to 25 nucleotide pairs with a two-nucleotide 3′-OH overhang.

The double-stranded fragments are handed over to a complex called RNA-Induced Silencing Complex (RISC), containing one of a family of Argonaute proteins. Argonautes are the effectors of the RNAi pathway and the specific Argonaute protein determines the target specificity of the RISC complex of which it is the key constituent. To carry out its function, the RISC complex needs a single-stranded RNA guide. The correct strand

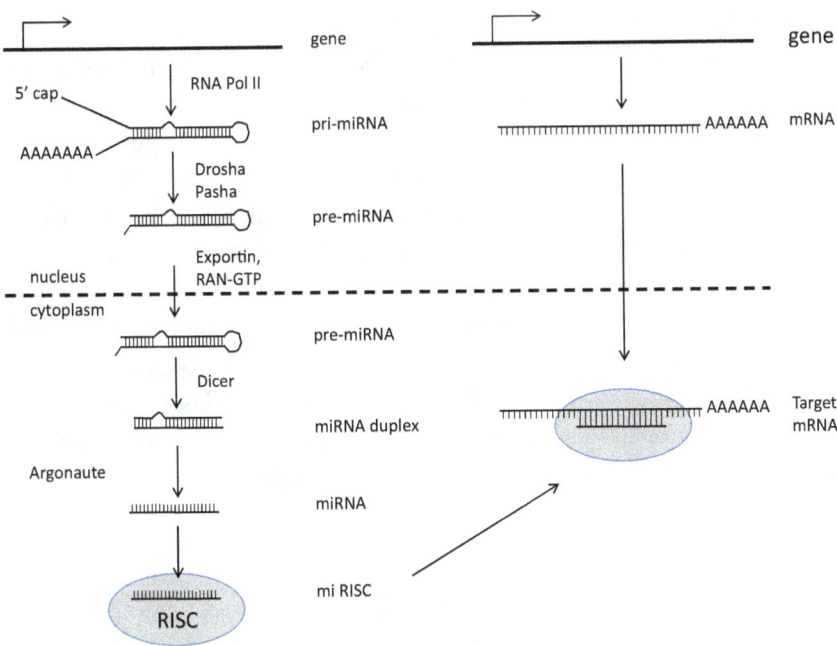

Figure 18. microRNA pathway. Specific primary gene transcripts containing the requisite fold-back structure are processed by nuclear endonuclease to a pre-miRNA and then transported out of the nucleus. In the cytoplasm, a Dicer endonuclease chops the pre-miRNA into short segments. An Argonaute protein binds the double-stranded fragments, selects the appropriate strand, and discards the other. The loaded Argonaute is the main constituent of the RISC complex that leads the single-stranded fragment, now acting as a guide RNA, to its target RNA transcript whose processing or translation it regulates.

of the double-stranded small RNA has to be selected and loaded on a specific Argonaute species, while the passenger strand is discarded. In *Drosophila*, AGO1 is involved in the miRNA pathway and AGO2 in the siRNA pathway but some organisms have multiple Argonaute proteins with multiple sequence and structural preferences to bind the correct small RNA, select the appropriate strand to be the guide strand, and degrade the passenger strand. The details of the strand selection are not entirely clear but they seem to prefer the strand with the least stably paired 5′ end and a preference for U at the 5′ end in the case of AGO1, for C in the case of AGO2. In mammals, however, no 5′ nucleotide preference for AGO loading has been found. Specific protein factors are probably also involved. In some cases, the 3′ end of the guide strand is methylated on the 2′OH, to further stabilize the guide RNA.

The mature RISC–guide RNA is now active. It uses the guide to associate with the target RNA molecule. For the miRNA pathway, which is exclusively cytoplasmic, the tasks are a variety of functions modifying RNA processing, stability, and translation, affecting the functional expression of a large number of mRNAs. In the case of siRNA pathway, the typical RISC function, mediated by Argonaute, is to recognize and cleave single-stranded RNA molecules containing a sequence complementary to the siRNA, a process called "slicing" (Figure 19). This mechanism of post-transcriptional silencing has been very extensively used in research as a way to selectively interfere with the function of specific genes in a

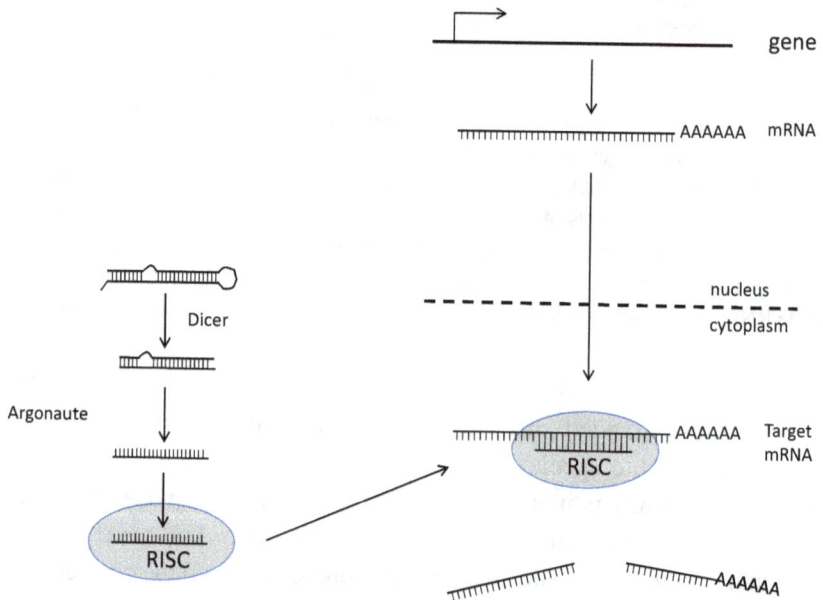

Figure 19.   The siRNA pathway. This pathway requires exact base pairing in the double-stranded RNA. The RNA is chopped into 21–24 bp fragments by a Dicer enzyme and captured by an Argonaute protein which discards the passenger strand and forms a RISC complex. The specific Argonaute for siRNA targets a complementary mRNA and "slices" it endonucleolytically.

kind of surrogate genetics. Use of a particular siRNAs to suppress the action of a gene is highly effective but the degree of suppression is variable, depending on the sequences involved, and is often referred to as "knock-down" of the gene, as opposed to the "knock-out" that would result from a gene deletion or loss of function mutation. In plants and even in lower metazoans such as the nematode *C. elegans*, this pathway is rendered more efficient by the possibility to amplify the siRNA through an RNA-directed RNA polymerase (RDRP), which can utilize single-stranded siRNA to prime RNA synthesis along a single-stranded RNA such as mRNA or an exogenous RNA. The resulting double-stranded RNA is then cut by Dicer to generate a large number of small RNAs directed against the same mRNA or viral RNA. RDRPs have not been found in *Drosophila* or in vertebrates and are not essential for RNAi mechanisms.

Transcriptional Gene Silencing by siRNA

It was at first very surprising when evidence began to accumulate in the 1990s showing that siRNA produced not only post-transcriptional effects through mRNA slicing but also repressive effects on the chromatin of the target gene itself. This process has been most thoroughly analyzed in the fission yeast *Saccharomyces pombe* and occurs co-transcriptionally. That is, the RISC complex in the nucleus is targeted to nascent transcripts by the guide RNA and itself recruits chromatin silencing complexes that inhibit transcription of the target gene. In fission yeast, RNAi mechanisms using small RNAs from the pericentromeric region are necessary for the formation of heterochromatin. These small RNAs are derived from bi-directional transcription of pericentromeric repeats, after processing by a pathway similar to the siRNA pathway described above. Fission yeast possesses an RdRP and can further amplify the small RNAs produced by Dicer. The equivalent of the RISC complex is called the RNA-induced Transcriptional Silencing (RITS) complex. RITS includes the fission yeast AGO1 with its bound siRNA and a chromodomain protein that binds to histone H3K9me3 like HP1. The RITS complex is recruited to the target nascent transcript by base pairing with the guide siRNA and to the surrounding chromatin that bears or will bear H3K9 methylation.

The RITS complex recruits a complex containing Clr4, the fission yeast's homolog of the Su(var)3-9 H3K9 methyltransferase, which provides the H3K9 methylation that stabilizes the binding of the RITS complex itself (Figure 20). The H3K9 methylation also recruits heterochromatin proteins Swi6 and Chp2, homologs of the metazoan HP1 heterochromatin protein. These proteins in turn recruit histone deacetylases and produce the typical heterochromatic transcriptionally repressed and condensed structure. In fission yeast, nematodes, and other organisms but not higher metazoans, Swi also recruits the RNA-dependent RNA polymerase, which uses the siRNA to produce additional double-stranded RNA to enter the Dicer/ RITS cycle and amplify the whole silencing process.

In principle then, siRNA can mediate both post-transcriptional and transcriptional silencing, in fact generating heterochromatin, at least in fission yeast. There is an apparent paradox in that transcription of repetitive sequences, providing both the siRNA and the nascent transcript target, is required to ultimately silence that same transcription. How are those RNAs produced then to maintain the silenced heterochromatic state from one cell cycle to the next? The most likely answer is that the

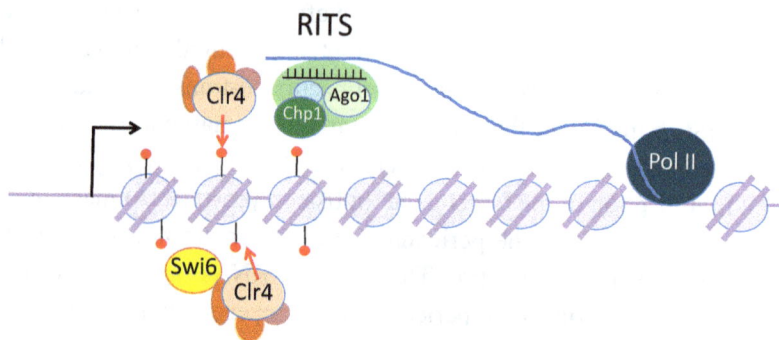

Figure 20.   RNA-mediated transcriptional silencing in fission yeast. A RITS complex containing Argonaute 1 and siRNA base pairs with a cognate transcript as it is transcribed by RNA Pol II. A complex containing the histone methylase Clr4, homologous to Su(var)3-9, which trimethylates H3K9. A chromodomain protein Swi6 (homologous to HP1) binds H3K9me3 and recruits Clr4 to maintain the methylation independently of transcription. The RITS complex also contains a chromodomain protein Chp1, which contributes to repeat the transcription-dependent chromatin methylation. Higher metazoans lack a Chp1 homolog.

silencing is not uniform throughout the cell cycle. In fission yeast, the production of siRNA takes place in M phase, peaking in early S phase, when DNA replication occurs. Similarly, the binding of HP1 to heterochromatin peaks shortly after that, peaking in G2, which represents about 70% of the cell cycle. In fact, a transient decondensation of heterochromatin occurs in M phase, initiated by phosphorylation of histone H3S10 by the Aurora kinase. This phosphorylation places a large, negatively charged phosphate next to the methylated H3K9, interfering with the binding of HP1. This is the so-called "phospho-switch" by which the effects of histone methylation can be transiently neutralized. Release of HP1 causes decondensation of heterochromatin and allows transcription, peaking as DNA replicates in S phase. This is when the siRNA mechanism is necessary to ensure H3K9 methylation of newly replicated chromatin. After DNA replication, H3S10 is dephosphorylated, allowing HP1 to bind again and restore the repressive condensed heterochromatin.

The piRNA Pathway

RNA-dependent silencing mechanisms have been persuasively demonstrated in fission yeast and in the nematode. Evidence for transcriptional silencing by siRNA is much less extensive in *Drosophila* and in vertebrates but the essential components of the RNA-mediated transcriptional silencing pathway are well conserved in these organisms. In addition, much evidence shows that at least part of heterochromatin formation is dependent on RNA-dependent mechanisms. The most persuasive evidence is that for the piRNA pathway which is dedicated to transcriptional silencing of transposable elements.

The piRNA pathway was originally discovered for its most important role in silencing transposable elements in *Drosophila* germ line cells, critical to avoid transmission of mobilized transposons to the progeny. piRNAs are 24–31 nucleotides long, slightly longer than miRNAs or siRNAs. The source of the piRNAs is different and surprising. It comes from transcription of certain genomic sites that contain strings of sequences derived from transposable elements. These sites, called piRNA clusters, serve as a sort of protective memory, an inventory of earlier transposon invasions. piRNA clusters are transcribed from multiple promoters to produce long single-stranded RNAs studded with transposable element motifs, usually representing the strand complementary to that of the normal transposable element transcript. Some piRNA clusters contain transposon sequence in either orientation and may be transcribed bi-directionally. If a new invasive transposon enters the genome and inserts in a piRNA cluster in the appropriate orientation, it will therefore create the piRNA sequences needed to repress that new transposable element. There is a certain similarity here between piRNA clusters and bacterial CRISPR arrays (see CRISPR-Cas Genome Editing, Chapter 13) although the mechanisms are very different. In both cases, sequence elements derived from previous genome invasions (bacteriophage or transposable elements, respectively) are stored in an array from which they can be retrieved to provide a defense against subsequent attacks. piRNA clusters both one-directional and bi-directional are found in mammals as well as in *Drosophila*, but their transcription and piRNA production have been better characterized in the fly, as described in the discussion that follows (Figure 21).

The primary transcripts from piRNA clusters are exported to the cytoplasm and trimmed by endo- and exonucleases although the details of what specifically identifies them as piRNA precursors are not very clear. In *Drosophila*, where this pathway was originally identified, the major processing enzyme is called Zucchini and is associated with the surface of mitochondria. The maturation process produces piRNAs that have preferentially a U at the 5' end and include a 2'-O methylation at the 3' end. The piRNA then binds to the PIWI protein to form a PIWI-piRISC complex. Piwi, an Argonaute family protein, is a cytoplasmic protein and only enters the nucleus in the form of a PIWI-piRISC complex. In the nucleus, the PIWI-piRISC complex targets nascent transposable element transcripts, recruiting Su(3)-9 and HP1 and directing histone H3K9 methylation in the corresponding chromatin much in the way siRNAs and RITS produce transcriptional gene silencing in fission yeast (see Figure 20). Note that the cytoplasmic processing and cleavage of target RNAs also cleaves primary transcripts from transposable elements and so inactivates them by post-transcriptional gene silencing just like siRNA.

Drosophila has two other PIWI-related proteins that can form corresponding piRISC complexes in the cytoplasm: Aubergine (Aub) with the antisense strand, like Piwi, and Ago3 with the transposon sense strand.

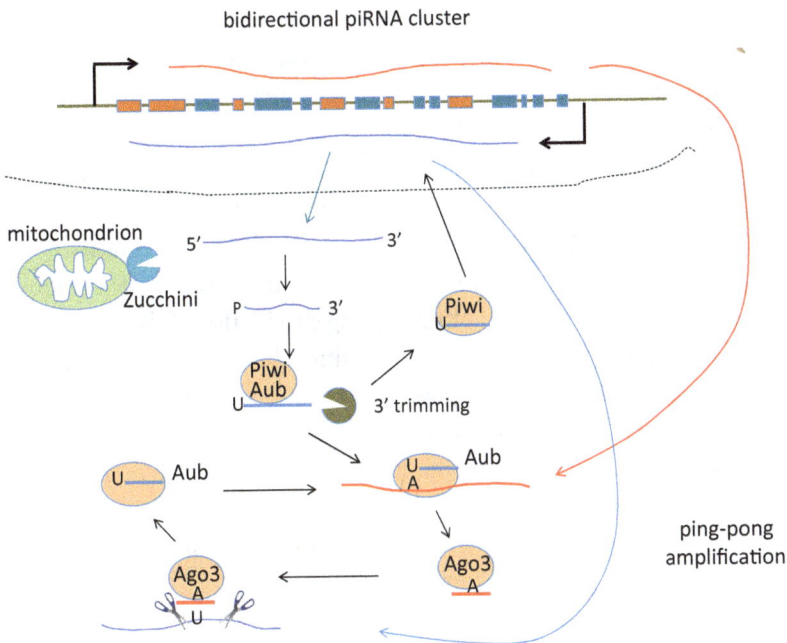

Figure 21. piRNA production and amplification. Bi-directional transcription of a piRNA cluster produces RNA transcripts complementary to transposon sequences (blue) and transcripts with sense sequences (red). Both are exported to the cytoplasm where the Zucchini endonuclease, bound to mitochondria, chops the blue transcripts, Piwi and Aubergine, further cut to produce 5′ ends enriched in' U. After trimming, these Piwi-bound fragments can re-enter thee nucleus for transcriptional silencing of transposable elements. In association with Aubergine, the same fragments can enter a ping-pong amplification cycle in which they target the red transcripts at complementary sites, producing fragments complementary to blue transcripts, directing cleavage by Aubergine into fragments that re-enter the cycle.

Much as in the ordinary siRNA pathway, Ago3-piRISC and Aub-piRISC can target transposon RNA and cleave it by their slicer action. In the *Drosophila* germ line, primary piRNA can also be produced from piRNA clusters transcribed from both strands and this seems to be the case also for the mammalian germ line. In this case, some primary transcripts may also be processed by the Argonaute pathway common to siRNA.

Once the primary piRNA production is under way, the Aub-piRNA or Ago3-piRNA complexes in the cytoplasm use their slicing action to cleave the antisense and sense transposon transcripts, respectively. This initiates a secondary pathway of piRNA production, the so-called ping-pong mechanism (Figure 21). This pathway is exclusively cytoplasmic and, in germ line cells, produces a fuzzy perinuclear structure called nuage, where the factors involved in piRNA production accululate. The slicer activity of Aub-piRISC cuts the target RNA at a position 10–11 nucleotides from the 5′ end of the piRNA. Since piRNA has a U at the 5′ end, the slicer activity produces an RNA with A at the position 10 nucleotides from its 5′ end, characteristic of ping-pong production. It is not very clear what produces the 3′ end, possibly Zucchini. This small RNA binds Ago3 and can target antisense transposon RNA for slicing, producing more Aub-piRNA, which re-enters the cycle. The result of the ping-pong cycle is to increase the consumption of transposon RNA while amplifying the production of piRNAs. Transcriptional silencing of transposable elements and heterochromatin formation take place by mechanisms similar to those described in fission yeast (Figure 20).

Transcription of piRNA Clusters

As described above, transposable element transcripts are subject to both post-transcriptional and transcriptional silencing. This raises the question of how piRNA clusters remain able to be transcribed to maintain the silencing. In fact, the transcripts of piRNA clusters are very unusual. They do not have specific 5′ ends, they lack the normal 5′ cap, they are not spliced, and they tend to be very long and lack specific termination. Furthermore, piRNA clusters have a distinct heterochromatic character and are rich in H3K9 methylation, as might be expected from the action of Piwi-piRISC. It is this heterochromatic histone mark, rather than sequence features, that guides transcription initiation in piRNA clusters. In *Drosophila*, the initiation complex is recruited by a HP1-related protein called Rhino, whose chromodomain binds to H3K9me2,3 and recruits Moonshiner, a relative of a core TFIIA component, which in turn recruits TBP-Related Factor2 and RNA polymerase II. In addition, Rhino-dependent recruitment of Deadlock and Cutoff proteins prevents 5′ capping, splicing, polyadenylation, and antagonizes termination of the transcript. It remains unclear how Rhino-dependent transcription is limited to piRNA clusters and does not occur in typical heterochromatin. Mammals have a set of Piwi-related proteins, called MIWI and MILI in mouse and HIWI, and HILI in humans, and corresponding but less well-characterized processes take place during spermatogenesis.

Somatic piRNA Role

Piwi and piRNA functions were first characterized in *Drosophila* male germ line cells but it was soon found to play a role in the somatic cells of the ovary as well. Loss of Piwi causes male sterility and defective ovaries. Further evidence showed that the piRNA pathway acts also in other somatic tissues although it is not well understood how they generate piRNAs. For example, mutations in Piwi have a strong effect on position-effect variegation of the *white* gene in the eye. Most conclusive evidence for the functioning of Piwi-dependent mechanisms in somatic tissues is the detection of Piwi in the nuclei of somatic cells. Piwi binds to polytene chromosomes with a localization similar to that of HP1a. In fact, Piwi binds to HP1a and is required for heterochromatic PEV. Both Piwi and HP1a binding to chromatin are RNA-dependent and are lost upon RNase treatment of nuclei. Furthermore, the Piwi-HP1a complex also recruits Su(var)3-9 (Figure 22). This Piwi-dependent binding accounts for most but not all HP1a/Su(var)3-9 binding sites, suggesting that the piRNA mechanism is a major but not the only pathway to heterochromatin formation. In agreement with this, Piwi mutations cause a decrease but not a total loss of H3K9 methylation. Piwi-dependent binding and transcriptional silencing affect many but not all transposons. Certain transposon families are also silenced by recruitment of HP1a and H3K9 methylation but by mechanisms not involving Piwi or piRNAs.

Transcription is required for transcriptional gene silencing. Non-transcribed genes do not become silenced, do not bind Piwi, and are not enriched in H3K9 methylation. It may seem paradoxical that silencing requires some level of transcription but it is consistent with evidence showing that heterochromatic silencing is not absolute and some transcription takes place at some stage in the cell cycle. In the fission yeast

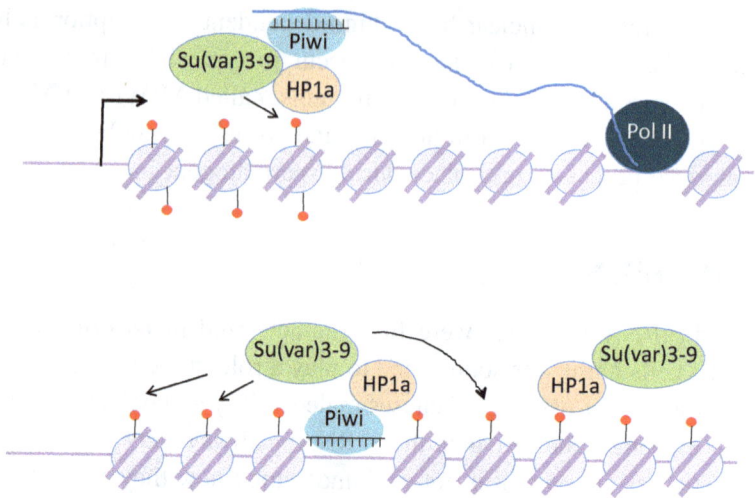

Figure 22.   piRNA-chromatin silencing. piRNA-mediated targeting of nascent transcripts brings HP1a and Su(var)3-9 H3K9 methylation and transcriptional silencing. In hetero-chromatin (below), Piwi may be targeted by base pairing directly to DNA and maintain H3K9 methylation and heterochromatic silencing. HP1a-Su(var)3-9 binding to densely methylated chromatin may also take place independently. In the *Drosophila* female germ line, dSetdb1 may replace Su(var)3-9 as the H3K9 methyltransferase. Numerous addi-tional factors are not shown in this simplified model.

Saccharomyces pombe, a distinction has been made between H3K9me2 domains, which effectively silence genes but do not completely abolish transcription, and H3K9me3 domains, which are fully silent. The differ-ence in the two chromatin states is presumably due to different efficien-cies in recruiting silencing complexes. Whether this is true for higher eukaryotes is unclear, particularly in mammals, where heterochromatic silencing is complicated by the involvement of DNA methylation.

The piRNA pathway is primarily targeted to transposable elements, whose sequences produce the piRNAs. However, it may affect the expres-sion of normal euchromatic, single copy genes in several ways. Insertion of a transposable element in the vicinity of a euchromatic gene may affect that gene's expression as chromatin silencing may spread from the trans-poson. In other cases, transcription of the transposable element extends into an adjacent euchromatic gene so that that gene's sequences become included in the piRNA repertoire. This has been shown to result in the down-regulation of certain genes during development.

In conclusion, RNA-mediated pathways have been found to be responsible for at least part of heterochromatin formation and heterochromatic silencing. But heterochromatin is not all the same and no known pathway can account for all heterochromatin. Although the piRNA mechanisms explain much of the behavior and properties of pericentric heterochromatin, there remain some aspects that are not affected by mutations inactivating these mechanisms. This implies the existence of other heterochromatin pathways about which remarkably little is known. Some heterochromatin may be produced by Dicer-dependent siRNA transcriptional silencing instead of piRNA mechanisms, as has been reported for a chicken cell line. DNA-binding proteins may, in some cases, recruit heterochromatic complexes and establish a heterochromatic state. In fact, some satellite sequences bind sequence-specific DNA-binding proteins and some evidence suggests that preventing that binding suppresses PEV. Unfortunately, this aspect has not been followed up by researchers so far.

Further Reading

Bartel DP (2018). Metazoan microRNAs. *Cell.* **173**, 20–51.

Bernstein BE, Mikkelsen TS, Xie X, Kamal M, Huebert DJ, Cuff J *et al.* (2006). A bivalent chromatin structure marks key developmental genes in embryonic stem cells. *Cell.* **125**, 315–326.

Czech B, Munafó M, Ciabrelli F, Eastwood EL, Fabry MH, Kneuss E *et al.* (2018). piRNA-guided genome defense: From biogenesis to silencing. *Annu Rev Genet.* **52**,1545–2948.

DuPraw EJ (1968). *Cell and Molecular Biology.* Academic Press, Inc.: New York.

Elgin SCR and Reuter G (2013). Position-effect variegation, heterochromatin formation, and gene silencing in *Drosophila. CSH Perspect Biol.* **5**, a017780.

Ernst C, Odom DT and Kutter C (2017). The emergence of piRNAs against transposon invasion to preserve mammalian genome integrity. *Nat Comm.* **8**, 1411.

Fanti L, Giovinazzo G, Berloco M and Pimpinelli S (1998). The Heterochromatin Protein-1 prevents telomere fusions in *Drosophila. Mol Cell.* 527–538.

Ipsaro, JJ and Joshua-Tor L (2015). From guide to target: molecular insights into eukaryotic RNA-interference machinery. *Nat Struct Mol Biol.* **22**, 20–28.

Jacobs SA and Khorasanizadeh S (2002). Structure of HP1 chromodomain bound to a lysine 9-methylated histone H3 tail. *Science.* **295**, 2080–2083.

Keenen MM, Brown D, Brennen LD, Renger R, Khoo H, Carlson CR *et al.* (2021). HP1 proteins compact DNA into mechanically and positionally stable phase separated domains. *eLife.* **10**, e64563. doi: 10.7554/eLife.64563.

Larson AG, Elnatan D, Keenen MM, Trnka MJ, Johnston JB, Burlingame AL *et al.* (2017). Liquid droplet formation by HP1α suggests a role for phase separation in heterochromatin. *Nature.* **547**, 236–240.

Martienssen R and Moazed D (2015). RNAi and heterochromatin assembly. *CSH Perspect Biol.* **7**, a019323.

Riddle NC, Minoda A, Kharchenko P., Alekseyenko AA, Schwartz YB, Tolstorukov MY *et al.* (2011). Plasticity in patterns of histone modifications and chromosomal proteins in Drosophila heterochromatin. *Genome Res.* **21**, 147–163.

Ross RJ, Weiner MM and Lin H (2014). PIWI proteins and PIWI-interacting RNAs in the soma. *Nature.* **505**, 353–359.

Shin Y and Brangwynne CP (2017). Liquid phase condensation in cell physiology and disease. *Science.* **357**, 1253.

Sienski G, D'nertas D and Brennecke J (2012). Transcriptional silencing of transposons by Piwi and Maelstrom and its impact on chromatin state and gene expression. *Cell.* **151**, 964–980.

Tsang B, Pritišanac I, Scherer SW, Moses AW and Forman-Kay JD (2020). Phase separation as a missing mechanism for interpretation of disease mutations. *Cell.* **183**, 1742–1756.

Wallrath LL and Elgin SCR (1995). Position effect variegation in *Drosophila* is associated with an altered chromatin structure. *Genes Dev.* **9**, 1263–1277.

Wang L, Gao Y, Zheng X, Liu C, Dong S, Li R *et al.* (2019). Histone modifications regulate chromatin compartmentalization by contributing to a phase separation mechanism. *Mol Cell.* **76**, 1–14.

Yasuhara JC and Wakimoto BT (2008). Molecular landscape of modified histones in *Drosophila* heterochromatic genes and euchromatin-heterochromatin transition zones. *PLoS Genet.* **4**, e16.

Chapter 6

Transcription

Introduction

Genomes contain the sequence information that specifies proteins. A fundamental requirement of genomes is the apparatus that reads this information. In the case of DNA-based genomes (all organisms except certain types of virus), this means transcribing the DNA sequence into RNA, which can eventually be translated into protein by the ribosomes. While bacteria and archaea have a single RNA polymerase, eukaryotes have generally three RNA polymerases, each specialized for a particular type of gene: RNA pol I transcribes ribosomal RNA genes; RNA Pol II transcribes protein-coding genes into precursors that are then processed to form messenger RNAs; RNA pol III transcribes t-RNA genes and a number of small RNAs that are components of various enzymatic machineries in the cell. Plants have additional RNA polymerases that also produce various small RNAs. In this review of transcription, we will deal primarily with RNA pol II and focus on the aspects that are of particular relevance to chromatin and epigenetic mechanisms.

RNA Polymerase II

Eukaryotic RNA polymerases are highly sophisticated multicomponent machines whose basic function is enzymatic: they take nucleotide triphosphates and add nucleotides to the 3′ end of a growing chain of RNA. They do so by copying the DNA, that is, the nucleotide to be added must fit in a pocket where it matches the template DNA base. The energy that drives the formation of the new phosphodiester bond comes from the hydrolysis of the nucleotide triphosphate and release of the diphosphate. This energy also drives the powerful molecular motor that makes RNA polymerase advance relative to the DNA and simultaneously unwind it. The rate of advance in chromatin varies depending on the circumstances and the chromatin region because it requires mechanisms to displace or get around nucleosomes and varies also with the sequence but generally attains a brisk 10–100 nucleotides per second. If 10 nucleotides correspond to 3.4 nanometers of double helix length, this means 12–120 micrometers of DNA per hour. The average human gene is about 20 kb long, which takes some 3–30 minutes to transcribe. But genes range enormously in size from 100 nucleotides to the 2.5 Mb of the extraordinarily long *dystrophin* gene. The primary transcript of the *dystrophin* gene could therefore take days to transcribe by a continuously advancing RNA polymerase. RNA polymerase is also able to correct itself if it has incorporated a nucleotide that does not match the template. It does so by backtracking to remove the wrong nucleotide before proceeding with elongation.

The RNA Pol II complex is a large assembly that is highly conserved from yeast to man. It contains 12 subunits in mammals, named in order of descending size. Thus, the largest subunit is RBP1 of 217 kD. RPB1 contains the catalytic activity and a critical C-terminal domain (CTD) consisting of a heptapeptide YSPTSPS repeated, with small variations a large number of times. The CTD is essential for transcriptional activity and the number of repeats increases from 26 in yeast to 52 in vertebrates. Reducing the number of repeats by deletion has a strong effect on the transcriptional activity. Deleting the CTD altogether renders the polymerase inactive. RPB1 forms a large cleft and one of the two jaws that capture the DNA template and a clamp that opens and closes the cleft (Figure 1). RPB2, at 133.9 kD the second largest subunit, forms the other jaw and mediates continued contact with the active site, the DNA template, and the nascent RNA. During transcription, a helical domain from RPB1 runs across the catalytic site in the cleft and moves like a ratchet to translocate the DNA–RNA hybrid after the addition of each nucleotide.

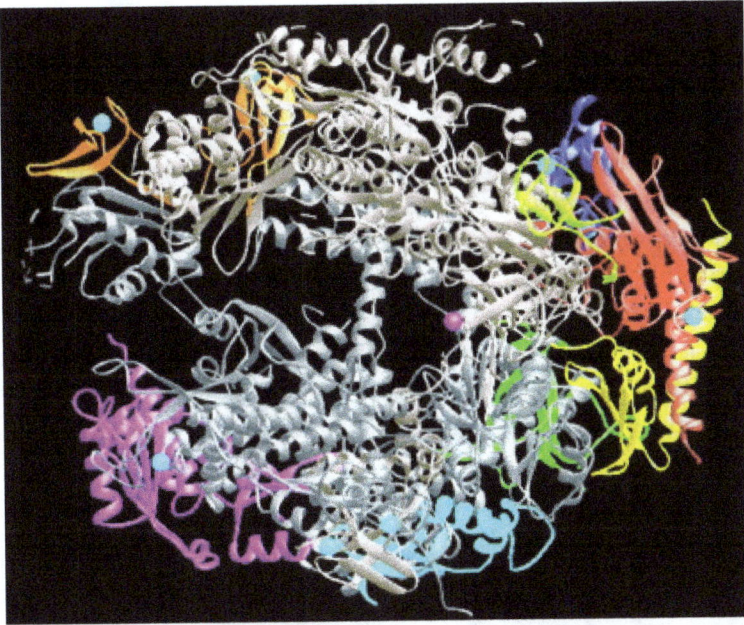

Figure 1. Structure of yeast RNA Pol II. The gray-colored structure represents RBP1 and the white structure is RBP2, forming the jaws between which is the cleft that houses the DNA template strand and nascent RNA. The other colors mark the smaller polymerase subunits.

Source: Cramer *et al.* (2001).

The Promoter

The first problem, however, is to find the correct site to begin transcription: the Transcription Start Site (TSS). Random transcription can occur but is much less favored because it lacks a mechanism to displace nucleosomes, to assemble the numerous general transcription factors that promote transcription starts and the strategically placed enhancer elements that help recruit the polymerase and configure the initiation complex. Transcription of a gene typically initiates at a well-defined site, the promoter, where RNA polymerase is recruited by general transcription factors. These multiprotein complexes help recognize core promoter sequence elements, position RNA polymerase correctly, and facilitate the formation of the Pre-Initiation Complex (PIC). Most mammalian genes have more than one TSS spread over 50–100 bp, and TSS choice and activity are often determined by regulatory inputs, that is, by the transcription factors that bind proximal and distal *cis*-regulatory elements.

The most detailed studies of core promoter sequences were done in budding yeast (*Saccharomyces cerevisiae*) and then extended to mammalian and *Drosophila* promoters. Several motifs were identified in a region from roughly 35 bp upstream to 35 bp downstream of the transcription start site (TSS) (Figure 2). Different promoters may have different selections of features, resulting in different activity or efficiency. And in some types of promoters, different factors might play a more important role than core promoter elements in determining the TSS. The core promoter

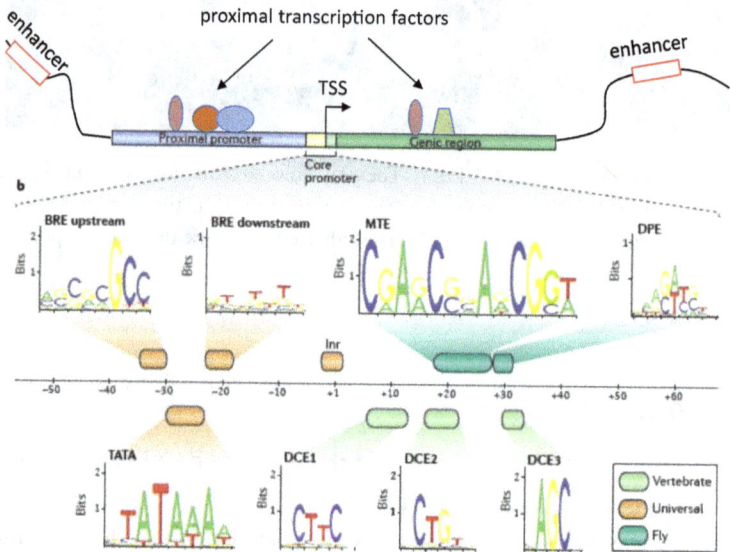

Figure 2.   Promoter regulation. The region around the transcription start site (TSS), both upstream and downstream, can bind proximal transcription factors that help recruit the RNA Pol II and activate transcription. Distant regulatory elements that may be hundreds of kb upstream or downstream are called enhancers. Immediately adjacent to the TSS are frequently found sequence motifs shown in boxes based on the JASPAR database. Most promoters have only one or a few of these motifs. BRE: B recognition element; MTE: motif ten element; DPE: downstream promoter element; DCE: downstream core element.

Source: Lenhard *et al.* (2012).

elements include the B recognition element (BRE), downstream core element (DCE), DNA recognition element (DRE), motif ten element (MTE), which replaces the DCEs in *Drosophila*, TATA box, and Initiator (Inr). While these motifs are all short and somewhat variable., the Initiator is probably the most variable in sequence and length, consistent with the variety and range of promoter activities, properties, and strengths and with the fact that recruitment of the transcriptional machinery to promoters involves not only sequence recognition but multiple chromatin features.

What roles do these promoter features have? Effective initiation of transcription by RNA Pol II requires the functions of a set of general transcription factors (GTFs) that position the polymerase, help it to open the DNA double helix, and regulate its transitions. These GTFs are the factors that are cooperatively assembled by the sequence features of the core promoter elements. The key role is played by Transcription Factor IID (TFIID), which in itself is a large complex containing TATA-binding protein (TBP) and numerous TBP-associated factors (TAFs). Needless to say, TBP binds to the TATA box. Table 1 lists the GTFs, their key roles, and the core promoter elements with which they associate.

Table 1. General transcription factors and promoter elements

General Transcription Factors	
TFIIA:	Stabilizes TFIID binding to DNA. Not essential for PIC assembly
TFIIB:	Helps select TSS. Binds to BRE
TFIID:	Contains DNA-binding TBP. Contains numerous TAFs
TFIIE:	Recruits TFIIH to PIC
TFIIF:	Recruits RNA Pol II to PIC
TFIIH:	Contains helicases that unwind DNA at the TSS
Core Promoter Elements	
TATA box:	Binds TBP and TFIID
Inr:	Binds TAF1 and TAF2
DPE:	Binds TAF6 and TAF9
MTE:	Helps recruit TFIID
DCE:	Binds TAF1
BRE:	Binds TFIIB

In addition to the core promoter elements, metazoan promoters generally have proximal promoter regulatory elements, sites that bind additional factors that help the core promoter to assemble the PIC. Proximal promoter elements are considered those that lie less than 1kb from the TSS. A different class of regulatory elements lie further distal and can be upstream as well as downstream of the TSS. These include enhancers, silencers, or more complex regulatory hubs. When a core sequence element such as the TATA box is not discernible in a given promoter, it does not mean that the corresponding GTF is not present. It means that it is recruited passively by the multiple interactions with the other GTFs or with help from proximal transcription factors. Not surprisingly, most of the core promoter elements interact with TAFs, which are components of TFIID. In the absence of a TATA box, for example, TFIID may not be recruited by TBP but instead by the interactions of other component TAFs with other core promoter elements or histone modifications. In some cases, help may come from factors bound more distantly, such as enhancer factors. In addition, TFIID recognizes histone marks, particularly on the first nucleosome downstream of the TSS. H3K4me3 is detected by the PHD finger of TAF3 and acetylated H4 through a double bromodomain in TAF1. The chromatin features of the promoter region are important elements of the recruiting process. Here, sorting out the causes and the consequences becomes more difficult, as some chromatin features both help recruitment and may in turn be produced by the recruited complexes (see the following).

Types of Promoters

The advent of massively parallel or Next Generation Sequencing of the transcriptome allowed the systematic study of TSSs and promoter sequences surrounding them in the whole genome. A particularly valuable technique to identify and map TSSs was Cap Analysis of Gene Expression (CAGE), with which transcript initiation sequences are selected by biotin-tagging the cap structure at the 5′ end. Although metazoan promoters are highly variable, they could be grouped into three main classes differing largely in their content and distribution of CpG dinucleotides and whether they have a broad spread of TSSs or a more sharply defined TSS. In humans, some 70% of promoters are found at CpG islands and artificially introduced CpG-rich regions behave like promoter regions.

Type I promoters

These promoters are generally found in tissue-specific genes of differentiated cells in adults and therefore need to be activated by tissue-specific factors. They are generally not enriched in CpG content and have a sharp, specific TSS. The TSS is frequently at a defined distance from the TATA box and specified by the presence of the Initiator sequence. In the inactive state, the promoter region is generally covered by arrays of disordered nucleosomes and may be dependent on nucleosome remodeling for accessibility. *Cis*-regulatory elements that bind activators are generally closely associated with the promoter and help recruit GTFs though without resulting in positioned nucleosomes.

Type II promoters

These are associated with CpG islands, regions of several hundred nucleotides enriched in CpG content. The density of CpGs, as we will see, results in a lower tendency to form nucleosomes and higher tendency to initiate transcription, resulting in multiple, broadly distributed TSSs in an ~50 nt region. These promoters often lack TATA boxes, rely more on DREs, and tend to correspond to "housekeeping" genes.

Type III promoters

These are found in developmentally controlled genes, often master regulators that determine cell identities in development and differentiation. They tend to have broad or even multiple CpG islands that may extend into the gene body but transcription initiates in tightly defined TSSs controlled by a Inr or Inr plus DPE. These genes are often targets of silencing mechanisms such as Polycomb repression, that control their cell and developmental specificity.

This classification is not strict and some promoters have mixed features. In *Drosophila*, which lacks CpG islands, this three-fold classification is maintained on the basis of the distribution of TSSs.

Accessing the Promoter: Nucleosome Positioning

Core promoter sequence features such as the TATA box are important to help recruit components of the promoter complex but access to the DNA sequence depends on the presence and positioning of nucleosomes. Therefore, the chromatin aspects of promoter architecture are essential to understand promoter function. Many features are involved in making promoter sequences accessible. Their relative importance varies from one promoter to another and, in general, many aspects cooperate or act simultaneously.

There has been considerable debate about the degree to which promoters may be sites where the nucleotide sequence is either unfavorable for stable nucleosome formation or preferentially positions nucleosomes so as to permit promoter-proximal factors to bind to DNA. In general, sequence features that facilitate nucleosome formation include GC dinucleotides spaced at intervals of 10 bp, interspaced with AA or TA dinucleotides at 10 bp intervals. This periodic alternation favors the formation of the sharp bends needed to wrap the DNA around the histone core (see also Chapter 2). Conversely, stretches of As or Ts are stiffer and are preferentially found in linkers between nucleosomes. The extent to which sequence features determine nucleosome positioning at promoter regions depends on the individual gene. In mammals and vertebrates, in general, it appears that CpG islands are particularly suited to act as promoters. They are in fact relatively depleted of nucleosomes and less prone to nucleosome assembly. This is surprising since we know that A/T-rich sequences are the ones structurally unfavorable to nucleosome assembly but the evidence indicates that CpG-rich sequences promote nucleosomes at their boundaries but become more depleted internally. The longer the CpG-rich region, the more it becomes nucleosome-depleted. As a result, CpG islands are most suited as promoters of housekeeping genes that are needed in all tissues. For the same reason, though, they will have a degree of impreciseness in the position of the promoter and tend to have multiple TSSs. This is the situation of Type II promoters.

In proliferating cells, the recruitment of the general transcription factors is generally in competition with the formation of nucleosomes at the replication fork, particularly when distinct core promoter sequences are present. Promoter access can be modulated in many ways: it can be blocked by repressors, chromatin silencing processes, and DNA methylation. It can be facilitated by chromatin remodelers, histone marks, and protein–protein contacts. The majority of Pol II promoters are not active in all cells but depend on cell-type-specific transcriptional activators to allow the recruitment or activity of RNA Pol II. These factors may bind to proximal regulatory sites near the promoter itself or distant sites sometimes several hundred kb from the promoter in either direction in vertebrates. These distant sites are generally called enhancers and the mechanisms that allow them to contact their respective promoters and regulate their activities are the object of intense study. We will discuss these processes at length later. It is clear, however, that, if promoter factors can recruit appropriate nucleosome remodeling machines, the assembly of the PIC will displace nucleosomes from the region immediately preceding the transcription start site. Overall then, access to the DNA may be provided by DNA sequences unfavorable to nucleosome formation or by the binding of key factors that recruit remodeling machines, or by the GTFs themselves, or combinations of these, depending on the promoter. One key feature of functional promoters that is not determined by the DNA sequence is the position of the first nucleosome after the TSS and, to a lesser extent, the position of the first nucleosome upstream of the TSS. The positioning of these nucleosomes reveals the involvement of nucleosome remodeling machines (see Chapter 2). Mutations affecting these machines cause loss of positioning of the critical nucleosomes and of the nucleosome array following them. In the absence of remodeling, sequence features, histone marks, and protein contacts must do the work.

But where does the information come from that allows nucleosome remodeling machines or histone modifying complex to select where to do their work in situations where the core promoter sequence features are either absent or not accessible? The answer at present seems to be that some information is always available, at least transiently, and different bits of information can cooperate to allow promoter opening. In addition, histone modifications play an important role in helping to recruit GTFs, chromatin remodelers, and other coactivators. For example, TAF1

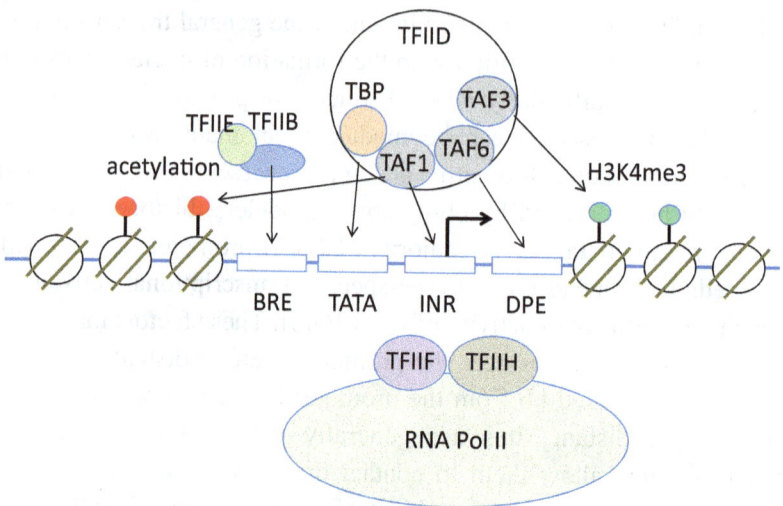

Figure 3.   Recruitment of the Pre-Initiation Complex. Various components of the Pre-Initiation complex are targeted by sequence features of the core promoter and assisted by histone marks such as acetylation and H3K4 methylation.

contains a double bromodomain that binds to diacetylated histone H4. TAF3 has a PHD finger that recognizes H3K4me3 (Figure 3). These marks are important to recruit TFIID and their loss results in reduced transcriptional activity.

Enhancers

Most regulated genes require the action of one or more enhancer elements. These are regions containing binding sites for transcription factors or similar complexes that either stimulate or repress a promoter. Enhancers have been identified and characterized in the whole genome by combinations of techniques. Sequence analysis can identify motifs associated with the binding of known enhancer factors. Chromatin immunoprecipitation (ChIP) can map sites to which specific factors bind. Functional identification of enhancers has relied on transgene constructs in which potential enhancers are placed next to a reporter gene to look for the ability to promote transcriptional activity. Chromatin marks associated with enhancers, such as H3K4me1 and H3K27ac (see the following), have also been useful to identify enhancers. However, the most common feature that identifies active enhancers (and promoters) is the presence of nucleosome-free regions, needed to allow access to DNA-binding factors (see the following). These methods have led to estimates of the total number of enhancers in the human genome that range from about 20,000 to one million. The only safe bet at this time is that the 20,000 estimate is much too low.

Cis-regulatory regions near promoters help assemble the PIC. However, developmentally regulated genes are generally governed by multiple, often partially redundant, enhancers that are typically located at a distance upstream or downstream of the promoter. In some cases, the distance can be of the order of megabases but more typically it is tens to hundreds of kilobases. How enhancers can affect the functioning of one or more promoters at such distances has been much debated but, at least in most cases, it is now shown to result from the physical looping of the intervening chromatin so that the enhancer can be brought to bear on the promoter and its transcriptional machinery, generally with the help of the Mediator complex (see the following). Enhancers are generally bi-directional, in the sense that they act on target promoters independently of their orientation. The fact that they act at a considerable distance raises the question of how they can be specific and avoid inappropriate looping and activation of the wrong genes. This question is related to the mechanisms that determine genome architecture and will be discussed later (see Chapter 8).

Multiple enhancers can act on the same promoter either concurrently or alternatively with the result that a given gene can have complex patterns of expression within a tissue or in different tissues or different developmental stages or in response to different external signals. This is one of the reasons why highly complex functional patterns in higher metazoans can be produced by a number of genes that have not increased much more than two-fold from unicellular or lower eukaryotes to higher eukaryotes with a large number of differentiated tissues and organs.

In recent years, there has been a trend to see much more symmetry between enhancers and promoters than originally imagined or thought possible. First, many, perhaps most, promoters have, in addition to the classical TSS and PIC, another TSS and PIC on the upstream side of the nucleosome-free region and transcribed on the opposite strand.

The resulting transcripts, called promoter upstream transcripts (PROMPTS), are generally shorter than 500 bp and are degraded by the exosome exonuclease. These transcripts terminate due to the presence of polyadenylation sites and the lack of 5′ splice sites (see the following), features that are respectively selected out of and selected for in normal mRNA-transcribed regions. On the side of enhancers, it has been noted that in many cases nucleosome-free regions containing the binding sites of enhancer factors assemble divergent PICs much like those found at promoters and often initiate transcription of enhancer RNAs (eRNAs) in divergent directions. These eRNAs are relatively weakly transcribed and degraded by the exosome. Figure 4 summarizes the similarities and

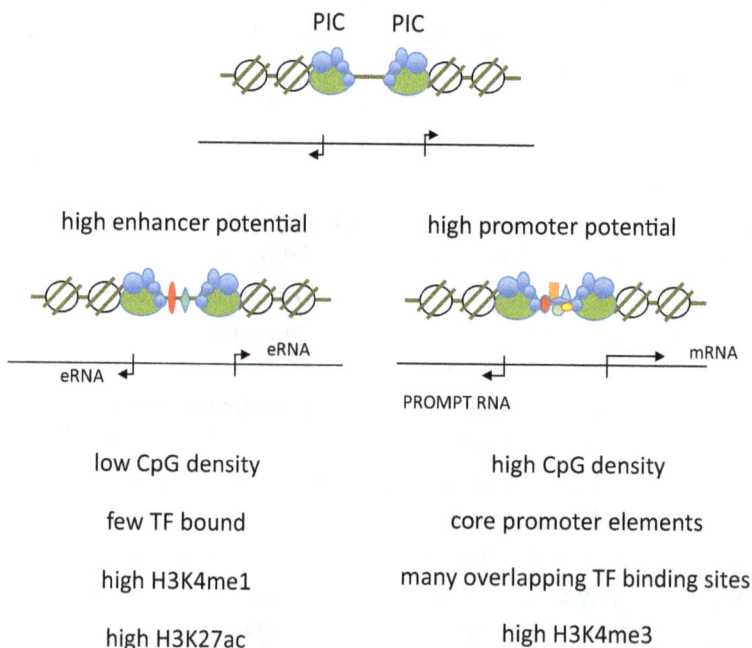

high enhancer potential

high promoter potential

low CpG density

few TF bound

high H3K4me1

high H3K27ac

high CpG density

core promoter elements

many overlapping TF binding sites

high H3K4me3

Figure 4.   Comparison of RNA Pol II sites at enhancers and promoters. A basic regulatory element has a nucleosome-depleted region that recruits bidirectional RNA Pol II and can form PICs. In principle, such a site can act as a promoter or as an enhancer and, in fact, often both. Features that are associated with strong mRNA transcribing promoters on one hand or strong enhancer activity on the other hand are listed.

Source: Andersson and Sandelin (2020).

differences between enhancers and promoters. Part of the difference is due to the presence of core promoter sequences and distribution of binding factors at promoters stimulating a higher level of transcription in the correct, mRNA-transcribing direction. Recent results demonstrate that the enhancer–promoter contacts are mediated by the interactions between factors bound to both sites, facilitated by the loading of cohesin and cohesin-dependent loop extrusion (see Chapter 8).

Pioneer Factors

Chromatin presents a fundamental difficulty to all access to the underlying DNA. Enhancer factor binding encounters the same problem as promoter regions in competing with the assembly of the DNA into nucleosomes. In general, therefore, nucleosomes need to be displaced to allow the binding of transcription factors. CpG islands are more accessible than bulk chromatin but many enhancers and promoters, especially when tissue-specific, tend to be wrapped in nucleosomes and their sequences are not easily read by DNA-binding proteins. Two kinds of mechanisms may help open a DNA region to tissue-specific factors and activators. One is a random, transient action by histone acetylases, which acetylate histone tails and attract chromatin remodeling machines that displace or partially unwind nucleosomes. A more targeted approach is due to the role of tissue-specific pioneer factors. Unlike most DNA-binding proteins, which are unable to bind to nucleosomal DNA, pioneer factors can compete with linker histone H1 and access DNA. Pioneer factors binding to nucleosomes may also distort the nucleosomal DNA wrapping, facilitating access to additional sequences or preventing higher-order interactions among nucleosomes. Most importantly, as in the case of tissue-specific enhancers, pioneer factors can recruit histone acetylases such as CBP/ p300, histone H3K4 methylases, and nucleosome remodelers, partially unwinding or altogether displacing nucleosomes and exposing additional DNA-binding sites to other transcriptional activators (Figure 5) (see also super-enhancers).

Mapping of histone modifications at known enhancers showed early on that a common chromatin signature was H3K4me1, later shown to be produced by the Trr histone methyltransferase complex in *Drosophila* and

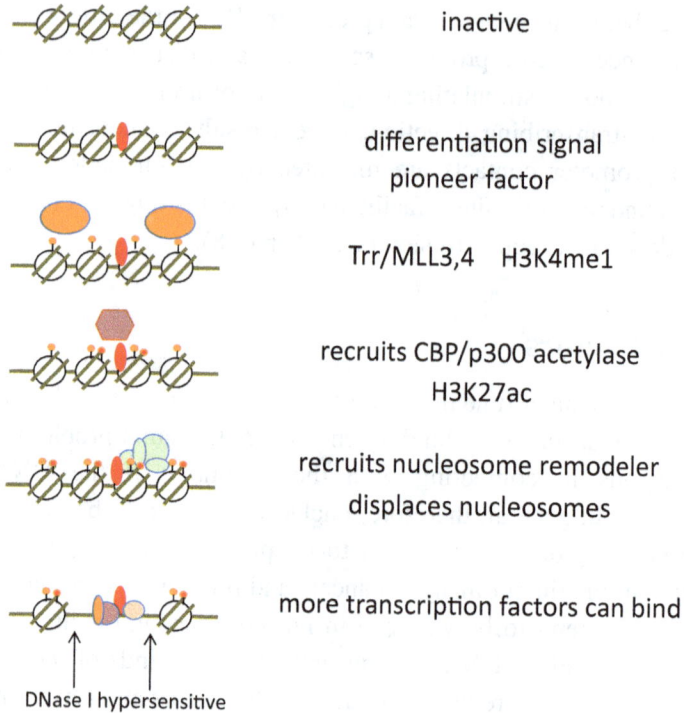

Figure 5.   Schematic of enhancer opening and activation. It is not clear what the initial differentiation signal might be but it would make sense if this signal is a pioneer factor, able to bind to nucleosomal DNA. In that case, a pioneer factor would recruit a histone methylase Trr in *Drosophila*, MLL3,4 in mammals to monomethylate H3K4. The methylation helps the pioneer factor recruit the CBP/p300 acetylase, which acetylates H3K27. This in turn recruits nucleosome remodelers to displace nucleosomes, creating nucleosome-free regions. Additional enhancer factors can now bind to newly accessible DNA.

its homologs MLL3 and 4 in mammals (see Chapter 7). This mark preceded the binding of CBP/p300 and the acetylation of H3K27. Together, these two marks can predict more than 80% of known enhancers but there remain some that lack these marks or contain H3K4me3 instead. Furthermore, while H3K4me1 and H3K27ac enhancers are associated with transcriptionally active genes, known enhancers marked with H3K4me1 but not H3K27ac in embryonic stem cells correspond to differentiation-specific genes. These enhancers acquire H3K27ac upon differentiation and their associated genes become transcriptionally active. H3K4me1 was therefore considered to be the mark of poised enhancers that were not yet activated. In embryonic stem cells, such enhancers and their associated promoters were also marked with H3K27me3, the mark of Polycomb repression (see Chapter 7; also Chapter 9). The H3K27 methylation explains why they could not be acetylated at that site.

Once a nucleosome-free site is produced, further action by different nucleosome remodeling machines comes into play. Analyses of nucleosome-free sites in different organisms show that histone replacement at the flanking nucleosomes tends to enrich them for the histone H2A variant H2A.Z, often in combination with the histone H3 variant H3.3. These changes, especially in combination, make those nucleosomes less stable, more susceptible to turnover or displacement (see Chapter 2), and thus tend to maintain the nucleosome-free region.

Mapping Nucleosome-free Regions

The production of nucleosome-free regions makes chromatin more accessible to enzymes that act on DNA. It has been known for a long time that transcriptionally active chromatin is much more sensitive to nucleases than silent chromatin. In particular, DNaseI, a DNA-specific nuclease, is a somewhat larger protein than micrococcal nuclease and less able to attack chromatin. It is better able, therefore, to distinguish nucleosome-free regions from normal linker regions and has been widely used to map such regions in the genome. Genome-wide analyses in many different cell types showed the presence of a very large number of DNaseI hypersensitive sites, many of which were cell-type specific. Only a few percent of these sites corresponded to the promoters of active genes. A much larger number were found in transcribed intronic regions and in intergenic regions and tended to correspond to known enhancers and regulatory regions. Within a nucleosome-free region, sites bound by DNA-binding factors are protected against DNaseI digestion, a feature that may be used to characterize transcription factor binding sites. In such cases, the DNA flanking the binding site is often distorted by the binding, becoming more sensitive to DNaseI cleavage and producing a DNaseI hypersensitive site.

Another approach to map genomic regulatory sites takes advantage of the fact that nucleosome-bound DNA tends to be soluble in phenol while naked DNA is more soluble in the aqueous phase. The technique, called formaldehyde-assisted isolation of regulatory elements (FAIRE) uses formaldehyde to crosslink and stabilize nucleosomes, which are much more easily crosslinked than transcription factors binding to DNA. After phenol extraction, the nucleosome-free genomic fraction is found in the aqueous layer (see Chapter 13). This approach identifies many of the same sites also identified as DNaseI hypersensitive sites but a fraction of sites are found with one but not the other method.

The method of choice today exploits the binding and DNA cleavage properties of the transposase enzyme from a bacterial transposon (see Chapter 13, ATAC Assay). Since the transposase binding requires access to DNA, this assay for transposase-accessible chromatin (ATAC) also detects nucleosome-free sites and has become widely used for its ease of application with minimum manipulations that might alter native chromatin.

Mediator

The DNA region containing the core promoter elements and the TSS may assemble a preinitiation complex and even initiate transcription but is generally not sufficient for more than a minimal level of activity. Additional upstream sequences nearby or more distant enhancers include binding sites for a class of transcriptional regulators that contain transcriptional activator domains. Some enhancer factors can activate transcription by direct contact with RNAPII or with one of the general transcription factors bound to core promoters, helping to recruit or stabilize the components of the PIC. This, however, is usually limited to enhancers that are very close or adjacent to promoters. In most cases, enhancer factors act through a large multiprotein complex called the Mediator (of RNA Pol II transcription). Mediator is a large complex with a highly variable composition with as many as 30 constituents, depending on conditions. It is recruited by enhancer-binding factors, which interact with one or more of its many subunits. Chromatin looping, driven by cohesin (more about this in the Genome Architecture chapter), then brings the distant enhancer, through the Mediator, in contact with the promoter and the GTFs (Figure 6). Mediator is generally required for PIC assembly. Mediator interacts with many general transcription factors and with RNA Pol II itself, helping to recruit them, stabilize their binding, and assemble the PIC. In this role, Mediator is a molecular bridge between the enhancer factors and the promoter complexes. The size and complexity of Mediator allow it to interact with multiple enhancer factors and multiple promoter factors at the same time, integrating the effects of many activators and promote, facilitate, and stabilize PIC formation. Mediator structure is highly flexible and variable. Many of its subunits have amino acid sequences that are predicted to form Intrinsically Disordered Regions (IDRs), whose three-dimensional structure is loose and able to enter into multiple, individually weak interactions with similar domains found in many enhancer factors (more about IDRs in the Genome Architecture chapter). Binding of Mediator to such proteins can cause major structural

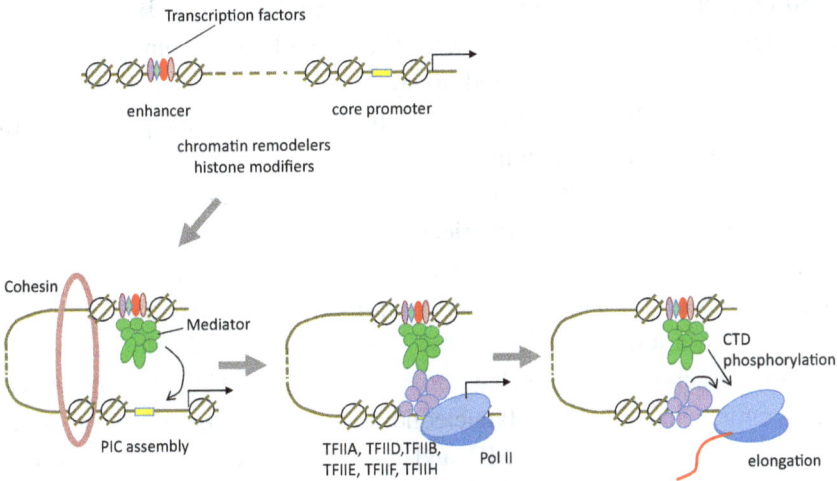

Figure 6. Role of the Mediator. The enhancer region binds transcriptional activators. These recruit chromatin remodelers and histone modifiers that act on chromatin structure. Mediator binds to various transcription factors and, with help from cohesin, forms a loop to contact the promoter region, where general transcription factors are assembled. Mediator promotes PIC assembly and recruitment of RNA Pol II. Mediator helps the CDK7 component of TFIIH phosphorylate the Pol II CTD at serine 5, required for release from the promoter and beginning of elongation.

changes that affect its function and interactions with other factors. Mediator interacts with the RNA Pol II C-Terminal Domain (CTD), a key structure in determining the subsequent steps of the polymerase. These multiple functions make it clear that Mediator is not merely a bridging factor but plays an active role in many of the steps involved in productive transcription initiation.

Assembly of the Pre-initiation Complex

Binding TFIID is the first and critical step in assembling the pre-initiation complex. If a TATA box is present, TFIID is recruited by TBP binding to the TATA box. If a well-defined TATA box is absent, other features of TFIID and constituent TAFs must do the work. The binding of TBP to DNA produces a sharp bend in the DNA through a conformational change of the TFIID complex. TBP interacts with TFIIA and stabilizes the binding. TBP also interacts with TFIIB, which helps RNA Pol II and TFIIF to bind correctly to the promoter region. The binding of TFIIE and TFIIH completes the PIC. TFIIH includes ATPase and helicase functions which twist the DNA causing unwinding by about one turn and forming the transcription bubble. The DNA strand that will act as a template binds to the polymerase cleft containing the catalytic site.

The polymerase, with the help of the general transcription factors critical for correct positioning and orientation, selects a transcription start site (TSS), binds an appropriate nucleotide triphosphate, and initiates the first nucleotide bond formation. Transcription initiation may be abortive since a chain of just a few nucleotides is too short to prime stable elongation and promoter escape so the short chains may be released and initiation attempted again until a chain of about 10 nucleotides is reached. Now, the RNA Pol II must be released from the PIC and move forward from the promoter. TFIIA/B/E/H leave once RNA elongation begins. TFIID and the Mediator remain with the polymerase until elongation is finished. The elongating RNA chain remains associated with the template DNA for 8–9 nucleotides within the polymerase cleft. At each step, the next DNA base pair is separated, moving forward the transcription bubble, while at the same time, one base pair of the 5′ end of the DNA–RNA hybrid is separated, allowing the template DNA strand to reanneal with the other DNA strand.

Transcription Factories

The preceding account of promoter selection, recruitment of the PIC, and transcription initiation follows the classical narrative, which is based on the historical sequence of largely *in vitro* experiments that elucidated transcription initiation. While much of the ground-breaking mechanistic analysis of the process is not in question, more recent *in vivo* studies of RNA polymerase and transcriptional activity have shown that both are highly clustered in the nucleus. Active genes often co-localize in space even though they may be very distant in the genome. These clusters of transcriptional activity are called transcription factories. In growing cultured cells, RNA Pol II factories are estimated to number about 8,000 and contain on average eight polymerases each, usually transcribing eight different genes. What associates these transcribing polymerases is not clear but, as each must involve GTFs, transcription factors, and associated machinery, it is possible that the physical properties of these proteins might play a role. Many of these factors contain intrinsically disordered regions (IDRs), which are thought to favor a multiplicity of loose and weak non-specific interactions that cause them to associate forming a stable condensate, in some cases even resulting in a liquid phase transition that excludes other kinds of proteins. The concept of transcription factories inverts the terms of the classical description of promoter activation. Instead of the promoter region recruiting GTFs, enhancer factors RNA Pol II and assembling a transcription complex, we need to think of the promoter region, after some initial steps in PIC assembly, being recruited to a transcription factory and taking its turn to be incorporated in an initiation complex. Several examples suggest that genes that are co-regulated or share transcriptional activators might have a higher tendency to be found at the same transcription factory. This, however, is a preference and not an absolute requirement: physical association of co-regulated genes is found in only a few percent of the cells.

The C-terminal Domain of RNA Pol II

The RNA Pol II C-terminal domain (CTD), in reality the C-terminal domain of the largest subunit RPB1, plays a key and essential role in the release from the promoter-associated PIC and in productive transcription elongation. The CTD consists of a seven amino acid peptide, YSPTSPS, highly conserved in evolution, repeated, with some variation, many times, ranging from 26 copies in budding yeast to 52 copies in mammals (Figure 7). This repetitive domain forms a highly flexible tail that serves as a scaffold, contacting and receiving inputs from enhancer factors, Mediator, and PIC components and in turn recruiting to the polymerase a variety of factors necessary for transcription elongation, mRNA capping, splicing, and 3′ end formation. The number of repeats is essential for CTD effectiveness. Mouse cells whose polymerase has had the number of copies reduced to 26 do not survive. Similar experiments have also shown that too many consensus copies are also deleterious. The number of repeats facilitates the interactions with regulatory factors and also amplifies the resulting ability to bind to subsequent factors. The structure and function of the CTD are highly dependent on its phosphorylation. When unphosphorylated, the CTD forms a compact spiral and when highly phosphorylated, it spreads broadly to a diameter much greater than that of the core enzyme. The repeat unit contains five amino acids that can be phosphorylated to convey specific signals. The first to be phosphorylated are Serine5 and Serine7 by the cyclin-dependent kinase CDK7, a component of the general transcription factor TFIIH. Serine5 phosphorylation, which also requires the involvement of Mediator, is essential for promoter release of the polymerase. The role of serine7 phosphorylation is unclear but it is known not to be essential. Not all of the copies of the CTD repeat are phosphorylated and it is not clear how many must be phosphorylated at Serine5 for promoter release. Mediator is also involved in the next step. After release from the promoter, polymerase synthesizes 20–60 nucleotides and then pauses, requiring additional signals (Figure 8). Many genes in fact contain a polymerase paused promoter-proximally, allowing much transcription regulation to occur at this level. At heat shock promoters, for example, RNA polymerase is already present and transcriptionally engaged but paused. Heat shock signals the release from pausing.

Transcriptional Pausing

Pausing is not just a cautious hesitation before committing to transcription elongation. It is found in most highly expressed genes and is important for

S. Cerevisiae (budding yeast)	D. rerio (zebra fish)	H. Sapiens (human)
FSPTSPT	YSPTSPA	YSPTSPA
YSPTSPA	YEPRSPGGG	YEPRSPGG
(YSPTSPS) 3~16	YTPQSPG	YTPQSPS
YSPTSPA	(YSPTSPS) 4~5	(YSPTSPS) 4~5
(YSPTSPS) 18~21	YSPTSPN	YSPTSPN
YSPTSPN	(YSPTSPS) 7~21	(YSPTSPS) 7~21
(YSPTSPS) 23	(YSPTSPS) 22	YSPTSPN
YSPTSPG	YSPTSPN	YSPTSPN
YSPGSPA	YTPTSPS	YTPTSPS
(YSPKQDE) 26	(YSPTSPS) 25	(YSPTSPS) 25
QKHNENENSR	(YSPTSPS) 26	YSPTSPN
	YSPTSPN	YTPTSPN
	YTPTSPN	(YSPTSPS) 28
S. Pombe (fission yeast)	(YSPTSPS) 29~30	(YSPTSPS) 29~30
	YSPSSPR	YSPSSPR
	YTPQSPT	YTPQSPT
YGLTSPS	YTPSSPS	YTPSSPS
YSPSSPG	YSPSSPS	YSPSSPS
YSTSPA	YSPTSPK	YSPTSPK
YMPSSPS	YTPTSPS	YTPTSPS
(YSPTSPS) 5~8	YSPSSPE	YSPSSPE
YSATSPS	YTPTSPK	YTPTSPK
(YSPTSPS) 10~29	YSPTSPK	YSPTSPK
	YSPTSPK	YSPTSPK
	YSPTSPT	YSPTSPT
	YSPTTPK	YSPTTPK
	YSPTSPT	YSPTSPT
	YSPTSPT	YSPTSPV
	YTPTSPK	YTPTSPK
	YSPTSPT	YSPTSPT
	YSPTSPK	YSPTSPK
	YSPTSPT	YSPTSPT
	YSPTSPKGST	YSPTSPKGST
	YSPTSPG	YSPTSPG
	YSPTSPT	YSPTSPT
	(YSPA---) 52	(YSLTSPA) 52
	ISPDDSDEENN	ISPDDSDEEN

Figure 7. Structure of the C-terminal tail. The CTD of the large subunit of RNA Pol II is compared among four eukaryotes. The heptad repeats are shown with the C-terminal-most at the bottom. Consensus heptads are shown in red and amino acids that differ from the consensus in the human CTD are in blue. The zebrafish and human CTDs are almost identical, with the differing residues in yellow. This confirms that the presence and positioning of the divergent heptads are not random but evolutionarily conserved.

Source: Hsin and Manley (2012).

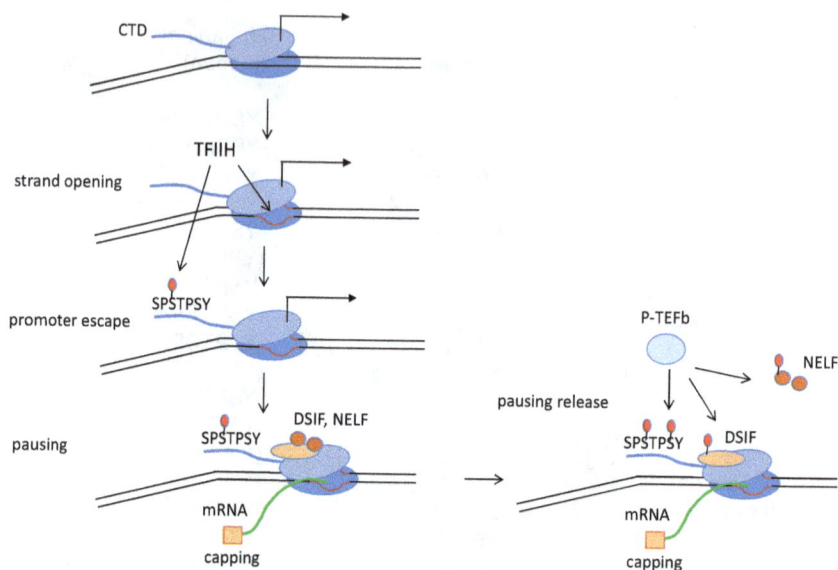

Figure 8.   Promoter escape, pausing, and elongation. After assembly of the PIC, the heli-case associated with TFIIH unwinds about 10 nucleotides of the DNA bound to the RNA polymerase, forming the transcription bubble. The CDK7 kinase, also part of TFIIH, phosphorylates serine 5 of the CTD, necessary for promoter escape. After transcribing 30–60 nucleotides, the DSIF and NELF factors bound to the polymerase cause pausing. The capping enzyme caps the nascent RNA with 7me-G. Pause release occurs when P-TEFb complex is recruited, with help from the Mediator. P-TEFb phosphorylates serine 2 of the CTD, NELF, and DSIF. This releases NELF and converts DSIF into an elongation factor.

effective regulation. The presence of the polymerase just downstream of the promoter has also been shown to keep the promoter itself open and nucleosome-free. This readies the core promoter for the recruitment of the next RNA polymerase and another round of transcription. Pausing is induced by the binding to RNA Pol II of Negative Elongation Factor (NELF) and DRB Sensitivity-Inducing Factor (DSIF), also known as SPT5-SPT4. The nascent RNA is thought to play a role in recruiting DSIF, which binds to the RNA exit channel of the polymerase. NELF interacts with the polymerase interface with SPT5. The polymerase slows down, probably affected by the conformation and sequence of the DNA–RNA hybrid. Release from pausing that allows effective elongation occurs when a complex called Positive-Transcription Elongation Factor b (P-TEFb), which includes Cyclin-Dependent Kinase9 (CDK9), is brought to the paused polymerase. P-TEFb can be recruited in various ways, depending on the gene and, ultimately, on the transcription factors and Mediator, which remain in contact with the polymerase at least until pause release. Two common mechanisms involve bromo-domain protein 4 (BRD4), which binds to acetylated histones and recruits P-TEFb or the super elongation complex (SEC), various forms of which bind P-TEFb. Chromatin looping and interaction between enhancer factors and promoter is generally involved in the release from pausing, making the release from pausing a key regulatory step. P-TEFb has three main targets. It phosphorylates NELF and DSIF, causing them to dissociate from the polymerase. Crucially, it phosphorylates the CTD at serine2. This is necessary for the recruitment of elongation factors that allow transcription to proceed.

At different stages in initiation and elongation, the CTD recruits numerous activities important for productive transcription. One of the earliest of these, after Serine5 phosphorylation, is the enzyme that caps the 5′ end of the nascent RNA. The cap protects the RNA and is also important for later RNA processing, export from the nucleus, and translation. Capping attaches the 5′ end of a 7-methyl guanosine to the 5′ triphosphate of the nascent RNA, forming a 5′ to 5′ triphosphate linkage (Figure 9). As polymerase moves from Ser5 phosphorylation to Ser2

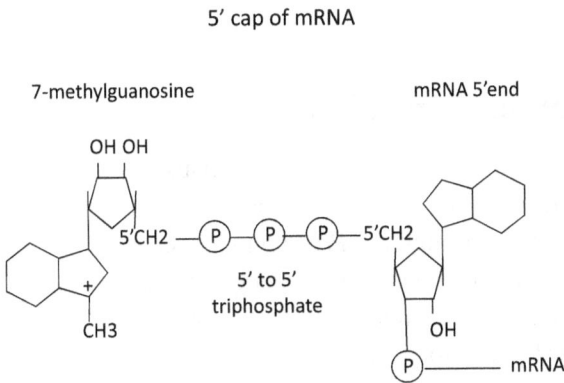

Figure 9. 5′ cap of mRNA. A capping enzyme adds 7-methyl guanosine to the triphosphate at the 5′ end of the nascent RNA.

phosphorylation, it recruits Set1 (Set1A,B in mammals), a histone methyltransferase that produces the H3K4me2 and me3 that are characteristic of the promoter region of active genes. H3K4me3 helps recruit components of the general transcription factor TFIID and therefore stimulates repeat initiation of new RNA Pol II. Highly transcribed genes tend to have a prominent peak of H3K4me3 just downstream of the transcription start site. In certain genes, H3K4 trimethylation is part of the initiation process, necessary to overcome repressive activities. In these cases, different methylases are involved, Trx in *Drosophila* and MLL1 and 2 in mammals (see Chapter 7). These methylases produce H3K4me2,3 around the TSS and upstream region. MLL1,2 also bind to the CTD phosphorylated at Serine5 and continue to stimulate transcription.

In addition to the DSIF- and NELF-induced promoter-proximal pausing, RNA Pol II has to contend with the transient pausing resulting from the intrinsic difficulties of elongating through nucleosome-packaged DNA. To ensure its ability to elongate transcription reliably and robustly and to handle the growing RNA transcript, the polymerase must now assemble a number of transcription elongation factors. In higher eukaryotes, the first nucleosome is positioned around 140 bp downstream from the TSS. As the polymerase moves towards the first nucleosome, the dissociation of NELF makes available a binding site for Polymerase-Associated Factor 1 (PAF1). The PAF complex mediates histone modification marks and recruitment of factors that handle the nascent RNA.

Transcription Elongation

Productive elongation after release from pausing occurs with gradually increasing speed. In fact, phosphorylation of serine2 of the CTD increases progressively and, through the PAF complex, causes additional factors to be recruited to the elongating polymerase, including the exosome RNA degrading complex that digests prematurely released RNA in a 3' to 5' direction. Ser2 phosphorylation of the CTD together with the PAF complex recruit enzymes that mono-ubiquitylate histone H2BK120 (Figure 10). This is a prerequisite for the recruitment through the PAF complex of several other chromatin-modifying activities in the gene body. These

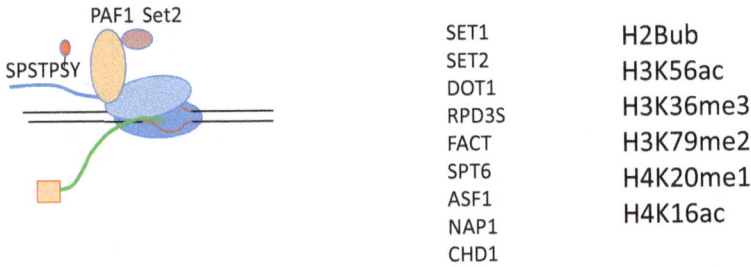

Figure 10.   The elongating RNA polymerase. The Ser2 phosphorylation of the CTD and the binding of the PAF complex result in the recruitment of numerous activities that promote transcription elongation and the processing of the RNA transcript. These include H2BK120 ubiquitylation, prerequisite for recruitment of methyltransferases SET1 (H3K4me3), SET2 (H3K36me3), DOT1 (H3K79me2), FACT (displaces H2A-H2B), and RPF3S (histone deacetylase), as well as histone chaperones and chromatin remodelers such as ASF1, NAP1, and CHD1.

include H3K56ac, H3K79me2, and H4K20me1. PAF recruitment of the SETD2 methyltransferase produces H3K36me3, whose abundance increases further in the gene body. H3K36me3 methylation in turn recruits to the gene body the MRG15-KDM5B demethylase to remove H3K4me3 and the Rpd3S histone deacetylase. Together, these remove the transcription-associated histone methylation and acetylation, reducing the tendency to make the gene body a target for inappropriate RNA polymerase binding and transcription initiation within the coding region. This effect would then be similar to that of gene body DNA methylation (see Chapter 3) and would prevent the deleterious production of partial protein products. This is an enduring risk because transcription elongation involves the recruitment of histone chaperones and chromatin remodeling complexes that aid RNA polymerase to transcribe through nucleosomes. In the process, nucleosomes are partially destabilized and heavily transcribed genes tend to lose some of the nucleosomes in the transcribed regions. Nucleosomes can be reassembled in these regions but doing so independently of DNA replication means that they utilize the histone variant H3.3, as is normally the case in regions with high nucleosome turnover. An example of such factors is FAcilitates Chromatin Transcription (FACT). FACT recruitment is also dependent on H2B ubiquitylation and competes with nucleosomal DNA for binding to H2A-H2B dimers thus partially unwinding the nucleosomal DNA. This is important to facilitate transcription elongation by the RNA polymerase. The displaced H2A-H2B dimer can, in principle, be restored to the nucleosome after the passage of the polymerase and removal of H2B ubiquitylation by deubiquitylases. Deubiquitylation is required for the effective recruitment of splicing factors.

Elongation rates are also dependent on the DNA sequence. Lower CG content and low-complexity sequence, typical of intronic sequences, favor higher rates. Though relatively rare in lower eukaryotes, introns, generally multiple introns, are the rule for protein-coding genes in higher eukaryotes and mammals in particular. Exons tend to have higher CG content and higher nucleosome occupancy, as well as higher levels of H3K36me3, while they have lower levels of H3K79 methylation and H2B ubiquitylation. Removal of H2B ubiquitylation is in fact required for effective recruitment of splicing factors. Transcript elongation slows down in exons, which is helpful to recruit the splicing machinery to initiate splicing as the RNA is being transcribed. At the same time, the higher levels of H3K36me3 help recruit more Nucleosome Destabilizing Factor (NDF), an ATP-dependent remodeler that partially unwinds nucleosomes. Many of the factors involved in transcription elongation vary in different tissues, contributing to the choices of splicing factors, splicing sites, exon skipping, or alternative splicing. More details about splicing can be found in the Genome Organization chapter and the Aging chapter.

Transcription termination is initiated when the polymerase transcribes a polyadenylation signal sequence AAUAAA (Figure 11). This signal is recognized by a cleavage and polyadenylation complex that binds at the AAUAAA and a GU-rich site downstream. An endonuclease in the complex then cleaves the RNA transcript between the two sites, usually within 30 nucleotides of the AAUAAA signal, while a poly(A) polymerase activity in the complex begins to add the poly(A) tail. This releases the pre-mRNA but does not stop the RNA Pol II polymerase, which continues to transcribe but now produces RNA with an uncapped 5′end. An exonuclease XRN2 attacks the unprotected 5′ end, degrading the nascent transcript until it catches up with the polymerase. This releases the polymerase from the DNA and terminates transcription at distances of hundreds of nucleotides from the polyadenylation signal.

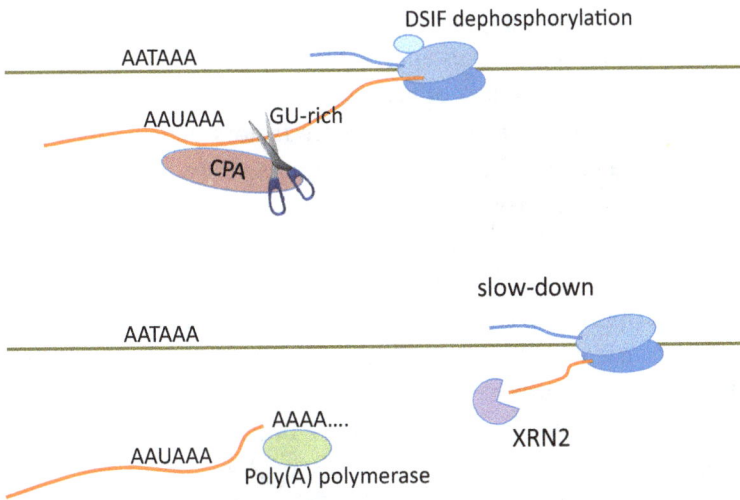

Figure 11.   Transcription termination. When Pol II transcribes a AATAAA polyadenyla-tion signal, the Cleavage And Polyadenylation (CPA) complex binds to the AAUAAA and a GU-rich region downstream and cleaves the RNA between the two. The exonuclease XRN2 attacks the 5′ end of the nascent RNA, which is no longer protected by a cap and degrades the RNA progressively. Traversing the AATAAA signal also triggers the dephos-phorylation of the SPT5 component of DSIF, This results in a deceleration of transcription and allows XRN2 to catch up with the polymerase and causes transcription termination.

Transcriptional Bursting

Descriptions of transcriptional activation generally give the impression that, once activated, transcription proceeds continuously, with new poly-merases recruited to the promoter continuously re-initiating. In fact, stud-ies with single cells show that transcription in eukaryotes occurs in bursts, with several rounds of initiation interspersed with quiescent periods. Gene activity is therefore the product of the frequency of bursts and the burst size (the number of transcripts produced per burst). Various models based on different promoter states have been proposed to fit experimental burst-ing data but they seem artificial models without mechanistic coherence. Single-gene and genome-wide studies have suggested that the burst size is largely determined by core promoter elements while the burst frequency is determined by enhancers with bursts initiated by enhancer-promoter looping. In strongly transcribed genes, activity is regulated by modulating the burst size while weakly transcribed genes vary their burst frequency. This view may not fit all genes and is still far from providing a mechanistic account even when it does apply.

Most likely, during a burst, promoter factors and Mediator remain associated but a critical factor controls the assembly. Dissociation of the limiting factor would then signal the end of a burst. It is not clear which would be the critical factor. This may vary from one promoter to another. The formation of these assemblies is certainly favored by the tendency of many transcription factors, including Mediator, to form aggregates through intrinsically disordered amino acid sequence domains (see Chapter 8). Such aggregates may partition into a separate liquid phase, such as an oil droplet in an aqueous medium. The formation of such aggregates is often favored by the presence of RNA molecules and by the three-dimensional organization of the genes and chromatin in the local nuclear environment (see Chapter 8).

Further Reading

Akhtar J, Renaud Y, Albrecht S, Ghavi-Helm Y, Roignamt J-Y, Silies M *et al.* (2021). m6A RNA methylation regulates promoter- proximal pausing of RNA polymerase II. *Mol Cell.* **81**, 3356–3367.e3356.

Allen BL and Taatjes DJ (2015). The Mediator complex: A central integrator of transcription. *Nat Rev Mol Cell Biol.* **16**, 155–166.

Andersson R and Sandelin A (2020). Determinants of enhancer and promoter activities of regulatory elements. *Nat Rev Genet.* **21**, 71–87.

Cramer P, Bushnell DA, Fu J, Gnatt AL, Maier-Davis B, Thompson NE *et al.* (2000). Architecture of RNA polymerase II and implications for the transcription mechanism. *Science.* **288**, 640–649.

Cramer P, Bushnell DA and Kornberg RD (2001). Structural basis of transcription: RNA polymerase II at 2.8 angstrom resolution. *Science.* **292**, 1863–1876.

Fernandez Garcia M, Moore CD, Schulz KN, Alberto, O, Donague G, Harrison MM *et al.* (2019). Structural features of transcription factors associating with nucleosome binding. *Mol Cell.* **75**, 921–932.e926.

Furlong EEM and Levine M (2018). Developmental enhancers and chromosome topology. *Science.* **361**, 1341–1345.

Hsin J-P and Manley JL (2012). The RNA polymerase II CTD coordinates transcription and RNA processing. *Genes Dev.* **26**, 2119–2137.

Jonkers I and Lis JT (2015). Getting up to speed with transcription elongation by RNA polymerase II. *Nat Rev Mol Cell Biol.* **16**,167–177.

Lenhard B, Sandelin A and Carninci P (2012). Metazoan promoters: Emerging characteristics and insights into transcriptional regulation. *Nat Rev Genet.* **13**, 233–245.

Ng HH, Robert F, Young RA and Struhl K (2003). Targeted recruitment of Set1 histone methylase by elongating Pol II provides a localized mark and memory of recent transcriptional activity. *Mol Cell.* **11**, 709–719.

Pavri R, Zhu B, Li G, Trojer P, Mandal S, Shilatifard A *et al.* (2006). Histone H2B monoubiquitination functions cooperatively with FACT to regulate elongation by RNA polymerase II. *Cell.* **125**,703–717.

Schilbach S, Albara S, Dienemann C, Grabbe F and Cramer P (2021). Structure of RNA polymerase II pre-initiation complex at 2.9 Å defines initial DNA opening. *Cell.* **184**, 4064–4072.e4028.

Schoenfelder S and Fraser P (2019). Long-range enhancer-promoter contacts in gene expression control. *Nat Rev Genet.* **20**, 437–455.

Williams SK and Tyler JK (2007). Transcriptional regulation by chromatin disassembly and reassembly. *Curr Opin Genet Dev.* **17**, 88–93.

Yang F, Tanasa B, Micheletti R, Ohgi KA, Aggarwal AK and Rosenfeld MG (2021). Shape of promoter antisense RNAs regulates ligand-induced transcription activation. *Nature.* **595**, 444–449.

Yang Y, Li W, Hoque M, Hou L, Shen S, Tian B *et al.* (2016). PAF complex plays novel subunit-specific roles in alternative cleavage and polyadenylation. *PLoS Genet.* **12**, e1005794.

Zhu B, Zheng Y, Pham A-D, Mandal SS, Erdjument-Bromage H, Tempst P *et al.* (2005). Monoubiquitination of human histone H2B: the factors involved and their roles in HOX gene regulation. *Mol Cell.* **20**, 601–611.

Chapter 7

Polycomb Mechanisms

Introduction

No account of Polycomb mechanisms can start without an outline of homeotic genes, whose genetic analysis in *Drosophila* first revealed the role Polycomb mechanisms play in some of the most important developmental processes. We now know that Polycomb functions are not limited to the expression of homeotic genes but affect in some way most of the fundamental activities of chromatin. We start here with homeotic genes or *Hox* genes and their roles in the organization of body structures in higher metazoans. During development, certain genes control not simply specific cellular or tissue functions but whole patterns of expression of other genes in a way that regulates the formation of entire body structures. A particularly fundamental pattern of body organization is that based on repeated segmental units that are then further modified or specialized through developmental decisions.

In earthworms, for example, most of the body is constructed of essentially identical segments. More sophisticated segmental structures are found in insects, where body segments in anterior, thoracic, or abdominal regions have become modified and have acquired additional structures. Anterior segmental structures have become modified to form head, antennae, and mouth parts while thoracic segments have developed legs and, in some cases, wings together with powerful muscles to drive them. Segmental structures are still detectable in vertebrate body plans, from the repeated pattern of somites to the vertebral column and its associated muscles and nerves. Here too, each segmental unit is not identical to the others but is differentiated in a regular anterior/posterior order. In all these cases, developmental decisions must be made to tell individual cells or tissues that they must grow and differentiate in a way that is segment-specific. All segments differentiate tissues such as muscle, nerve, and skin but in different amounts, distributions, and shapes. It is mainly the pattern of these tissues that varies from one segment to another. The master regulatory genes that coordinate these segment-specific patterns of gene expression are the homeotic genes, a class of transcription factors first discovered in *Drosophila* but highly conserved in all higher organisms.

Homeotic genes first came to notice for the remarkable morphological effects produced by some of their mutations in which one body part is replaced by another. Mutations that convert insect antennae into legs were first called homeotic mutations by the geneticist William Bateson in his 1894 work *Materials for the study of variation*. Such mutations, affecting the consequently named gene *Antennapedia*, are clearly regulatory mutations, causing the expression of the gene in an inappropriate body segment or developmental stage (Figure 1). Genetic and structural analysis of the

The Antennapedia mutant

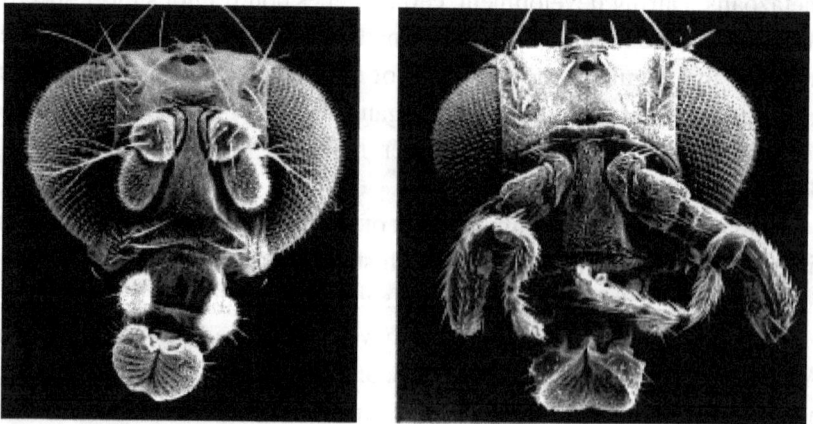

Figure 1.   The Antennapedia homeotic transformation. The head of a normal fly is shown on the left. The head of a dominant Antennapedia mutant fly shows the transformation of the antennae to legs.

Source: F.R. Turner (Indiana University).

homeotic genes, now called *Hox* genes for short, began in the 1960s and 1970s. *Drosophila* geneticist E.B. Lewis followed by T.F. Kaufman and his group and W.J. Gehring and his group showed that they are a set of genes encoding closely related transcription factors that are arranged in two clusters in *Drosophila* and are expressed co-linearly in a segmentally specific pattern such that the anterior-most genes (the most 3′) are also expressed most anteriorly in the embryo (Figure 2). More posterior genes are repressed in the more anterior segments. In this way, each homeotic gene becomes active and specifies the identity of the segment in which it is most strongly expressed. Inappropriate expression of a homeotic gene in a more anterior segment causes a homeotic transformation. Thus, the *Antennapedia* gene (*Antp*) is normally expressed in the thoracic segments

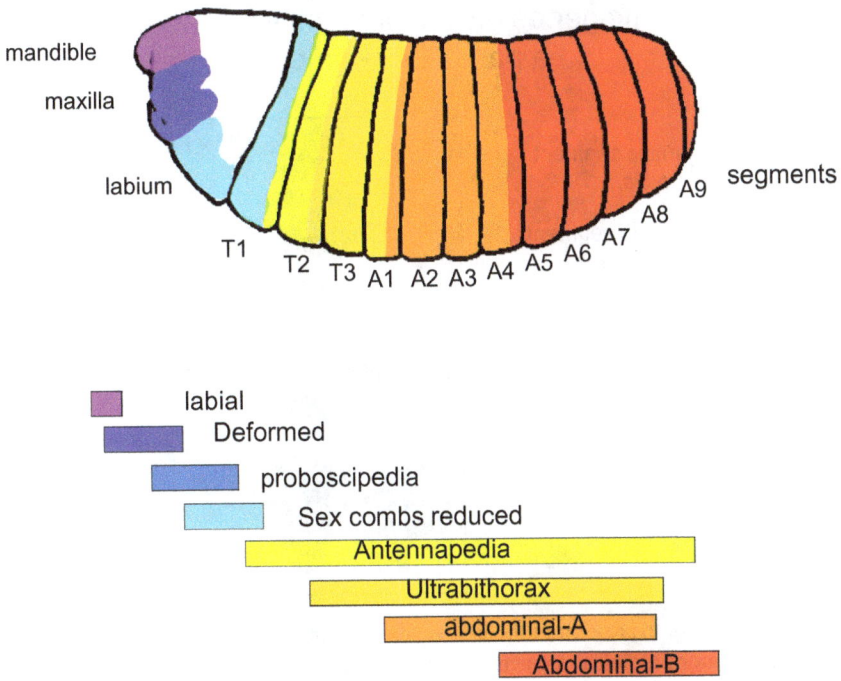

Figure 2. Homeotic genes and domains of expression. The domains of expression are color-coded to indicate the relevant homeotic genes. Note that the genes are expressed in parasegmental units, which correspond to the posterior half of an anatomical segment plus the anterior half of the following segment.

and is repressed in the head segments. Inappropriate expression of *Antennapedia* in the head causes the conversion of head structures such as the antennae into thoracic structures such as legs (Figure 1). Similarly, the *Ultrabithorax* gene (*Ubx*) is normally expressed in the posterior thoracic segment and is repressed in the mesothorax and more anterior segments. Insufficient expression of *Ubx* in the posterior thorax causes its transformation into mesothorax. This is a very dramatic transformation because the mesothorax produces wings and the correspondingly large muscles necessary to drive them while the posterior thorax is very small and, instead of wings, it normally develops small knoblike halteres. Regulatory mutations that reduce expression of *Ubx* in the posterior thorax, as shown by E.B. Lewis, result in flies with two sets of wings, the eponymous bithorax phenotype (Figure 3). Conversely, the inappropriate expression of *Ubx*

Homeotic genes give their identity to the cells of a particular segment

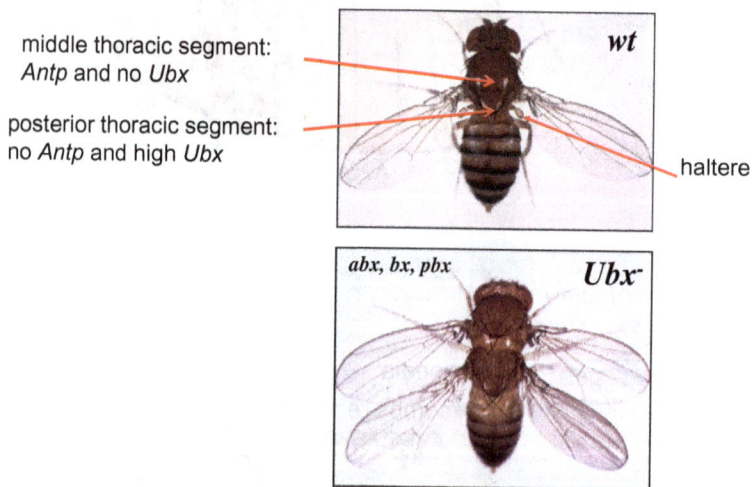

middle thoracic segment: *Antp* and no *Ubx*

posterior thoracic segment: no *Antp* and high *Ubx*

wt

haltere

abx, bx, pbx

Ubx⁻

Figure 3.   Loss of expression of the *Ubx* gene in parasegment 6 (posterior thoracic segment and anterior abdominal segment), where its expression is normally strongest, causes the transformation of the corresponding structures, which are normally very small (upper figure) into a second middle thoracic segment, which is normally large, bearing large wings instead of tiny halteres and the powerful flight muscles.

Source: E.B. Lewis and P. Lewis, California Institute of Technology Archives http://archives-dc. library.caltech.edu/islandora/object/ct1%3A8798.

in the mesothorax, more anteriorly than normal, suppresses the development of wings and results in a very small mesothorax with halteres instead of wings, resembling the posterior thorax (Figure 4).

Hox gene products are DNA-binding proteins, containing a highly conserved DNA-binding domain called the **homeodomain** (Figure 5). The homeodomain belongs to the helix-turn-helix family of DNA-binding domains, so called because of the protein-structural organization of the amino acid sequence that interacts with the nucleotide sequence it recognizes. This domain is now found in many transcription factors but, more than 500 million years ago, one of these factors became tandem-duplicated several times, with small changes in each copy. Together with a complex regulatory region, the entire gene cluster assumed the role of defining the antero-posterior structure of the early ancestor of all

Expression of Ubx in the middle thoracic segment transforms wings to halteres

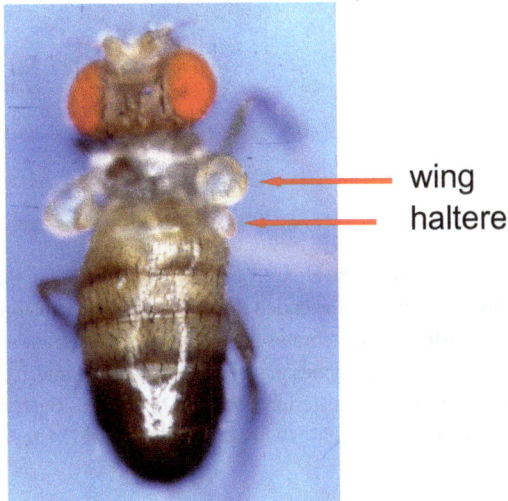

Figure 4.   Expression of *Ubx* in the middle thoracic segment transforms wings to halteres. This fly illustrates the opposite phenomenon: the *Ubx* gene is made to express one segment more anterior than normal. This causes a transformation of the middle thoracic segment to posterior thorax, which is very small and the wings are transformed to halteres.

Source: V. Pirrotta.

Consensus Homeodomain

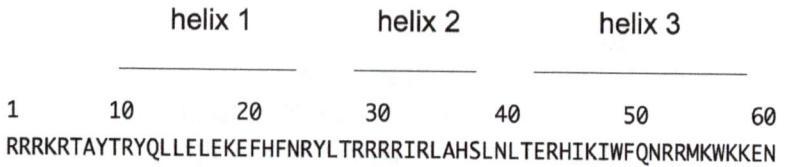

helix 1	helix 2	helix 3

```
1       10        20        30        40        50        60
RRRKRTAYTRYQLLELEKEFHFNRYLTRRRRIRLAHSLNLTERHIKIWFQNRRMKWKKEN
```

Figure 5.   The homeodomain is approximately 60 amino acids long and forms a typical helix-turn-helix DNA-binding domain. The first two helices are antiparallel and stabilize the third, the DNA-binding helix, roughly perpendicular to the first two. The third helix lies in the major groove of DNA and interacts with the bases. For an example of a helix-turn-helix domain binding to the DNA double helix, see Chapter 1.

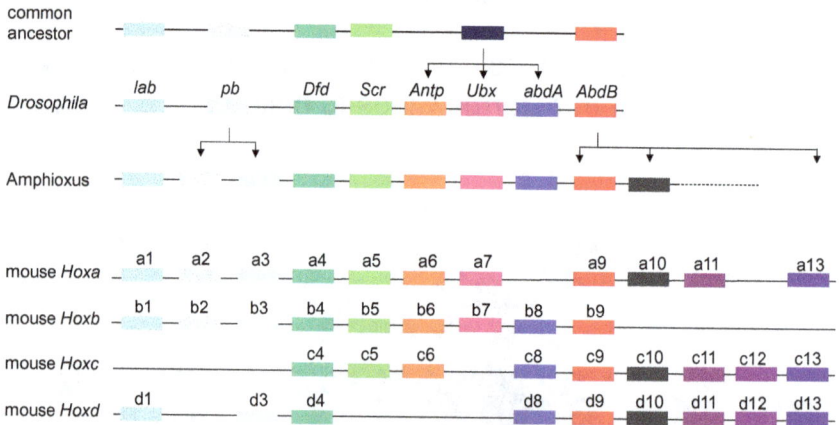

Figure 6.   Conservation of the Hox genes in *Drosophila* and in mammals. *Drosophila* has one set of homeotic genes (color-coded to correspond to the anatomical domains of expression anterior to posterior). Vertebrates have duplicated this set twice in the course of evolution. In each cluster, some genes have been lost and some have been duplicated and diversified but the anterior/posterior domains of expression have been preserved. The arrows do not imply that Amphioxus is descended from *Drosophila*. Both derive from a common ancestor.

bilaterian animals (Figure 6). The ancestral set of *Hox* genes was organized in a single co-linear cluster in which the linear structure of the gene cluster reflects the anterior/posterior axis of the body structure it regulates. This organization or the *Hox* genes is essential for the mechanisms that regulate their expression. The *Hox* gene acting most anteriorly is at the 3′ end of the cluster and the most posterior gene is at the 5′ end. In *Drosophila*, the cluster has split into two, separated by several megabases. In the vertebrate ancestor, it was still a single cluster of genes highly homologous to the corresponding *Drosophila Hox* genes. During the evolution of vertebrates, the cluster underwent two duplications and internal differentiation so that modern vertebrates have four *Hox* clusters, *Hoxa, Hoxb, Hoxc,* and *Hoxd*, each of which is slightly different, some of the clusters have lost some components or have diversified other components. In mammals, the four clusters have partially overlapping functions, but the basic principles of co-linearity and anterior/posterior hierarchy and timing of expression are preserved in all four clusters: the more 3′ genes are expressed more anteriorly and earlier in embryonic development, the more 5′ genes function more posteriorly and later in development. In vertebrates, the *Hox* genes have acquired an additional role in the development of the proximo-distal axis. That is, in the limb buds that give rise to the vertebrate appendages, the more proximal (closer to the body axis) structures are dependent on the more anterior *Hox* genes and the more distal structures are controlled by the more posterior *Hox* genes (Figure 7). In humans, for example, the shoulder blade and shoulder are specified by *Hox9*, the upper arm by *Hox10*, the forearm by *Hox11*, the wrist bones

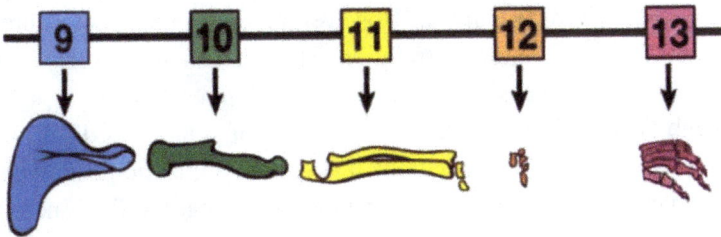

In vertebrates, Hox genes have acquired in addition a function to specify the limb proximo-distal axis

Figure 7.   The proximo-distal axis. In vertebrates, *Hox* genes have acquired a new function to specify the limb proximo-distal axis. Hox cognate genes from more than one *Hox* cluster collaborate to specify different segments of the proximo-distal axis in the vertebrate limb.
Source: Davis *et al.* (1995).

by *Hox 12*, and the fingers by *Hox13*. A mutation in *Hoxd13* causes poly-dactyly, the development of extra fingers (or toes) in the hand (or foot).

Key to the functioning of the *Hox* clusters in *Drosophila* as in mammals are the mechanisms that silence the expression of more posterior *Hox* genes in more anterior regions of the embryo. These mechanisms were discovered in *Drosophila* through the homeotic phenotypes caused by mutations disrupting their repressive functions, one of the first of which was a mutation called *Polycomb* (*Pc*). Insufficient Polycomb repression of posterior *Hox* genes allows them to be expressed more anteriorly, therefore tending to transform anterior segments to a more posterior identity. Homeotic genes are a classical example of master regulatory genes that are controlled by Polycomb mechanisms. Many other master regulatory genes activate pathways of differentiation, define cell identity, regulate cell proliferation, and in most cases are under Polycomb control.

Polycomb Group Genes and Mutations

The expression of the homeotic genes is determined by the segmentation genes expressed during early embryonic development of *Drosophila*. In particular, some of the segmentation genes acting as repressors set the boundaries of the domains of expression of each homeotic gene. A particularly well-studied example is the case of *Ubx*. Expression of *Ubx* is, in principle, activated in each embryonic segment but it is repressed by the *Hunchback* (*Hb*) gene in the anterior region and in the posterior-most region of the embryo (Figure 8). However, the *Hb* gene ceases expressing in this pattern shortly after gastrulation. The maintenance of the repressed state of homeotic genes in subsequent development is the task of the Polycomb Group of genes (PcG). This group of genes was discovered in the search for *Drosophila* mutations that caused homeotic phenotypes but did not map to homeotic genes. Genetics shows that the PcG includes at least a dozen genes whose mutations give very similar phenotypes of homeotic derepression. This indicates that the PcG genes act together to produce their repressive function. Loss of function of one PcG gene inactivates the whole PcG repressive mechanism. For example, embryos lacking the function of the prototypical PcG gene *Polycomb* fail to maintain the

The Hunchback repressor defines the Ubx expression domain

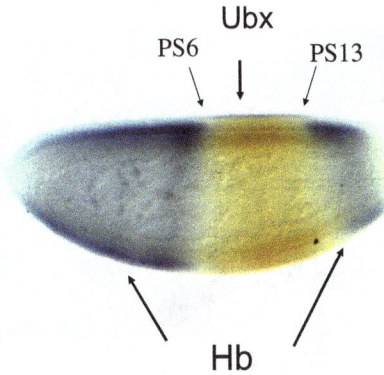

Figure 8. The Hunchback repressor defines the *Ubx* expression domain. In the very early *Drosophila* embryo, expression of the *Ubx* gene is repressed by the maternal repressor Hunchback (Hb) in the region anterior to parasegment 6 and posterior to parasegment 13. Hb stained in blue and Ubx in brown.

Source: V. Pirrotta.

repressed state of *Ubx* in embryonic domains where it is initially repressed by *Hb* (Figure 9). In fact, in *Pc⁻* embryos, all the homeotic genes are derepressed in all the cells. When all the *Hox* genes are functioning at the same time, the most posterior *Hox* gene is predominant and represses the more anterior genes. This means that all the segments are transformed into the most posterior segment (Figure 10). Such an embryo has a disorganized nervous system, disorganized muscles, disorganized gut, etc. The cells are alive and well but the organism cannot survive as a whole because its body segments are not appropriately structured and differentiated.

In most cases, even a heterozygous loss of function mutation already shows some derepression: like the *Su(var)* genes, the PcG functions are sensitive to PcG gene dosage. This means that even reducing the amount of a PcG protein by half causes some detectable homeotic derepression. One of the first signs of homeotic derepression is the transformation of the second and third legs into the first leg. In male flies, the first leg has a row of thicker and darker bristles called the **sex comb** (Figure 11).

Polycomb Group (PcG) and trithorax Group (trxG) genes are respectively required to maintain the repressed and active state of homeotic genes

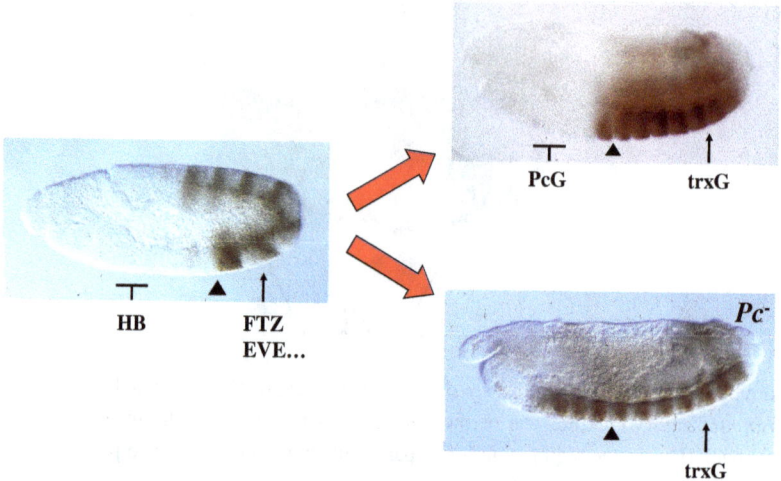

Figure 9.   Regulation of *Ubx* expression by Polycomb repression and Trithorax stimulation. Shortly after gastrulation, Hb expression fades and Polycomb repression sets in. Note that the embryonic segments first expand posteriorly and curl over the dorsal side (left figure), later they retract (figures o the right). Polycomb repression maintains the *Ubx* gene off where it had been repressed by Hb but allows continued expression where *Ubx* had been active. In a Pc⁻ mutant embryo, Polycomb repression fails and the Ubx gene is expressed in all segments.

Source: V. Pirrotta.

In heterozygous PcG mutants, sex combs are often seen on the second and even the third leg as well as the first. This characteristic dominant phenotype of *Polycomb* and other PcG mutations is responsible for many of the PcG gene names: *Polycomb (Pc)*, *Posterior sex combs (Psc)*, *Sex combs extra (Sce)*, *Sex combs on midleg (Scm)*, and *extra sex combs (esc)*. Other PcG genes are named for the way they modify the *zeste* effect, a pairing-dependent repression of the *white* gene by a particular mutant of the *zeste* gene: *Enhancer of zeste [E(z)]*, *Suppressor of zeste2 [Su(z)2]*, and *Suppressor of zeste12 [Su(z)12]*.

Sometimes, other kinds of dominant effects are seen in heterozygous PcG mutants: clumps of disorganized cells appear in the head. In cases when

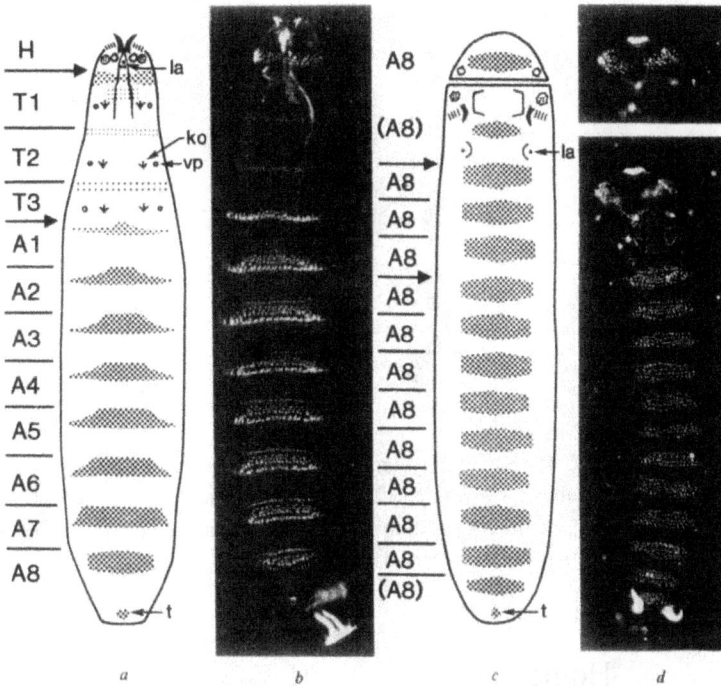

Figure 10. Hox genes in *Drosophila* embryos. On the left is shown a wild-type embryo at the end of embryonic development and a schematic representation of its segmental pattern. On the right is shown an embryo entirely lacking both maternal and zygotic function of the Polycomb Group gene *extra sex combs* (*esc*). As the cuticle pattern shows, all segments have been transformed to the posterior-most abdominal segment A8.

Source: Struhl (1981).

these clumps are large enough, it can be seen that they consist of cells that are forming thoracic structures, even a whole miniature wing can be seen arising from the top of the head (Figure 12). What has happened in these flies is that the PcG-repressed state of the homeotic genes is less stable. During early development, the homeotic genes in one or more cells of the head region have become derepressed conferring to that cell a more posterior identity. The derepressed state is transmitted to all the cellular progeny of that cell, producing a clone of cells that have a more posterior identity and therefore develop into a more posterior structure. This memory of a derepression event transmitted through multiple cell generations is highly reminiscent of the variegation phenotypes of heterochromatin mutants.

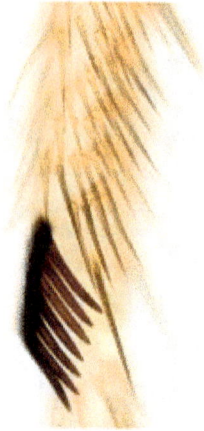

Figure 11.   The sex comb and the Polycomb phenotype. The sex comb is a row of thick black bristles found on the first leg of male flies. The second and third legs lack sex combs. The first sign of insufficient PcG function is often the appearance of sex combs on the second and third legs: they are transformed to the first leg.

Source: V. Pirrotta.

Homeotic "tumors" in Pc -/+ flies

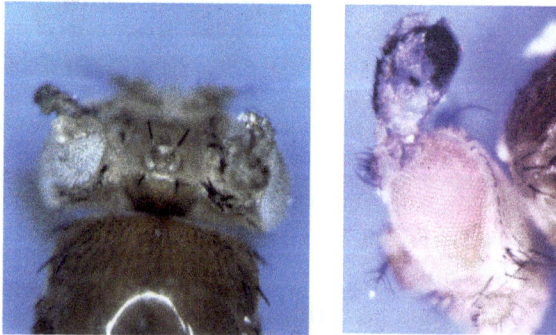

Figure 12.   Homeotic "tumors" in *Pc* –/+ flies. Insufficient *Pc* to ensure stable repression of Antp in the head region results in clones of cells with thoracic identity. When the clones are small, they look like disorganized "tumors" (panel left). When the clones are sufficiently large, they can be recognized as thoracic structures, a wing in the image to the right, small but with the correct triple set of sensory bristles at the anterior border, typical of the wing.

Source: V. Pirrotta.

The PcG Proteins

The PcG is not a family of related proteins. It is a group of structurally very different proteins. Biochemical analyses, pioneered by the group of Robert Kingston in the late 1990s, showed that PcG proteins form two distinct multiprotein complexes: Polycomb Repressive Complex 1 (PRC1) and PRC2. The Polycomb protein Pc, a component of PRC1, contains a structural domain with strong homology to a domain found in the hetero-chromatin protein HP1. This was called the **chromodomain**. The PRC2 component Enhancer of zeste, E(z), was found to contain a domain with strong homology to two other proteins then known: the heterochromatin protein Su(var)3-9 and Trithorax. This domain was therefore called the SET domain from the initials of the three proteins. After the discovery by the laboratory of Thomas Jenuwein in 2000 that Su(var)3-9 was a histone methyltranferase and that the SET domain was the catalytic active site, the similarity that had long been noticed between PcG silencing and hetero-chromatic silencing became clear. The PRC2 complex containing E(z) is also a histone methyltransferase that methylates H3K27, while Su(var)3-9 methylates H3K9. The amino acids surrounding the two methylation sites are very similar: QTARKS for H3K9 and KAARKS for H3K27. These sites can be mono-, di-, or tri-methylated (Figure 13). The higher methyla-tion states are recognized and bind to a corresponding chromodomain: the HP1 chromodomain in the case of H3K9 and the Pc chromodomain in the case of H3K27. In the epigenetics usage, the SET domain proteins are called "writers" of the methylation histone mark and the chromodomain proteins are "readers" of that mark (see Chapter 2).

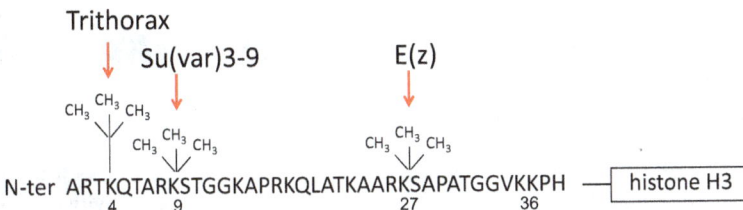

Figure 13.   Methylation of histone H3 by the first three SET domain proteins to be discovered.

The PRC1 and PRC2 complexes, as predicted by the genetics, generally work together to maintain the repressed state of their target genes. A survey of the *Drosophila* genome using chromatin immunoprecipitation with antibodies against various PcG proteins and against histone H3K27me3 shows that the genome contains hundreds of binding sites, not just at the *Hox* genes. At the vast majority of these sites, PRC1 and PRC2 proteins are found together and associated with chromatin containing the H3K27me3 histone mark. A handful of sites bind preferentially or exclusively to one complex or the other. At a typical target gene such as the *Ubx* gene, there is one, sometimes two, and occasionally several binding sites which correspond to the functionally defined Polycomb Response Elements or PREs. These were first identified by asking what small DNA region would be able to confer a sensitivity to PcG repression to test transgenes. To see how such a PRE operates, consider a transgene consisting of the *Ubx* promoter driving the expression of reporter gene such as the bacterial *lacZ* gene, which produces β-galactosidase (Figure 14). This is an enzyme that is not abundant in *Drosophila* embryos and can be readily visualized by staining embryos with a dye that detects the enzyme or

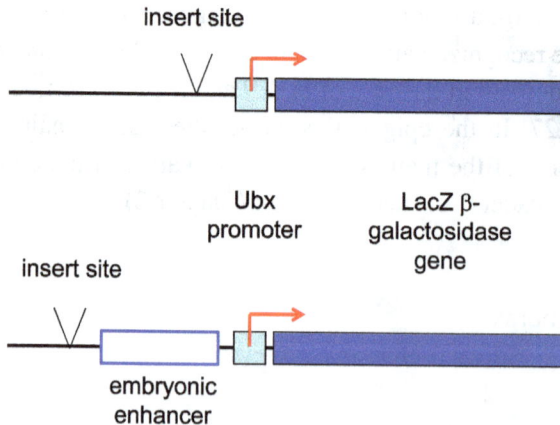

Figure 14.   Test constructs for regulatory activity. The diagram describes a transgene construct to assay genomic fragments of the *Ubx* gene for enhancer activity driving the expression of the bacterial *LacZ* gene from the *Ubx* promoter. The lower diagram is a construct to assay for fragments able to produce PcG-dependent silencing. The fragments to be tested are inserted in the insert site and the construct is introduced into the *Drosophila* genome by germ line transformation.

its enzymatic activity. With this reporter gene, fragments of the *Ubx* regulatory region could be tested to map enhancers that activate transcription in the embryo or in the imaginal discs (the precursors of adult segmental structures) (Figure 14).

The *Ubx* Regulatory Region

The *Ubx* gene, with a 75 kb transcript, is a fairly large gene by *Drosophila* standards. It has a long regulatory region of some 30 kb upstream of the promoter but also a downstream regulatory region contained within a large intron. These regions contain multiple embryonic enhancers that dictate expression in segmental domains (Figure 15) and, together,

Regulatory regions of the *Ubx* gene

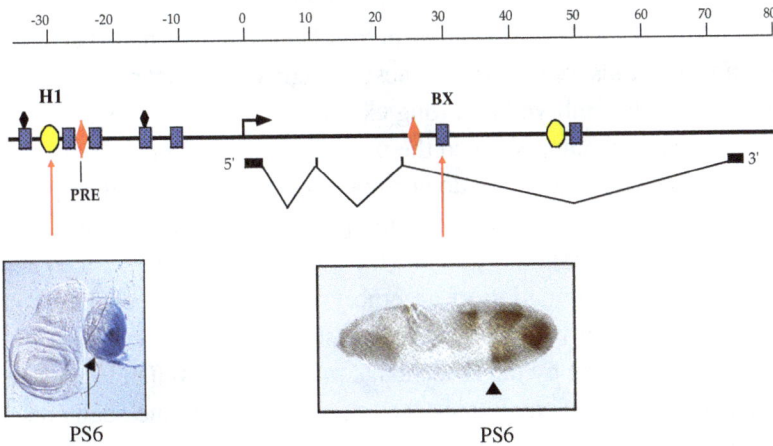

Figure 15.   The *Ultrabithorax* gene and regulatory elements identified by placing different fragments in a transgene construct expressing the bacterial beta-galactosidase gene. This approach identified several embryonic enhancers (blue rectangles), each expressing in part of the total pattern of the endogenous *Ubx* gene. Two enhancers expressing in the larval imaginal discs (yellow) were also identified. In addition, transgene constructs in which fragments were placed in a construct already driven by an embryonic enhancer identified Polycomb Response Elements (PREs), indicated by a red lozenge. The arrowhead labeled PS6 indicates the position of the boundary between parasegment 5 and parasegment 6.

Source: V. Pirrotta, S. Poux, and C. Kostic.

produce a segmental pattern of expression in the early embryo. Each of these enhancers contains binding sites for the Hunchback repressor, which suppresses expression in the head and posterior-most regions and confines expression to parasegments 6–12 of the embryo. This function of Hunchback ceases after gastrulation. Therefore, transgene constructs containing only these enhancers fail to maintain the repressed state after gastrulation and expression occurs in all segments. However, transgene constructs that contain a DNA fragment with PRE activity, in addition to the enhancer fragment, maintain the repression in the head and posterior-most region throughout embryonic development. PcG-dependent repressive activity prevents reactivation after gastrulation but does not prevent continued expression where this had been present in the early embryo (Figure 17). In other words, the Polycomb Response Element does not turn off an active gene but can maintain it in a silent state.

There are in addition two imaginal disc enhancers that become active late in embryonic development in the primordia of the imaginal discs that give rise to adult structures: the head-antenna discs, the wing discs, the haltere discs, as well as the three pairs of leg discs. When the reporter transgene contains only one of these imaginal enhancers, there is no expression in the embryo but strong expression in the imaginal discs.

Functional mapping showed the presence of a PRE in each of the two regulatory regions: one in the downstream region and one in the upstream region. A transgene construct containing just a PRE displays no expression in embryos or in larvae, just like the minimal transgene with no added enhancers. The combination of an embryonic segmental enhancer and a PRE produces a normal segmental expression repressed in the head and posterior-most region by the Hunchback protein (Hb). When Hb ceases to be expressed, the PRE maintains the repressed state in the segments initially repressed by Hb. Thanks to the PRE, expression of *Ubx* continues to be repressed in the anterior half of the body and in the posterior-most region (Figure 16). Importantly, while the PRE maintains the repressed state, expression continues in the segments where it was originally active.

When the transgene contains an imaginal disc enhancer and a PRE, however, no expression ever develops since the imaginal enhancer is not active in the early embryo when the PcG proteins establish the repressive function of the PRE. Therefore, the transgene is silenced in the embryo

Segmental enhancers

contain information about segmental specificity mediated by
the Hunchback repressor present in the anterior half of the early embryo

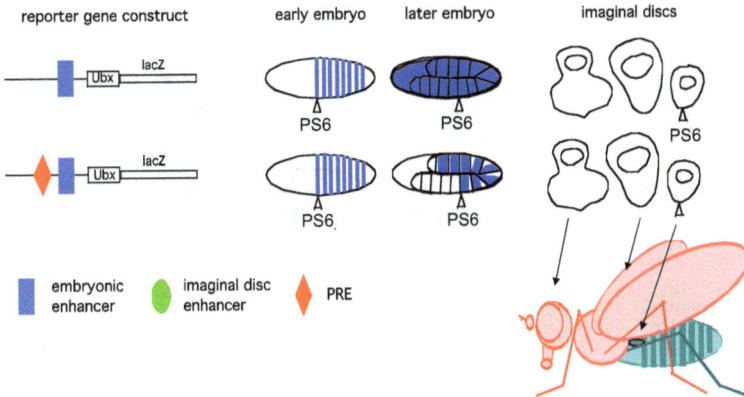

Figure 16. An embryonic enhancer from the *Ubx* gene drives expression in segmental stripes in the early embryo but is repressed by Hunchback in the anterior part of the embryo. In the later embryo, Hunchback is no longer present and expression expands to all segments. The embryonic enhancer has no activity in the larval imaginal discs, indicated here by the head, wing, and haltere imaginal discs. If a PRE is added to the transgene construct, expression in the late embryo is repressed by Polycomb in the anterior segments but remains active in the posterior segments where it was active earlier. The arrowhead indicates the parasegment 6 boundary.

and never turned on in the imaginal discs (Figure 17). In contrast, a transgene containing a combination of embryonic enhancer, imaginal enhancer, and PRE, simulating the endogenous *Ubx* gene, reconstitutes the normal segmental pattern of expression (Figure 18). The embryonic enhancer activates expression in the early embryo, regulated by Hb. The PRE maintains repression in the head and posterior regions but allows expression in the appropriate segmental domain, parasegments 6–12. Late in embryonic development, when the imaginal enhancer kicks in, expression is possible in these segments but repression mediated by the PRE prevents expression more anterior or more posterior than parasegments 6–12. As a result, expression is blocked in the head and wing imaginal

Imaginal enhancers

lack segmental specificity and function in head and thorax segments

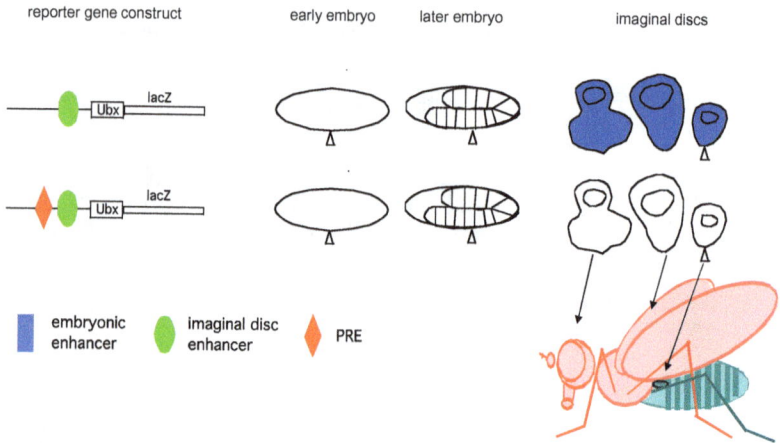

Figure 17.   The imaginal disc enhancer has no activity in the embryo but drives expression in all larval imaginal discs. If the PRE is added to the construct, there is still no expression in the embryo. This allows Polycomb silencing to set in so that expression is now silenced in all the imaginal discs. The arrowhead indicates the parasegment 6 boundary.

discs but is allowed in the posterior half of the haltere disc (parasegment 6). A parasegment, the unit composed of the posterior part of a physical segment and the anterior part of the next segment, is functionally a more meaningful unit than the anatomical segment and is the unit subdivision that controls *Hox* gene expression.

The PRE

In *Drosophila*, PREs are short genomic regions usually a few hundred base pairs long. They do not share a common sequence but they usually contain multiple binding sites for several DNA-binding factors but no single factor is present at all PREs. These factors are also present at hundreds of other genomic sites that are not PREs. This indicates that they act cooperatively to recruit PcG complexes, of which more will be discussed

The PRE

conveys the segmental specificity of the early enhancers
and maintains it in the imaginal enhancers

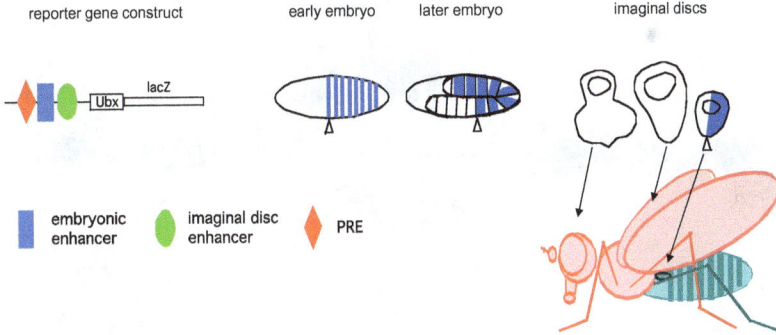

Figure 18. If all three elements are present in the transgene construct, expression in the posterior segments is maintained in the late embryo but is repressed by Polycomb in the anterior segments. Expression in the larva is silenced in the anterior imaginal discs, corresponding to the anterior segments but is allowed in the posterior part of the haltere disc, corresponding to parasegment 6, indicated by the arrowhead.

later. Together, however, their binding excludes the formation of nucleosomes. As a result, PREs tend to be depleted of nucleosomes and are instead DNase hypersensitive (Figure 19).

PREs work as repressive elements in combination with any promoter subject to the rules described above. Expression activated earlier than gastrulation is generally not repressed by most PREs. Polycomb repression becomes generally effective around gastrulation so that expression activated later in embryonic development is silenced. Expression that may be activated in between may be silenced in a variegated fashion. Some PREs are more strongly repressive than others. It should be noted, however, that a strong surge of activator can override even a strong PRE. For example, a transgene in which a PRE is flanked by a promoter inducible by the yeast GAL4 activator is totally derepressed with loss of PcG complexes when GAL4 is massively expressed.

Many interesting features of PRE-dependent silencing were first noticed using *Drosophila white* transgenes. The *Drosophila white* gene is

The *Ubx* Polycomb Response Element

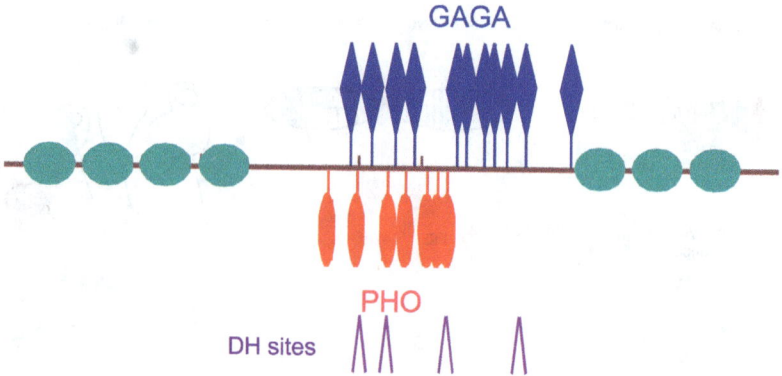

Figure 19.   The figure represents the *bxd* PRE, one of the two PREs in the *Ubx* gene. The green ovals indicate nucleosomes. The nucleosome-free region contains multiple binding sites for several DNA-binding proteins, two of which, GAGA Factor (GAF) and Pho, are indicated. The region contains several DNAse hypersensitive sites indicating sites that are hyperaccessible to DNase in chromatin that binds these factors and Polycomb complexes.

required for the bright red eye pigmentation of wild-type flies (Figure 20). The gene was in fact named *white* because it is needed to make the eye red. It may seem odd but it is typical in *Drosophila* genetics to name a gene after the phenotype of the mutant. So, loss of function mutations of *white* causes loss of pigmentation and white eyes. The eye pigmentation can be restored by introducing a *white* transgene. Adding a PRE to the *white* transgene can cause its total or partial silencing, the extent of which varies with the genomic site of insertion of the transgene. The variable silencing often varies also in different cells, giving rise to a variegated pigmentation, similar to that often seen in heterochromatic silencing of the *white* gene. In general, the effect of a PRE may be modulated by the genomic environment and by the physical environment. High temperature during larval development, for example, increases repression, contrary to the effects on heterochromatic variation. The genomic and nuclear environment can give rise to effects that were surprising and unexpected when

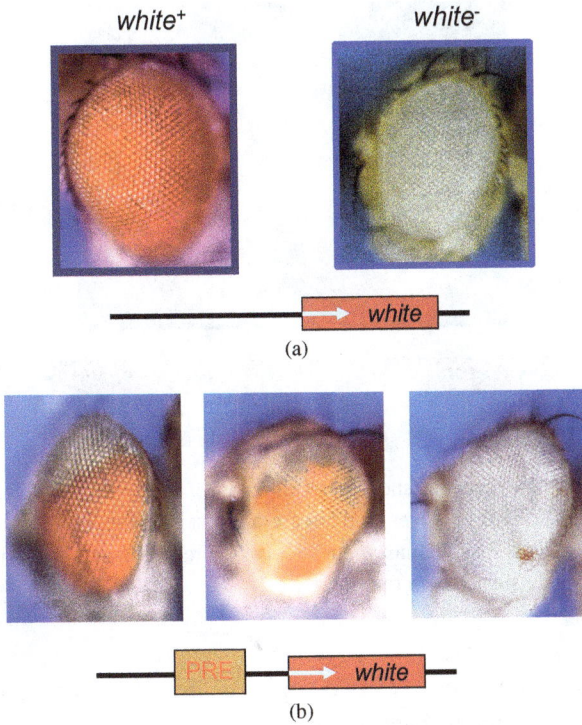

Figure 20. The *Drosophila white* gene as a reporter of Polycomb repression. (a) The *Drosophila white* gene is necessary for the bright red wild-type eye color. Loss of function of the *white* gene produces a white eye, after which the gene was named. A simple *white* transgene restores the red eye pigmentation to a *white⁻* mutant fly. A PRE can produce variegated repression. (b) Adding a PRE to a *white* transgene can result in total or partial (variegated) silencing. The variegated phenotype indicates that the *white* transgene is silenced in some cells but not in others, reminiscent of variegated heterochromatic silencing.

Source: V. Pirrotta.

they were first observed with genes regulated by Polycomb and with transgenes containing PREs. We may call them pairing and proximity effects.

Pairing effects were first noted with transgenes in which the *white* gene was placed next to a PRE. A partial or weak repression was often seen with one copy of the transgene. When the transgene insertion was made homozygous, instead of a stronger pigmentation, as would be

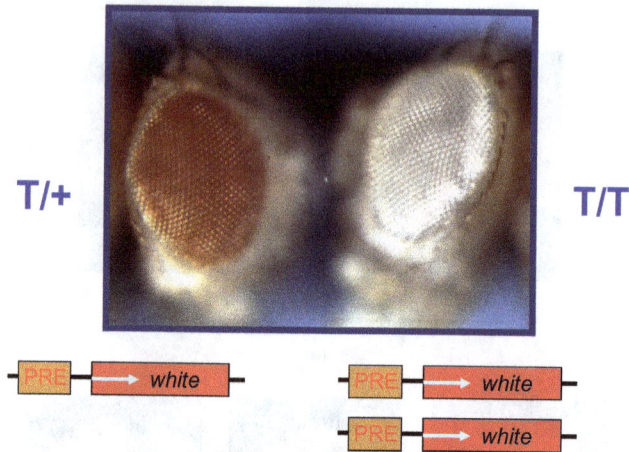

Figure 21.   Pairing-dependent silencing. One copy of the transgene T, containing the *white* gene and the PRE produces in this case a pigmented eye with slight variegation. When the transgene is made homozygous, the two paired PREs are much more effective and may completely silence both transgenes.

Source: V. Pirrotta.

expected from the presence of two copies of the *white* gene, the eye color became much lighter or even totally white (Figure 21). In other words, when two allelic copies of the PRE-containing transgene were present, the silencing effect became much stronger. In dipteran insects like *Drosophila*, homologous chromosomes pair up during interphase and the two transgene copies are therefore in close proximity to one another. This is known as pairing-dependent silencing and suggests that the Polycomb complexes are either more easily recruited by the two paired PREs or create a higher local concentration that results in stronger silencing. Interactions do not usually occur between non-allelic PRE-containing transgenes but are observed in some cases even between transgenes inserted on two different, non-homologous chromosomes. This observation suggested that chromosome folding in the nucleus and the tendency of PcG complexes to associate can result in physical clustering of PcG binding sites in the genome (Figure 22) (see Chapter 8).

That Polycomb complexes exert their action on genes in their physical proximity, even if on a different DNA molecule, was illustrated by another surprising phenomenon. This was found when the PRE present on one of

Polycomb "bodies"

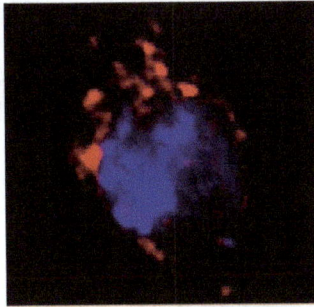

Figure 22. Polycomb "bodies". Polycomb binding sites in the genome have a tendency to come together resulting in the appearance of fewer but larger clusters, visualized here by staining a cell nucleus with an antibody against Polycomb (red).

Source: H.B. Li and V. Pirrotta.

the two homologous copies of the transgene was excised. This experiment is easily done if the PRE is flanked by FRT sequences, targets of a site-specific recombinase enzyme. When the recombinase gene is activated, for example, by a heat shock promoter, the PRE is excised. This makes it possible to construct flies in which a transgene containing a PRE can be homologously paired with a copy inserted at the homologous site but lacking the PRE. The surprising result was that the PRE on one copy on one chromosome can repress the transgene copy inserted at the homologous site but lacking the PRE. These results strongly suggest that PREs, and the PcG complexes they recruit, can act on a genomic site physically close in space even if that site is not on the same chromosome (Figure 23).

We now know that these effects are illustrative of the way in which epigenetic mechanisms function in the nucleus, not just Polycomb. The vicinity of repressive activity affects genes even if they are not on the same DNA molecule, simple physical proximity is sufficient. The same is true of activating mechanisms: an enhancer present on one allele of a gene can activate the other allele. Such effects had been observed in *Drosophila* genetics, often in circumstances involving Polycomb repression, and were referred to as **transvection** effects. This is why genomic architecture

Proximity-dependent repression

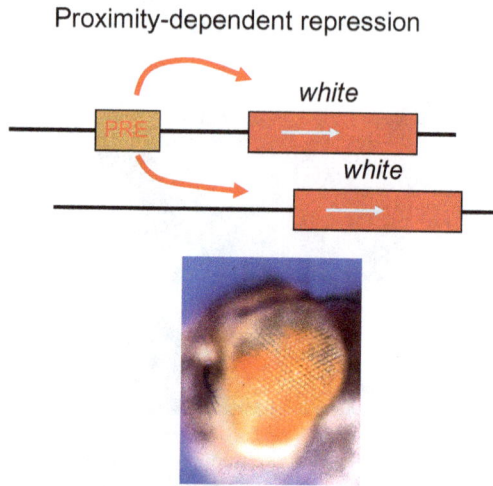

Figure 23.   Proximity-dependent repression. The transgene containing the *white* gene and the PRE was made homozygous but the PRE from one copy of the transgene was deleted. The remaining PRE on the allelic copy of the transgene can repress the *white* gene on both copies.

Source: C. Sigrist and V. Pirrotta.

seems to take special care to separate physically genes that should be repressed from genes that should be active (see Chapter 8).

Mapping of PcG proteins

Chromatin immunoprecipitation (ChIP, see Chapter 13) confirmed that PREs are indeed binding sites for PRC1 as well as PRC2 complexes. E(z), representing PRC2, and Pc or Psc proteins, representing PRC1, are found at the same sites (Figure 24). Their distributions form sharp peaks over PRE sites, with little presence over the promoter or enhancer regions. In contrast, the distribution of the H3K27me3 mark is broadly distributed over most or all of the silenced genes. However, the level of H3K27me3 dips to background values over the PRE itself. This is not surprising in view of the fact that the PRE is depleted of nucleosomes. This distribution raises several important questions. One is as follows:

Ubx gene

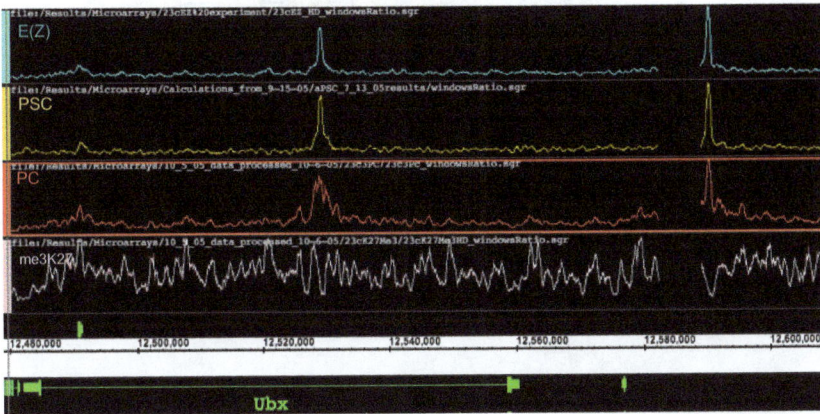

Figure 24.   PRC1 and PRC2 generally act together at target genes. The results of chromatin immunoprecipitation (ChIP) displayed on a genome browser for the *Ubx* gene. In green is the distribution of H3K27me3; in blue, E(z), a component of PRC2; in orange, Psc, a component of PRC1; in red, Pc, a component of PRC1. Note the sharp peaks of all three PcG proteins at the two Ubx PREs while the H3K27me3 distribution covers the entire region.

Source: Y. Schwartz, T. Kahn, and V. Pirrotta.

How is the H3K27me3 mark produced over such a broad region if the PRC2 complex is detected only at the PRE? One possible answer is that the PRC2 complex bound at the PRE can nevertheless loop over to contact and methylate flanking regions (Figure 25). Then, with help from the PRC1 and, in particular, from the Pc chromodomain, it can continue to loop over and continue to methylate more distant nucleosomes by a proximity-dependent interaction similar to that described in Figure 23. The affinity of the Pc chromodomain for already methylated nucleosomes may be responsible for the fact that the apparent Pc distribution is somewhat broader than that of the other PRC1 components such as Psc. The affinity does not seem to be strong enough, however, to cause stable binding of PRC1 to the entire methylated domain.

Another question raised by these results is as follows: How are PRC1 and PRC2 recruited? The fact that the Pc chromodomain binds to

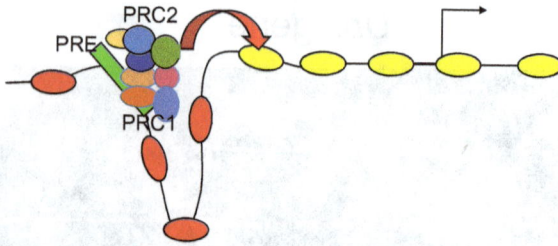

Figure 25.   Model for regional H3K27 trimethylation. The two Polycomb complexes are bound at the PRE, which loops to contact flanking regions to methylate nucleosomes (red). Once the region is trimethylated, the PRC1 complex with Pc and its chromodomain assist in contacting the already trimethylated region.

H3K27me3 suggested that PRC2 might be recruited first and PRC1 would be recruited subsequently by the H3K27me3 produced by PRC2. Remarkably, this scenario remained unaccountably popular and is still widely credited despite the fact that the PRE, where PRC1 is bound, is depleted of nucleosomes and thus of H3K27me3. In addition, PRC1 remains bound at the PRE despite the fact that the H3K27me3 is spread out over the rest of the target gene. More realistic experiments using cells in which either PRC1 or PRC2 is disabled have shown in fact that there is broad diversity among PREs. In *Drosophila*, most PREs can bind PRC1 in the absence of PRC2. This implies that PRC1 is not recruited by H3K27me3. In contrast, in the absence of PRC1, the majority of PREs suffer a substantial loss of PRC2 binding. A subset of PREs continues to bind expected amounts of PRC2 independently of PRC1, indicating that there are significant differences in the way different PREs function. The detailed mechanisms remain at present little understood but further in the following we will consider the role of some participating factors in helping the recruitment process and linking PRC1 and PRC2.

PRC2 and Histone H3K27 Methylation

The PRC2 complex has four core components: E(z), which contains the catalytic site, Su(z)12, Esc, and the histone chaperone Nurf 55 which is also involved in many other nucleosome transactions (Figure 26). Unlike many other histone methyltransferases, E(z) is not catalytically active

The PRC2 complex

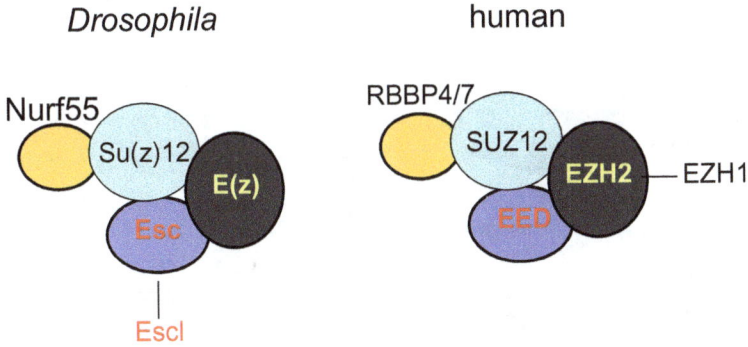

Figure 26.   The *Drosophila* PRC2 complex. E(z) is the core component containing the catalytic SET domain. PRC2 produces H3K27me1, -me2, and -me3. Methylation activity requires the other core components Nuer55 (also known as Caf1), Su(z)12, and Esc. Escl is a close relative of Esc that can take its place. On the right is a diagram of the human PRC2 core, indicating the human homologs of the *Drosophila* components.

unless complexed with at least Esc and Su(z)12. E(z) is wrapped around a core formed by Su(z)12 and Esc, which help structure and regulate the E(z) catalytic domain. Nurf 55 binds to Su(z)12. The mammalian PRC2 core is very highly conserved, relative to the *Drosophila* version. There are two alternative E(z) homologs: Ezh1 and Ezh2, of which Ezh2 is by far the more abundant and more catalytically active in most tissues. The mammalian Su(z)12 is called simply Suz12. The mammalian Esc is Eed, and Rbp48 (or RbAp48) is the histone chaperone homologous to *Drosophila* Nurf55.

Genomic ChIP analyses made it clear that, aside from the binding of the PRC complexes, the clearest indication of PcG repressive activity was the presence of the H3K27me3 mark. The PRC2 complex is the only H3K27 methyltranferase in *Drosophila* and in mammals. It operates step-wise rather than processively, meaning that mono-, di-, and tri-methyl H3K27 are produced separately and sequentially but, while the first two are produced rapidly, trimethylation is slower and much more difficult. Consequently, significant levels of H3K27me3 are generally found only

Distribution of H3K27 methylation

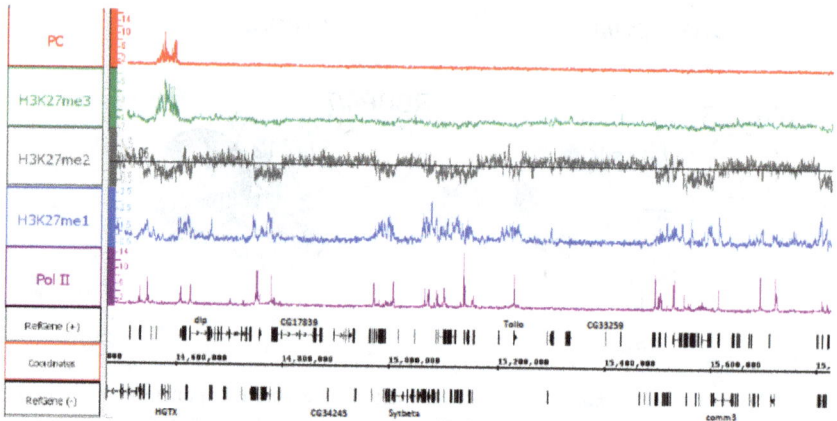

Figure 27.   Distribution of H3K27 methylation. The figure shows the results of ChIP in *Drosophila* cells, displayed by a genome browser. The two bottom lanes map the genes in the region. Genes in the upper of the two are transcribed towards the left. Genes in the bottom lane are transcribed to the right. H3K27me2 is almost in all regions where there is little transcription. H3K27me1 appears in actively transcribed regions. H3K27me3 is in just a few places that usually bind also Polycomb proteins belonging to PRC1 and PRC2 complexes. Pol II is RNA polymerase II; PC is Polycomb.
Source: Lee *et al.* (2015).

in regions that contain stable PRC2 binding sites (Figure 27). Instead, ChIP with antibody against H3K27me2 shows that this mark is far more widespread than H3K27me3. It is found at sites that have no stably bound PRC2 and, in fact, it is present in the genome everywhere there is no active transcription (except, of course, PRE-associated genes that have H3K27me3). This implies that the methylation activity associated with stably bound PRC2 is only a small fraction of the total genomic PRC2 activity. In fact, in flies and in mammals, some 60–70% of all histone H3 is dimethylated at K27. Only 7–10% carries K27me3. Surprisingly, H3K27me1 is found in transcribed genes, where its role is unclear. It may be an intermediate of demethylation. PRC2 is therefore principally a free, hit-and-run histone methyltransferase. It does not act equally on all chromatin, however. Structural and functional studies have revealed several mechanisms that steer its activity to chromatin regions that lack features of transcriptional activity. To see how this operates, consider the activity of PRC2 when chromatin replicates.

In the course of chromatin replication, old nucleosomes are disrupted but the core histone H3/H4 tetramer is approximately randomly redistributed to the two daughter DNA molecules (Figure 28). The newly replicated DNA therefore has half the complement of nucleosomes and new nucleosomes must be deposited to fill the gaps. As a result, the histone methyl marks present on the old chromatin become diluted two-fold. To restore the level of H3K27 methylation and to preserve the repressed state of genes that had been previously repressed, several feedback features modulate PRC2 activity and help steer it to specific chromatin targets. Components of PRC2 interact with surrounding nucleosomes and modulate the methylation activity of the catalytic component E(z) (Figure 29). A major role is played by the Su(z)12-Esc core around which E(z) is wrapped and which helps structure the catalytic domain. Su(z)12 interacts with nucleosomes containing H3K4me3 or H3K36me2/3, both marks associated with transcriptional activity, and the resulting allosteric shifts strongly repress the catalytic activity of E(z). Importantly, for the inhibitory effect, these two marks must be on the same H3 tail that contains the target H3K27 methylation site.

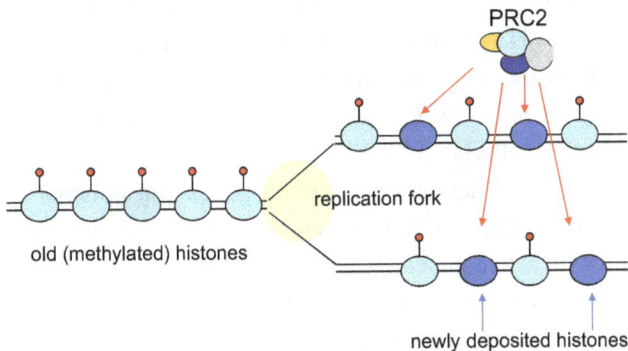

Figure 28.   Maintenance of methylation after replication. At the replication fork, the old, methylated H3-H4 core histones are transferred to the daughter DNA molecules roughly equally. New histones are deposited to fill in the gaps (darker blue ovals). This dilutes the old methyl marks by a half. PRC2 comes in to restore the methylation density, taking its cue from the flanking nucleosomes.

Stimulate

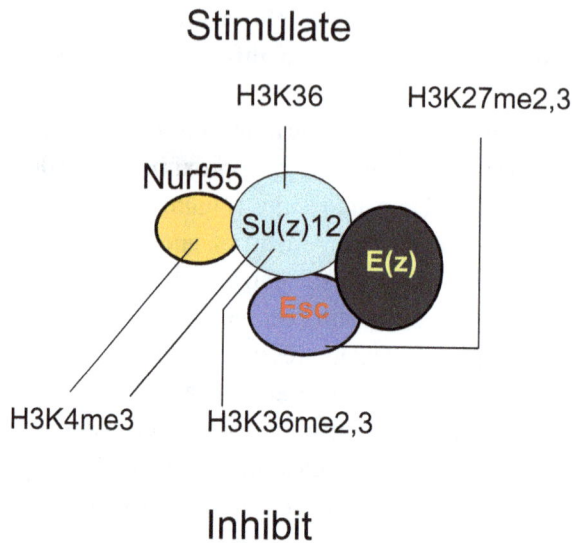

Figure 29.   Chromatin marks modulate PRC2 activity. PRC2 components Nurf55 and Su(z)12 contact H3K4me3 and inhibit H3K27 methylation. Su(z)12 detects H3K36me2,me3 and similarly inhibits catalytic activity. However, when H3K36 is not methylated, the effect is to stimulate methylation. Esc binds H3K27me2,3, which powerfully greatly stimulates methylation activity.

In contrast, Su(z)12 binds also to nucleosomes containing unmethylated H3K36 or even to H3 peptides containing an unmethylated K36. This inter-action stimulates methylation activity. As a consequence, genes containing a high density of nucleosomes (such as transcriptionally silent genes) are more effectively methylated by PRC2 while less nucleosome-dense chro-matin such as that of actively transcribed genes is a poorer PRC2 target. These mechanisms focus PRC2 on transcriptionally inactive chromatin and help explain why active genes are not silenced by the Polycomb complexes. A further and particularly important effect depends on Esc/Eed. This is a WD40-domain protein, a class of proteins to which Nurf55/Rbp48 also belongs. Such proteins contain a set of seven repeats of a domain of about 40 amino acids that terminate with a tryptophan and aspartate dipeptide (WD). The seven WD40 domains fold in a circular paddlewheel-like arrangement with the seven paddles arranged around a hollow core (Figure 30). Amino acids contributed by different WD40 repeats at the top of the hollow core combine to form an aromatic cage that binds very

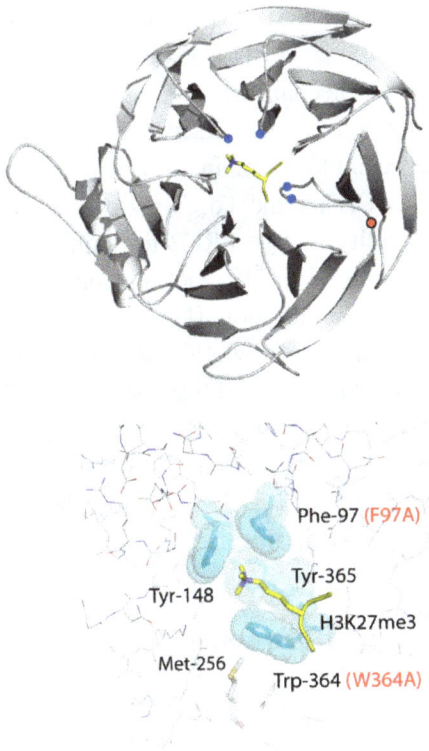

Figure 30.   The Eed/Esc protein binds H3K27me3. The WD40 paddlewheel structure of Eed/Esc forms a conical structure (shown here from the top) with a hollow core. Aromatic amino acid residues contributed by different WD40 repeats form a pocket at the top of the cone that binds methylated lysine (in yellow).

Source: Margueron *et al.* (2009).

effectively to trimethylated lysines. Binding to histone H3 or to peptides containing H3K27me3 is particularly effective and stimulates the E(z) catalytic domain to methylate histone H3 or an unmethylated nucleosome. The stimulatory effect is nearly 10-fold, less if the peptide contains H3K27me2 instead of me3. The result is that chromatin regions that already contain H3K27me3 are much better methylation substrates than unmethylated regions. This is just what is needed to facilitate the preferential remethylation of newly replicated chromatin, in which new nucleosomes are flanked by old, previously methylated nucleosomes. *In vivo* experiments in *Drosophila* show in fact that if the Esc aromatic cage is mutationally disrupted, the PRC2 is unable to establish normal levels of H3K27me3 or H3K27me2 and Polycomb silencing is lost.

With these several mechanisms available to help target PRC2 to untranscribed and previously methylated regions, it might be wondered whether PRC2 is sufficient to maintain an H3K27me3 domain once established, even when the PRE is removed. Experiments to test this hypothesis and to evaluate the ability of free PRC2 to maintain the repressed state found that, upon excision of a PRE, methylation is not diluted two-fold every cell cycle but significantly more slowly. This implies that PRC2 can, to some extent, replenish the methylation after replication even when the PRE is removed. The results showed that the rate of dilution depends on the chromatin environment, which may, to some extent, facilitate recruitment of PRC2. However, a few cell divisions after excision of the PRE, trimethylation is eventually lost. Significantly, however, repression is maintained as long as substantial trimethylation persists.

Accessory PRC2 Components

The core PRC2 complex is sufficient for enzymatic activity. In fact, some activity is retained by a minimal complex including just E(z), Su(z)12, and Esc. However, additional components are important for targeting, stimulating, and modulating PRC2 activity (Figure 31). In mammals, the

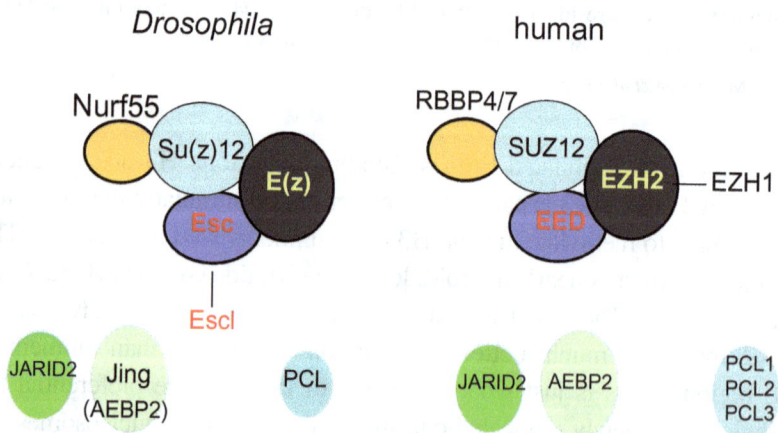

Figure 31. Accessory PRC2 components. They are called "accessory" because they are not needed for enzymatic activity but they are very necessary for correct function *in vivo*.

major optional components that have been reported are Adipocyte Enhancer Binding Protein 2 AEBP2 (*Drosophila* Jing), Jumonji AT-rich Interactive Domain JARID2 (*Drosophila* Jarid2), *Drosophila* Polycomblike Pcl or its mammalian homologs PHF1, MTF2, PHF17 (also known as PCL1,2,3), C17orf96, and histone deacetylase HDAC1 (Rpd3). Notably, the presence of AEBP2 is mutually exclusive with the presence of the PCL or C17orf96 cofactors. In fact, Pcl and its mammalian homologs are thought to stabilize a PRC2 dimer and increase its affinity for DNA, thus increasing its residence time and facilitating the step to trimethylation. AEBP2 and its *Drosophila* homolog Jing displace the Pcl homologs and stabilize the monomer structure. The role of JARID2 remained less clear but recent biochemical and structural work has shown that JARID2 is a major target of PRC2 methylation. The target is lysine 116, in an AQRKFAQ peptide context that resembles the AARKSAP surrounding histone H3K27. When the trimethylated JARID2 is incorporated in PRC2, the trimethylated lysine 116 binds to the Esc/Eed aromatic pocket and stimulates K27 trimethylation of nucleosomal H3 (Figure 32). This means that the PRC2 complex containing trimethylated JARID2 is now effective in trimethylating nucleosomes even in a previously unmethylated context. This PRC2 complex would therefore be effective to generate H3K27me3 *de novo* at genes that acquire Polycomb silencing in the course of development. Finally but significantly, both JARID2 and AEBP2 (as well as their *Drosophila* homologs) bind to histone H3 ubiquitylated at K119. This, as we shall see, can provide a further link between the PRC2 and PRC1.

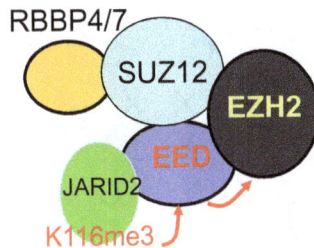

Figure 32.   Methylated JARID2. JARID2 is a major target of PRC2, which trimethylates JARID2 K116. When methylated JARID2 binds to the PRC2 complex, the K116me3 fits in the Eed binding pocket producing an allosteric shift that powerfully stimulates the catalytic activity of Ezh2.

The PRC1 Complexes

At most, but not all, of its target genes, Polycomb repression recruits and requires both PRC2 and PRC1 complexes. The structural core of PRC1 complexes is a heterodimer of two closely related proteins, both containing a structural motif called a RING domain. For example, the well-known breast cancer-related BRCA1 protein is a RING domain protein. Its partner protein is called BARD1. Don't look for a ring in the RING domain: it was so called because it was thought to be a Really Interesting New Gene when first described in 1991. The RING domain is a modified double zinc finger (Figure 33) commonly found in a class of proteins that function as E3 ubiquitin transferases that ubiquitylate specific lysine residues in their target proteins. The catalytic activity resides in the component of the heterodimer called Ring. In *Drosophila*, this is the product of the *Sce* gene. In mammals, there are two closely related proteins, Ring1 and Ring2 (earlier called Ring1b and Ring1a, respectively), but the former is the predominant one. The heterodimeric partner of Ring also contains a RING domain and is called generically Polycomb Group RING Finger Protein or PCGF (Figure 34). There are many possible PGCF partners. In *Drosophila*, there are two canonical alternatives: Posterior Sex comb (Psc) and Suppressor of zeste-2 [Su(z)2]. In mammals, there are at least six different PCGFs. The formation of the heterodimer allows the RING

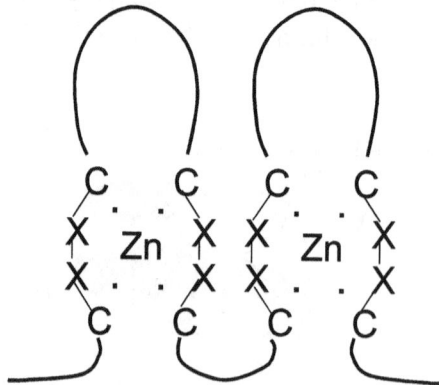

Figure 33.   The RING domain. The RING domain is a variety of double zinc finger each with a zinc ion coordinated by cysteines. It is found in a large variety of proteins, many of which have ubiquitin ligase activity.

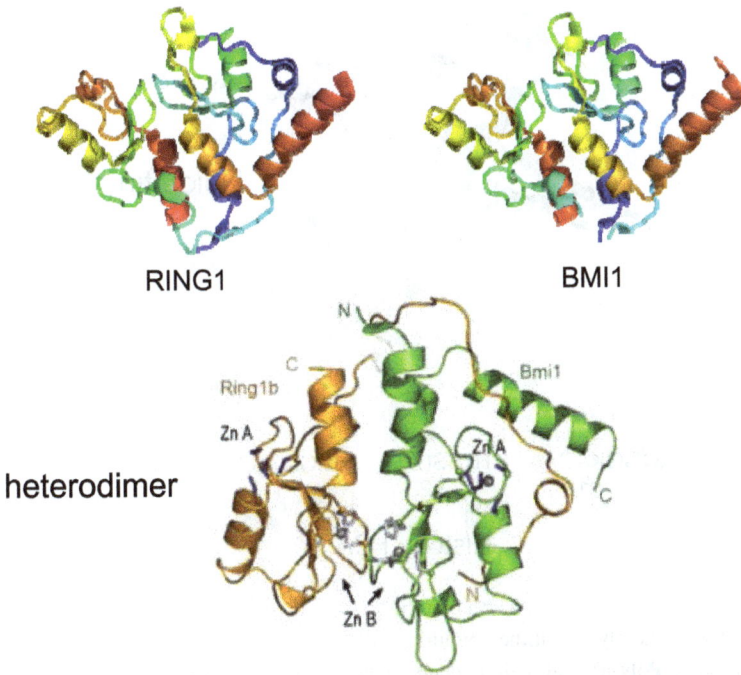

Figure 34. Structure of RING and PCGF proteins. The core structure of the RING and PCGF proteins though they might have sizable attached domains. BMI1 is now also called PCGF 4 and contains little more than the essential core with a very similar structure to that of RING1b. The RING domains of RING1b and PCGF proteins form heterodimers that are the core of PRC1 complexes. The formation of the heterodimer allows Ring1b to become catalytically active ubiquitylation histone H2AK119.

Source: Emw, Creative Commons Attribution (https://commons.wikimedia.org/wiki/File:Protein_ BMI1_PDB_2ckl.png, https://commons.wikimedia.org/wiki/File:Protein_RING1_PDB_2h0d.png). Heterodimer from Buchwald *et al.* (2006).

component to become catalytically active in ubiquitylating histone H2A at lysine 119 (or H2AK118 in *Drosophila*). Ubiquitin is a small protein of 76 amino acids (smaller than histone H2A: 129 amino acids) that can be attached to certain amino acid residues in a protein, most frequently to a lysine residue (Figure 35). Ubiquitin's most common role is to poly-ubiquitylate proteins that become thereby targeted for proteolytic distruc-tion by the proteasome. However, in many cases, such as that of histone

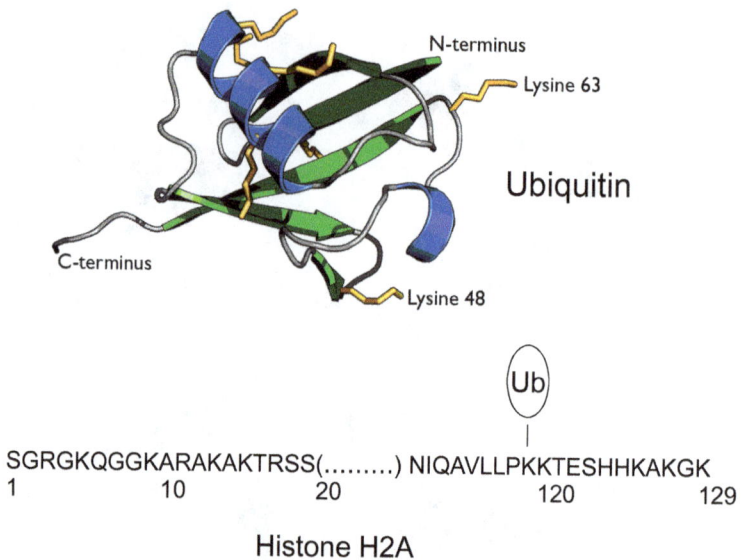

Figure 35.   Ubiquitin (top). The ubiquitin protein is usually attached by an isopeptide bond between the glycine at the ubiquitin C-ter to an acceptor site, usually lysine, on the target protein. Poly-ubiquitylation occurs by attaching additional ubiquitins to one of the ubiquitin lysines indicated in the figure. The amino acid sequence of histone H2A is shown, in part. Ubiquitylation by the Ring1 component of PRC1 occurs at K119.

Source: Ubiquitin structure figure by Rogerdodd, Creative Commons Attribution https://commons. wikimedia.org/wiki/File:Ubiquitin_cartoon-2-.png Histone H2A (bottom).

H2A and other chromatin proteins, only a single ubiquitin residue is attached. Mono-ubiquitylation is not a signal for destruction but the single ubiquitin acts as a recruiter or a framework for the binding of other proteins involved in chromatin regulation.

In addition to RING and a PCGF partner, the canonical PRC1 complex contains two other core components (Figure 36). One is the eponymous Polycomb protein, called Pc in *Drosophila*. In mammals, there are five alternative Pc homologs: the CBX proteins CBX2,4,6,7,8. Pc and its homologs contain a chromodomain, which, like the HP1 chromodomain, forms an aromatic pocket that binds trimethyl lysines (Figure 37). In the case of Pc, the lysine in question is histone H3K27, specified by interactions of the histone H3 N-terminal region that fits in a groove in the Pc

Canonical PRC1 complexes

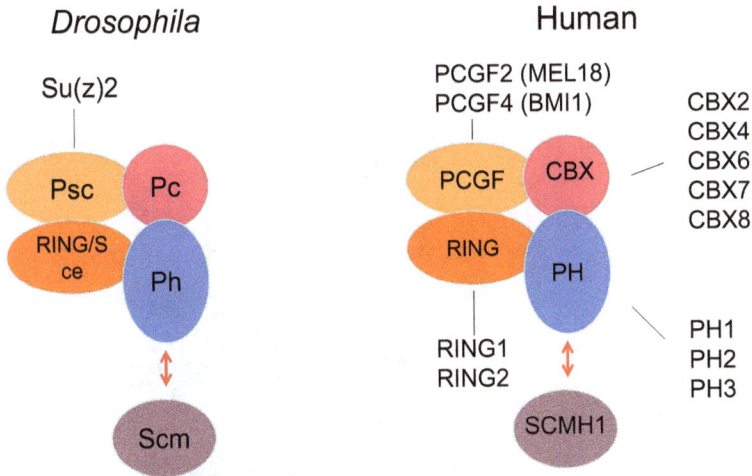

Figure 36. Canonical PRC1 complexes. The canonical *Drosophila* PRC1 complex is shown on the left and the canonical human PRC1 is on the right. By "canonical" it is meant that they contain a chromodomain component: Pc in *Drosophila*, one of the CBX components in the human case. The Scm component plays an important role but is loosely bound and is not a stable component of PRC1.

chromodomain. The specificity for H3K27me3 is much lower in the case of the CBX proteins, which also have high affinity for H3K9me3. The fourth canonical core component is Polyhomeotic (Ph) of which *Drosophila* has two homologs Ph-p and Ph-d while mammals have three (PH1,2,3). The Ph proteins contain a protein–protein interaction domain called the sterile alpha motif (SAM), also known as SPM, which, *in vitro*, mediates the formation of head-to-tail Ph oligomers. In principle, therefore, the Ph subunit can drive the association of many PRC1 complexes and has been said to be responsible for the formation of "Polycomb bodies" in the nucleus. The SAM motif can also interact with a similar domain found in an accessory protein called Sex Comb on Midleg (Scm), which is loosely associated with PRC1 as well as with PRC2. Scm contains a SAM domain as well as two MBT domains (Malignant Brain Tumor, a methyl lysine-binding domain that recognizes mono- and di-methyl lysine). As we will see, the Scm SAM motif turns out to be particularly important for the

Pc chromodomain

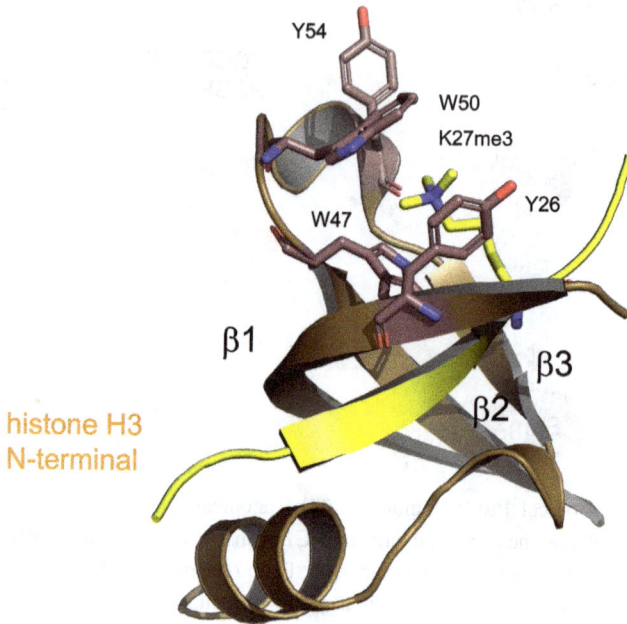

Figure 37.   Pc chromodomain. The structure of the Pc chromodomain is shown here bound to the N-terminal of histone H3K27me3 (in yellow). The lysine K27me3 fits in an aromatic pocket in the chromodomain. The aromatic residues Y26, W47, and W50 form the pocket into which fits the trimethylated nitrogen of K27me3. The N-terminal tail of H3 lies against three β strands forming interactions that help distinguish H3K27me3 from H3K9me3.

Source: Jinrong Min.

recruitment of Polycomb complexes. This combination of components constitutes a canonical PRC1 complex, whose key ability to recognize H3K27me3 links it to the action of the PRC2 complex.

PRC1-like RING complexes that lack a Pc component and therefore do not recognize H3K27me3 are commonly called non-canonical PRC1 complexes (see the following). They are more active ubiquityl transferases than canonical PRC1 and their functions usually depend on the choice of PCGF partner. The only non-canonical PRC1 reported in *Drosophila* contains a PCGF protein called L(3)73Ah and is responsible for much of the H2AK118 ubiquitylation in the fly genome.

Recruitment of Polycomb Complexes to PREs

As mentioned earlier, *Drosophila* PREs contain binding sites for multiple DNA-binding factors, such as GAGA binding Factor (GAF), Dsp1, Combgap (Cg), and Pleiohomeotic (Pho), that are thought to cooperate in recruiting Polycomb complexes although no one of them is found at all PREs and, individually, they are also found at many other non-PRE sites. The most interesting of these factors is Pho, the only one whose mutation causes a substantial weakening of Polycomb repression at many target genes. The Pho C-terminal region containing the DNA binding domain is highly homologous to the mammalian factor YY1. The PRE-binding Pho is in the form of a heterodimeric complex with Sfmbt, a protein containing four MBT domains as well as a SAM domain that interacts with the SAM domain of the PcG protein Scm. The SAM domains of Ph and Scm are able to interact head-to-tail to form homo- or hetero-oligomers. The Sfmbt SAM domain is sufficiently different that it cannot oligomerize. It does, however, interact with one end of the Scm SAM domain while the other end interacts with the Ph SAM domain. In this way, Scm is also a component of PRC1 although more loosely associated (Figure 38). Scm is also

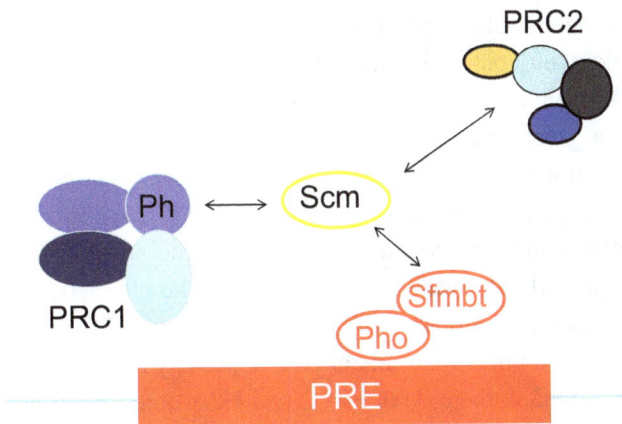

Figure 38. Cooperative binding at the PRE. The recruitment of PcG complexes is highly cooperative. No two PREs have the same sequence or exactly the same DNA-binding factors. These factors also bind individually to many other sites that are not PREs. A frequent PRE co-factor is the DNA-binding protein Pho, complexed with Sfmbt. Sfmbt has a SAM domain that interacts with the SAM domain of Scm, which in turn interacts with the SAM domain of Ph in PRC1. The three help each other bind to the PRE.

associated with PRC2, again more weakly than the core components. In the absence of PRC1 or PRC2, Scm is still found at most PREs, indicating that it has some independent yet unknown way of being recruited at these sites.

Scm is required for most PRC1 binding. It is likely that it serves a vital function by mediating the interactions of the Pho complex with PRC1 and PRC2 and at least one other DNA-binding recruiter and thus acts as the link that helps recruit and stabilize the several complexes. Since Scm interacts with PRC1 and with PRC2 as well as with the Pho complex, this appears to be the critical role of Pho in helping recruit PRC1 and PRC2. In turn, the interaction with Scm and the PRC1 complex helps to stabilize the binding of Pho to the PRE. This seems like a very rickety process and raises the question of why such a seemingly haphazard series of weak interactions have evolved to recruit and assemble the repressive complexes at the target genes. Why not, for example, simply endow a PRC1 component with a specific DNA binding domain to recruit to the PRE? Part of the answer is probably that the recruitment process cannot be so direct because, while Polycomb complexes are present in every cell, many potential target genes must not bind them. The repressive complexes are not recruited if the target gene is transcriptionally active: the recruitment must be made dependent on the chromatin state of the surrounding region. The details of the process that senses the chromatin state are still being worked out but it is clear that direct DNA-binding recruitment would be too blunt a process. At the same time, the recruitment process allows for a great variety of PREs and of detailed pathways of recruitment. For example, in the process just outlined, interventions could occur at different steps. Alternative ways to recruit Scm could cooperate with or bypass entirely the Pho-dependent step. At some sites, PRC2 might be recruited first and help bring in PRC1 through the interaction with Scm.

A key mutual relationship that links PRC1 and PRC2 is indicated in Figure 39. Each complex has an enzymatic activity that deposits a histone mark: H3K27me3 in the case of PRC2 and H2A ubiquitylation in the case of PRC1. Each complex also has a binding activity that recognizes the mark deposited by the other complex: the Pc chromodomain binds H3K27me3 and the AEBP2 and Jarid2 components bind ubiquitylated H2A. Each complex is both a "writer" of a histone mark and a "reader" of the mark written by the other complex. This reciprocal relationship contributes to the stability of the Polycomb-repressed state.

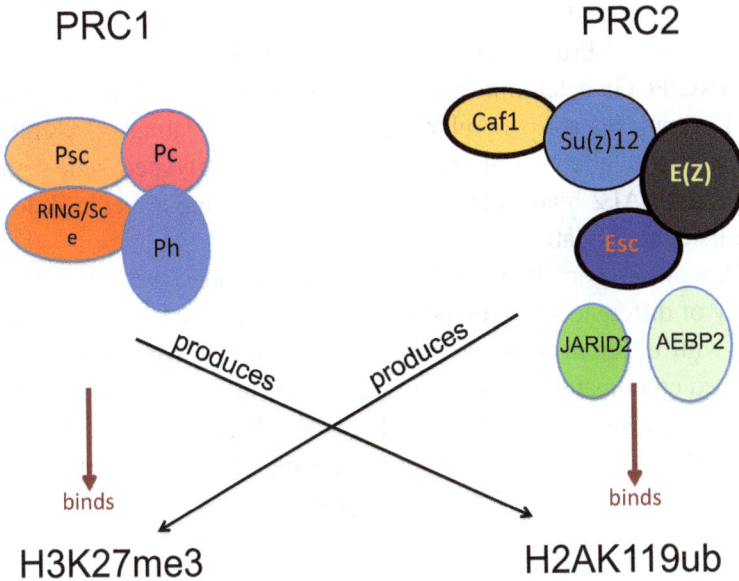

Figure 39. Mutual relationship between PRC1 and PRC2. Each complex is both a "writer" of a histone mark and a "reader" of the mark deposited by other complex.

Mammalian PRC1 Complexes

Mammalian PRC1 complexes are highly homologous to the *Drosophila* PRC1 but much more diversified (Figure 36). There are two RING proteins, RING1 and RING2 (formerly RING1a and RING1b), but RING2 is far more abundant and more active than RING1. Particularly important is a range of six PGCF partners, the choice of which largely determines what other components can be recruited. Two of these, PCGF2 and 4 (also known as MEL18 and BMI1), are the only ones that can assemble canonical PRC1 complexes. These include a CBX chromodomain component (one of CBX2,4,6,7,8); they also contain a PH homolog (one of PHC1,2,3) and a more loosely associated SCM component (one of SCMH1, SCML1, and SCML2). It is not clear what determines the choice of the homologs and how their functions differ but certainly the CBX alternatives vary widely in their specificity and affinity for H3K27me3 (as opposed to H3K9me3). PCGF2 and 4 can also assemble non-canonical PRC1 complexes. These are complexes that lack the chromodomain component as well as the PH and SCM components. They recruit instead RYBP (YY1 and PC-Binding Protein) or its close relative YAF 2 both of which bind to the RING/PCGF heterodimer. The non-canonical RYBP/YAF2-containing PRC1 complexes are particularly active in ubiquitylating H2AK119 and are especially effective at maintaining the ubiquitylated state because RYBP and YAF2 bind to H2AK119ub, thus creating a feedback loop to replenish ubiquitylation after DNA replication.

Complexes containing PCGF1,3,5,6 all include RYBP/YAF2 plus a variety of different other components that are thought to mediate interactions with different genomic sites. The multiplicity of alternatives and observed combinatorial possibilities gives rise to a vast number of variant PRC1 complexes (summarized in Figure 40). These complexes have been named PRC1.1, PRC1.2, etc. depending on which PCGF they utilize. What might be the role of this extensive collection of variants?

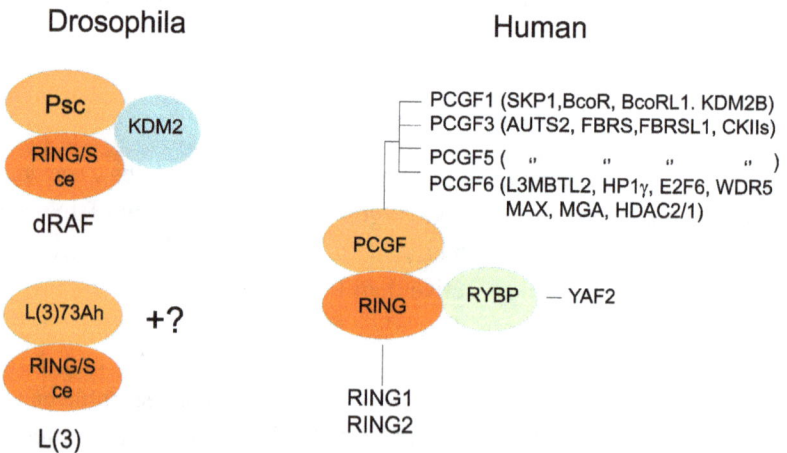

Figure 40.   Variant (non-canonical) PRC1 complexes. These variant complexes lack a chromodomain component but are very efficient at ubiquitinating histone H2A. The *Drosophila* non-canonical complexes are not well characterized but the complex containing L(3)73Qh seems to be responsible for most of the H2AK118 ubiquitylation. The structure of the mammalian non-canonical complexes depends on which PCGF they contain. That choice determines which set of other components they recruit.

It is clear in many cases that different variants might bind to the same genomic region. To begin to understand the roles played by these variants, we need to consider how Polycomb complexes are recruited to target sites in mammals. Intensive searches for mammalian PREs have shown that regulatory elements that behave like *Drosophila* PREs are rare in mammals and that the prevalent mode of recruitment is different. Although mammals have preserved SCM and MBT-containing proteins and the mammalian YY1 shares the C-terminal DNA-binding domain with *Drosophila* Pho, the interactions among these proteins have not been conserved. There is little relationship between YY1 and PRC1-binding sites in the mammalian genome and it is unlikely that YY1 plays a role similar to that of *Drosophila* Pho in helping recruitment. Instead, the majority of Polycomb complex binding sites correspond to CpG islands, regions of roughly 1 kb, high in CpG content that act as promoter regions for most regulated genes. In fact, it was soon found that any region with high CpG content will bind Polycomb complexes. Many transcription and regulatory factors bind to CpG islands through a modified zinc finger called the CXXC domain (see Chapter 3). A connection between CpG islands and some PRC1 complexes was made through KDM2B, a histone H3K36 demethylase that contains a CXXC domain. KDM2B is a component of the variant PRC1 complex called PRC1.1, assembled through the PCGF1 partner of RING (Figure 41). In principle, therefore all CpG islands are

The human variant PRC1.1 complex

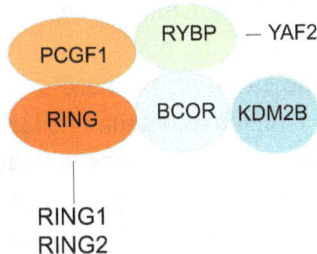

Figure 41.   The PRC1.1 complex. PCGF1 recruits BCOR, which in turn binds KDM2B, a H3K36 demethylase.

potential targets for PRC1.1 unless the chromatin is DNA methylated, pre-empted by binding other factors, or modified by transcriptional activity. In fact, blocking RNA Pol II activity is often sufficient to recruit PRC1 to CpG islands. It is clear therefore that, in general, genes must be turned off by specific regulators before Polycomb mechanisms can be established to maintain the silent state.

Once PRC1.1 is bound, a series of events have been shown to result in the recruitment of PRC2, of the canonical PRC1 complexes, and of stable Polycomb repression (Figure 42). The process begins with the ubiquitylation of histone H2AK119 in the CpG island by PRC1.1. The affinity of the PRC2 accessory components JARID2 and AEBP2 for H2A K119ub brings in PRC2 and its H3K27 trimethylation activity. The H3K27me3 in turn helps recruit canonical PRC1 complexes (containing the CBX chromodomain Polycomb homologs), which help extend and maintain the H3K27me3 domain. Whether this series of recruitment events depending on affinity for modified histones are sufficient to account for the formation of stable repressive states is not entirely clear but it is evident that it is at least part of the process that recruits Polycomb repression to a large number of genes. Recent results are not yet well digested into a coherent mechanistic model. They show that, at least in embryonic stem cells, loss of PRC2 does not result in gene derepression nor does loss of canonical PRC1. In these cells, PRC2 binds primarily to inactive promoters (the so-called bivalent promoters) (see Stem Cells). Most of the repressive activity in these cells is due to PRC1.1 and its ubiquitylating activity. Other experiments indicate, however, that both PRC2 and canonical PRC1 are needed for correct differentiation although at some genes either one is sufficient for repression. For recruitment, like the interaction of the CBX chromodomain with H3K27me3, the binding of PRC2 to ubiquitylated H2AK119 is not an absolute criterion. We need to take into account the fact that not all chromatin regions containing H3K27me3 bind PRC1 complexes and not all chromatin containing ubiquitylated H2A binds PRC2. There are in fact some chromatin regions that bind one Polycomb complex but not the other. What additional features are involved is not yet clear.

Current evidence suggests that some of the other variant PRC1s may function in a similar way though with different specificities. For example, PRC1.6, assembled with PCGF6, is targeted by specific transcription

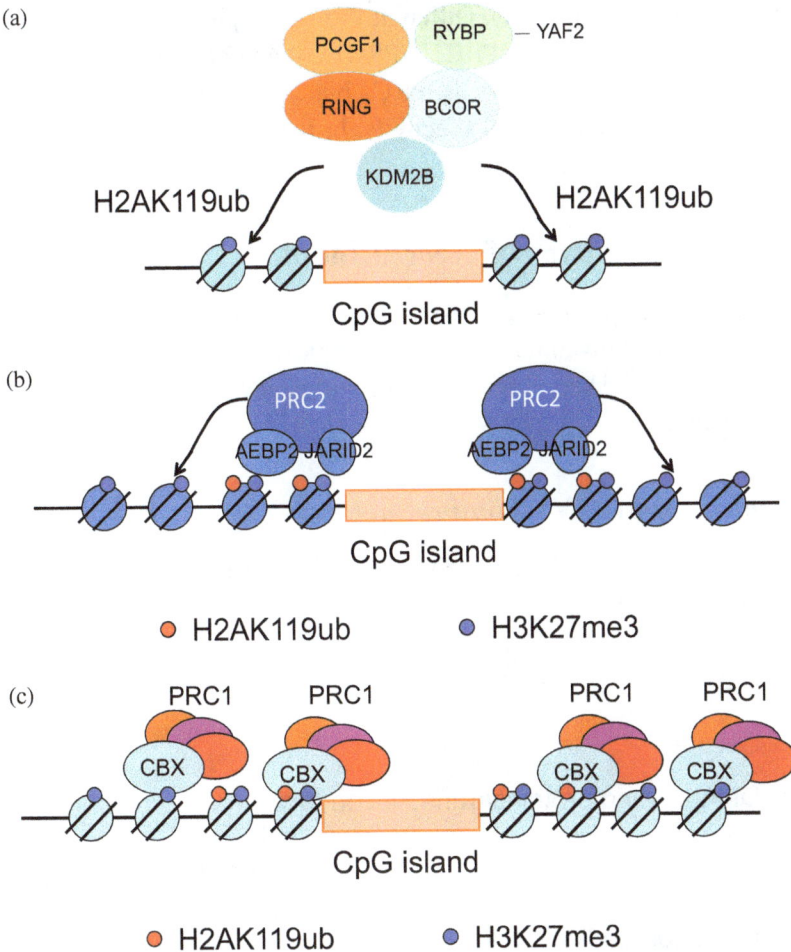

Figure 42. Targeting of Polycomb repression by variant PRC1 complexes. (a) Recruitment of PRC1.1 through the binding of KDM2B to CpG islands allows it to ubiquitylate histone H2A flanking regions. (b) Interaction with H2AK119ub allows the PRC2 complex to stay long enough to trimethylate H3K27. (c) The H3K27me3 is thought to recruit the canonical PRC1 through the chromodomain-containing CBX component.

Source: Blackledge *et al.* (2014).

factors MAX and MGA to germ cell-related genes in pluripotent embryonic stem cells. PCGF3 and PCGF5 assemble identical complexes with the same functional properties and are implicated in the recruitment of Polycomb silencing in the course of mammalian X chromosome inactivation (see Chapter 11). Different PRC1 complexes may bind to the same genes. This is true of PRC1.1/PRC1.2,4 and of PRC1.1/PRC1.2,4/ PRC1.6. In embryonic stem cells, PRC2 binds to CpG islands by default, unless prevented by RNA pol II activity. In fact, inhibiting RNA pol II is sufficient to recruit PRC2.

Other Mechanisms of Recruitment

Certain specific genomic processes have developed alternative mechanisms to recruit Polycomb repressive complexes. Some of these will be briefly summarized here (Figure 43) and will be invoked more specifically in later chapters.

Recruitment by DNA-binding factors

In some cases, DNA-binding complexes have been shown to act as recruiters of Polycomb complexes. Best known as a PRC-recruiting

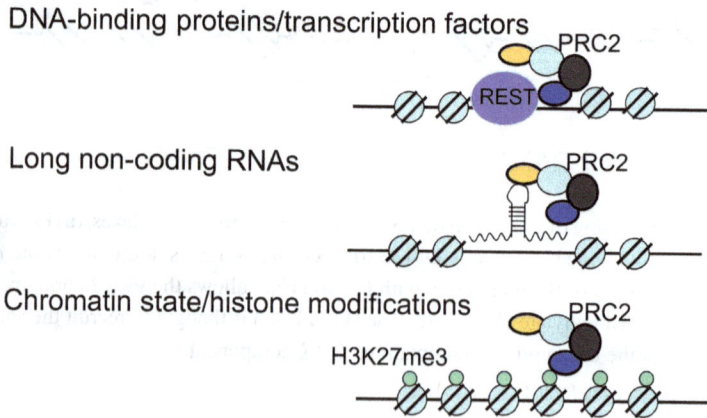

Figure 43.   Other PRC-recruiting mechanisms. Certain genes have acquired specific recruiting mechanisms such as association with specific DNA-binding proteins, for example, the REST factor. Long non-coding RNAs have been found to recruit PRC2 and in some cases also PRC1 complexes. Chromatin marks such as H3K27me3 can help bind PRC2 and canonical PRC1.

complex is probably the inhibitor of neuronal differentiation REST (RE1-Silencing Factor, also known as Neuron-Restrictive Silencer Factor NRSF). REST is a zinc finger factor that binds to a specific sequence called RE1 and represses pro-neural genes to prevent cells from entering the neural differentiation pathway. Chromatin regions containing a REST consensus binding sequence recruit both PRC1 and PRC2 and acquire H3K27 trimethylation.

Recruitment by lncRNAs

A recruiting mechanism whose importance is becoming increasingly apparent is one that employs long non-coding RNAs (lncRNAs). These are RNAs several hundred to several thousand nucleotides long and generally lacking significant open reading frames. lncRNAs have regulatory functions, often at the site of transcription where the nascent RNA binds protein complexes and regulates the surrounding chromatin. We will encounter many such lncRNAs in association with imprinted genes. A similar case is that of the *Xist* RNA, which controls mammalian X chromosome inactivation. A lncRNA of particular importance, because it involves a locus that regulates cell proliferation and is frequently mutated in cancer, is that of the *ANRIL* lncRNA and the *Ink4/Arf* locus (Figure 44). This complex locus encodes three distinct polypeptides: p16/CDKN2A, p15/CDKN2B, and p14/ARF. The first two are inhibitors of cyclin-dependent protein kinases and their expression blocks cell cycle progression and cell proliferation. p14/ARF has similar effects through a different pathway promoting the tumor suppressor p53. The three proteins have therefore similar effects in blocking cell proliferation. The locus produces also a lncRNA called ANRIL or rather a family of lncRNAs since the transcript is differentially spliced. Nascent ANRIL binds Polycomb complexes PRC1 and PRC2, causing the silencing of the entire locus, thus releasing the block to cell proliferation and allowing tumor growth.

How Polycomb Repression is Effected

This is still a hotly debated but unresolved question, despite many years of research, perhaps because there is not just one single mechanism of

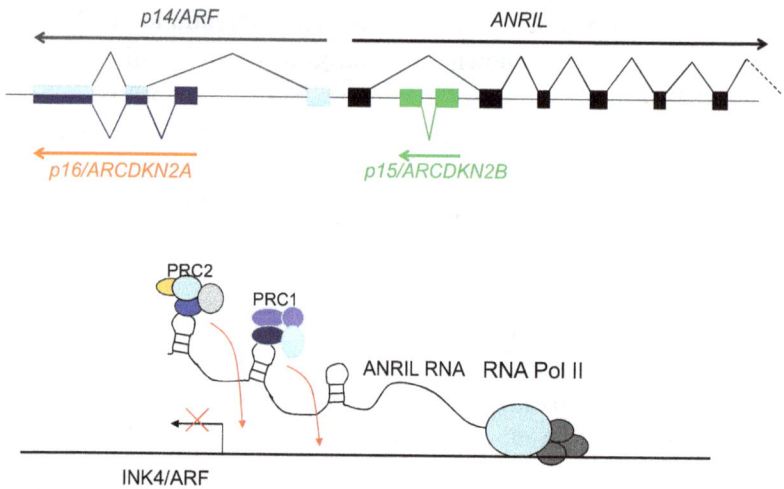

Figure 44.   Controlling cell proliferation. An important way to control proliferation is to prevent cell cycle progression by blocking the cyclin-dependent kinases. The INK4/ARF locus produces three proteins that do just this. Expression of the INK4A, INK4B, and ARF proteins arrests proliferation. Repression of the INK4/ARF locus promotes proliferation. They are therefore known as tumor suppressors. Their expression produces cellular senescence. A lncRNA called ANRIL is also transcribed from this locus. Nascent ANRIL RNA recruits both PRC1 and PRC2 complexes and represses the INK4 and ARF genes.

Polycomb repression (Figure 45). A common view is that Polycomb repression causes chromatin condensation and thereby prevents the binding of transcription factors and RNA polymerase. This is a holdover from the early days when heterochromatic silencing and Polycomb silencing were viewed as a process of coating and packaging chromatin in a way that rendered it impervious and inaccessible to transcription factors. More recent versions of this idea invoke the formation of liquid phase condensates that partition the chromatin into an inactive domain that prevents the entry of transcriptional activators. The tendency to form Polycomb aggregates in the nucleus is clearly demonstrable and it is also clear that, to some extent, this enhances Polycomb action and its silencing effects. We have already seen this in discussing pairing and proximity effects. Formation of aggregates is often thought to be a consequence of the ability of the SAM domain of the PH component of PRC1 to form head-to-tail oligomers. This is possible but the evidence for it is poor since, as we have

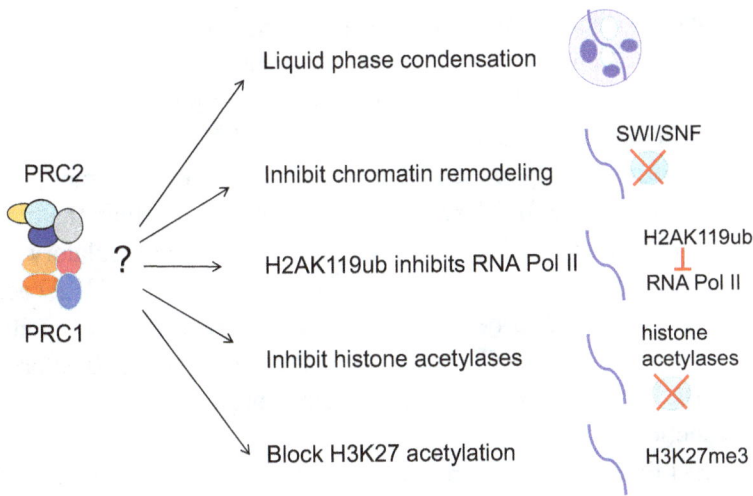

Figure 45. Mechanisms proposed for Polycomb silencing. These mechanisms act on the chromatin fiber and are not mutually exclusive.

seen, this domain is necessary for interaction with the SCM component and for recruitment. Therefore, disrupting this domain may prevent formation of aggregates but also of recruitment and therefore is not good evidence for the formation of aggregates.

Recent evidence shows that, although the density of Polycomb-repressed chromatin is somewhat higher than that of active chromatin, this is probably not sufficient to account for silencing and may be simply caused by the lack of transcriptional activity. *In vitro*, purified PRC1 complex inhibits the SWI/SNF nucleosome remodeling complex, which could prevent the access of activators and contribute to transcriptional silencing. However, *Drosophila* PREs, the major sites of PRC complex binding, are not themselves inaccessible; they are in fact DNase hypersensitive and sites of strong nucleosome turnover. *In vivo*, Polycomb repression does not prevent the binding of transcription factors and RNA pol II to a promoter but does prevent transcription initiation or elongation. This implies that Polycomb silencing involves some more specific action rather than just chromatin density.

Histone H2AK119 ubiquitylation by PRC1 has also been proposed to inhibit RNA polymerase but the evidence that this is a major mechanism of repression is inconclusive. There is, however, evidence that the ubiquitylating PRC1.1 complex can repress transcription. Clearly, however, if H2AK119ub recruits PRC2, ubiquitylation is an important contributor to repression. *Drosophila* Pc and its mammalian CBX homologs have been reported to bind directly to the CBP/p300 acetylases, the enzymes primarily responsible for H3K27 acetylation, thereby preventing their auto-acetylation. This auto-acetylation is part of an autoregulatory loop necessary to promote CBP/p300 enzymatic activity. In fact, H3K27 acetylation has been found to be closely involved in enhancer activation and promoter access (see also Chapter 6). By inhibiting CBP/p300 autoacetylation, PRC1 complexes would consequently prevent enhancer and promoter function.

Several lines of evidence point to H3K27 methylation as a major factor in Polycomb repression, possibly not just by helping to recruit PRC1. Any methylation of H3K27 would prevent its acetylation and, in fact, H3K27me2 or H3K27me3 is found at all transcriptionally inactive chromatin. Preventing H3K27 methylation increases the level of transcripts from all intergenic regions and inactive genes. It is clear that H3K27 methylation interferes with mechanisms that promote access to chromatin and transcriptional activity. Therefore, it appears that both PRC1 and PRC2 interfere with the access to and function of enhancers and promoters. Little has been reported in recent years about the involvement of histone deacetylases although loss of acetylation is a clear concomitant of Polycomb silencing. Overall, although we have many possible features that could contribute to transcriptional silencing, it has to be admitted that no convincing comprehensive account is yet available.

Additional Hints

More recent investigations of genes that modify Polycomb silencing in *Drosophila* have produced some additional hints about how they function. One set of mutations helped define another protein complex that is needed for efficient silencing of the homeotic genes of the Bithorax Complex. Surprisingly, this complex, containing the Calypso and Asx proteins, and its mammalian counterpart, containing the BAP1 deubiquitinase and the

ASXL1 or ASXL2 proteins, deubiquitinate histone H2A. This is unexpected and counterintuitive. In fact, however, while most Polycomb target genes are marked by H2AK119ub (H2AK118ub in *Drosophila*), deubiquitination is actually required for effective Polycomb silencing of some target genes. In *Drosophila*, the abdominal Hox genes *Ubx, abd-A,* and *Abd*-B are not ubiquitinated and Calypso mutations impair their repression by Polycomb. It is not clear why ubiquitination has to be removed at these genes for effective silencing: other Polycomb target genes, including other homeotic genes, are ubiquitinated when silenced. This clearly demonstrates that H2AK119 ubiquitination is not always required for silencing but leaves much to be explained.

Another activity that contributes to Polycomb silencing is that of the O-GlcNAc transferase OGT1. This enzyme adds an N-acetylglucosamine to hydroxyls of serine or threonine. In mammals, it is associated with the deubiquitinase complex. Several proteins are known to be substrates of this activity and it is not known which is the relevant target. Most suggestive, however, is the fact that the PH SAM domain is a target in *Drosophila* and in mammals. The acetylglucosamination blocks the head-to-tail polymerization of PH and therefore regulates the tendency of PRC1 complexes to form aggregates. This could be interpreted to mean that a little aggregation might be good but too much is countereffective for transcriptional silencing.

Derepression: H3K27 Demethylases

Another way to counter Polycomb repression is by erasing the H3K27 methylation marks. Two H3K27 demethylases are known in mammals, UTX and JMJD3, but only Utx in *Drosophila*. The two enzymes are at least partially redundant in their effects on target genes and on global H3K27me3 levels. These demethylases can reactivate genes repressed by Polycomb mechanisms when H3K27 methylation is decreased. Particularly important, however, are the global activities of UTX (Ubiquitously Transcribed tetratricopeptide repeat, X chromosome) and its non-enzymatic roles. *In vitro*, UTX is much more active in demethylating H3K27me1 and me2 and much slower against H3K27me3. In fact, it plays a much more general role in removing the mono- and di-methyl-ation that is otherwise pervasive in chromatin. This methylation needs to be removed in order to allow acetylation of H3K27 by CBP/p300 at enhancers, promoters, and transcription units. The *Utx* gene, as its name implies, is on the human X chromosome but it escapes silencing in the inactive X copy in females. Remarkably, a *Utx* homolog is found on the pseudoautosomal region of the human Y chromosome (the short region of residual homology between X and Y chromosomes) and is therefore called *Uty*. The product of the *Uty* gene, UTY, although 83% identical in amino acid sequence to UTX, has lost H3K27 demethylase activity. Surprisingly, however, it is able to partially complement the loss of *Utx* in embryonic development. This paradoxical result is due to the involve-ment of UTX/UTY in some important chromatin complexes that require their presence but not their enzymatic activity. One of these is the com-plex that includes MLL3/4, the enzyme that methylates histone H3K4 to poise enhancers for activation (see the following).

Derepression: The Phospho-Switch

We have seen that histone H3K27 methylation is important for Polycomb repression at least in part by binding the chromodomain of Pc protein or its mammalian Cbx homologs. As was first noted by Strahl and Allis in 2000, the methylation site H3K27 as well as the methylation site that marks heterochromatic silencing, H3K9, are followed by a serine residue (Figure 46). They pointed out that phosphorylation of H3S10 or of H3S28

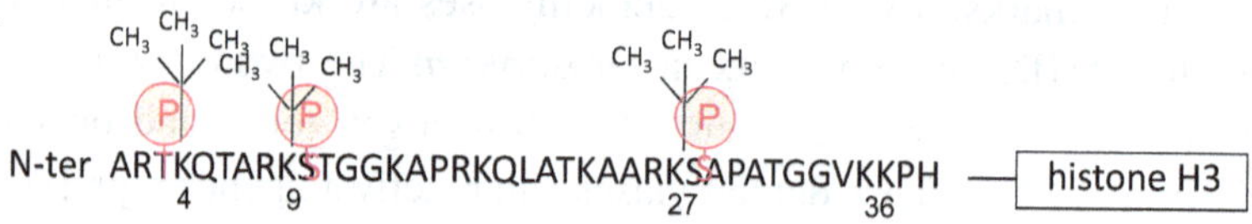

Figure 46. The phospho-switch. All three major methylation targets on the histone H3 N-ter tail, K4, K9, and K27 are immediately next to a phosphorylatable residue, serine or threonine. It is evident that the large, negatively charged phosphate interferes with recogni-tion of the trimethyl lysine by a chromodomain or PHD finger protein. Hence, phospho-rylation of the flanking amino acid prevents recognition of the methyl mark. This is a quick and flexible way to switch off the effect of the methyl mark without removing it.

would be likely to prevent the binding of the respective chromodomain proteins HP1 or Pc to the trimethylated lysine. Even the HK4 methylation site is immediately preceded by a potential phosphorylation target: threonine. Therefore, such phosphorylation would result in derepression of chromatin silenced by heterochromatic or Polycomb mechanisms and could be used as a switch for rapidly reactivating silenced genes. An example of this reactivation occurs upon stress signaling, when the MSK1/2 kinase phosphorylates histone H3S28 at stress-induced genes, displacing Polycomb complexes and reactivating gene expression. We do not know at this point how phosphorylation of H3S28 or of H3S10 is targeted, or how it reactivates silenced gene expression but this clearly is another mechanism to modulate two major chromatin silencing activities.

Trithorax and Anti-repressive Functions

We have seen that Polycomb mechanisms essentially maintain the silent state and are in general not able to initiate silencing of an active gene. In fact, the active state antagonizes the recruitment of PcG complexes through histone marks that inhibit the Polycomb hallmarks: H2A ubiquitylation and H3K27 methylation. Mechanisms that promote transcriptional activity are natural antagonists of Polycomb repression. The first gene to be identified as such was the *Drosophila trithorax* (*trx*) gene. The first mutation was identified by Ed Lewis in the 1960s and named *Regulator of bithorax* (*Rg-bx*). It was first characterized by Phil Ingham in 1983, who found independently a weak mutation that allowed the survival of flies showing partial transformation of the third and, to a lesser extent, the first thoracic segment towards the second thoracic segment. This phenotype was the opposite of that shown by *Polycomb* mutations: it caused decreased homeotic gene expression and, in fact, heterozygous *trx* mutations combined with heterozygous *Pc* mutations restored an almost normal phenotype. Analysis of mutant clones showed that not only homeotic genes were affected but also other genes such as *engrailed* that were known to be subject to Polycomb regulation. The *trx* product appeared to be necessary for such genes to maintain their activity and resist Polycomb repression.

In the 1980s and 1990s, systematic genetic screens were undertaken in *Drosophila* for activities that aggravated or improved the phenotypes of *Polycomb* or *Antennapedia* mutations. These screens revealed more than a dozen genes that were grouped with Trithorax under the name of Trithorax Group (TrxG) genes. Some of these genes encode components of the Trithorax complex or related complexes. Most TrxG proteins, unlike PcG proteins, are not functionally related in the sense of being involved in the same biochemical process. However, they are all involved in processes that facilitate transcriptional activity and, as such, they antagonize the effects of PcG activities on target genes. Among these are components of chromatin remodeling complexes such as Brahma (the *Drosophila* SWI/SNF homolog), required to make promoters and enhancers available. Some, like Trl/GAF or Mod(mdg4), are involved in chromatin conformation and architecture needed to bring enhancers to bear on promoter (see Chapter 8). In this discussion, we will focus only on those that are either components of Trithorax complexes or, Like Ash1, work in partnership with them.

What prevents active genes that are potential Polycomb targets from recruiting Polycomb complexes? The relationship between TrxG and PcG activities may be summarized as follows. A subset of genes, those containing a PRE in *Drosophila* and most CpG islands in mammals, can recruit Polycomb complexes provided they are not transcriptionally active or DNA methylated. TrxG functions produce epigenetic chromatin modifications that promote and maintain transcriptional activity and prevent the recruitment of PcG complexes. Different TrxG complexes accomplish this in different ways: Trithorax by methylating H3K4 and Swi/Snf by remodeling nucleosomes.

Drosophila Trithorax is a large protein (3726 amino acids) containing a SET domain and related to the Set1 protein first identified in budding yeast and the complex it forms was first characterized and named COMPASS (Complex Proteins Associated with Set1). Descendants of the yeast Set1 (*Drosophila* dSet1, mammalian SET1A, and SET1B) are still normally recruited by RNA Pol II to trimethylate H3K4 and facilitate transcription. They are responsible for most of the total H3K4me3 in the genome. *Drosophila* Trithorax and Trithorax-related (Trr) and their mammalian homologs, respectively, MLL1 and MLL2 and MLL3 and MLL4, assemble related COMPASS complexes that do not associate with RNA Pol II (Figure 47). The MLL1 and MLL2 complexes have functions similar to those of Trx in antagonizing Polycomb repression. At least in embryonic stem cells, MLL2 is required to trimethylate H3K4 at bivalent promoters while MLL1 acts at a small subset of genes that includes the HOX clusters. In contrast, Trr and mammalian MLL3 and 4 are involved in mono- and di-methylation of H3K4 at poised or active enhancers. How these complexes are recruited and what distinguishes the functions of MLL1 from MLL2 or MLL3 from MLL4 is unclear. The MLL name stands for Mixed-Lineage Leukemia not because this is the result of their loss of function but because MLL1 was first discovered in leukemias induced by MLL1 involvement in gene fusions in which the MLL N-ter region is fused to one of more than 70 different partners, usually transcriptional regulators. The resulting leukemias share features of both myeloid and lymphoid cancers, hence the name mixed-lineage leukemias.

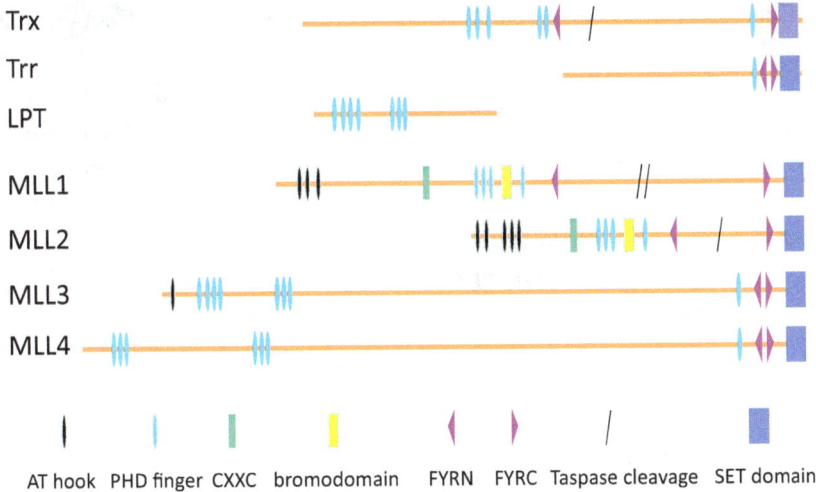

Figure 47. Structure of Trithorax, Trr, and MLL proteins. The different structural and functional domains are indicated. The Taspase cleavage sites are sites of proteolytic cleavage by Taspase, which cuts the Trx/MLL protein into a C-ter and an N-ter domain. The two remain associated through the FYRN and FYRC interaction domains. The *Drosophila* Trr protein has evolutionarily been separated into two nearby genes, which produce the Trr and LPT proteins. The two proteins, however, associate to reconstitute an MLL3-like structure.

The COMPASS complexes contain a core group of constituents essential for the enzymatic activity of their Trx component (Figure 48). This core consists of WDR5, RBBP5, DPY30, and ASH2 (called Wds, Rbbp5, Dpy30, and Ash2 in *Drosophila*). The first two are WD repeat proteins, so often involved in activities affecting nucleosomal histones. In fact, we have already encountered RBBP5 as a component of the PRC2 complex. ASH2 or rather its *Drosophila* homolog Ash2 was identified in a screen for functions required for normal development of imaginal discs. Its name derives from the loss of function phenotype of Absent, Small, or Homeotic discs, indicative of excessive silencing of Hox genes. It is not structurally related to Ash1, identified in the same screen, which we will discuss further down. Additional factors in the Trx and MLL1,2 complexes are HSF1 and MENIN, whose role is not clear. The Trr and MLL3,4 complexes include several additional proteins of which the most significant is the H3K27 demethylase UTX, which is essential for the function of the complex.

In *Drosophila*, loss of function of Trx has only a small effect on total H3K4 methylation. This implies that Trx must affect only a subset of genes. This subset appears to be genes that are regulated by Polycomb mechanisms. Trx is found in fact at all known *Drosophila* PREs, irrespective of whether they also bind PcG complexes or are in their repressive or active state. Trx appears therefore to be independently and constitutively recruited by PREs. In Polycomb target genes that are in the active state, Trx also binds to the promoter of the associated gene and is found also along the transcription unit. It is not known whether it moves along with

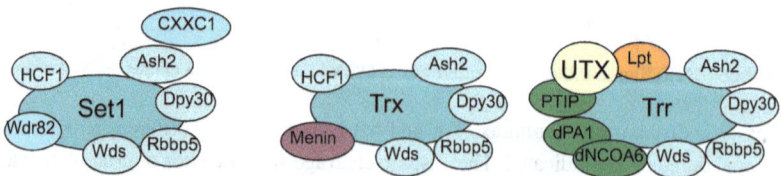

Figure 48.   Relationships among the Drosophila COMPASS complexes. Note that Wdr82 in the Set1 complex binds to RNA Pol II. Menin in the Trx complex binds to chromatin. UTX in the Trr complex is the histone H3K27 demethylase.

Source: Mohan *et al.* (2011).

the RNA Pol II but it is not physically associated with it. Whether it methylates H3K4 at the promoter has not been established, since in active genes the dSet1 complex is also associated with the polymerase. It is likely, however, that it is active in methylating H3K4 since it was found to produce H3K4me2 at the PRE. In addition, the mammalian MLL2 complex trimethylates the promoter of bivalent genes in embryonic stem cells although these genes are not actively transcribed. Both MLL1 and MLL2 contain a CXXC domain that binds to CpG-rich regions like CpG island promoters and is key to the generation of bivalent domains in embryonic stem cells. H3K4me3 antagonizes DNA methylation, promotes histone acetylation, and ultimately helps recruit chromatin remodeling machines such as the SWI/SNF complex. Nucleosome remodeling has been shown to not only open, remove, and displace nucleosomes but also to remove DNA-binding proteins that stand in their way. Suitably recruited, they could therefore interfere with the recruitment or the binding of Polycomb proteins. Although the mechanism has not been dissected, the SWI/SNF complex can both prevent the binding of Polycomb complexes *in vitro* and displace previously bound PcG complexes. In fact, systematic screens in embryonic stem cells have shown that the H3K4 methylating activity of MLL1,2 is not strictly essential to promote transcription but is needed to antagonize the repressive effects of DNA methylation, promoter occlusion, and Polycomb repression. If these are relieved by knockout or knockdown, transcription is restored even without the need for MLL1,2.

A separate activity that appears to be closely involved with Trx is that of Ash1 and its mammalian counterpart ASH1L. Like Trx, Ash1 is recruited to derepressed Polycomb target genes. It is not clear whether Trx recruits Ash1 but the two do not associate molecularly. Nevertheless, Ash1 is required for effective transcription of the derepressed genes. Ash1 also contains a SET domain and in fact it methylates H3K36 all along the transcription unit, where it either associates with or follows the RNA Pol II as it transcribes through the gene. The activity of Ash1 also results in extensive H3K27 acetylation by the CBP acetylase along the transcription unit. At this stage, it is not known whether Ash1 or the H3K36 dimethylation recruits CBP. H3K36 methylation inhibits PRC2, thus preventing H3K27 methylation and opening the way for H3K27 acetylation. Combined with the action of the Trx/COMPASS complex, these Ash1 activities could account for the anti-silencing functions that prevent Polycomb complexes from repressing their targets once they are activated by their appropriate enhancer factors.

Trr/MLL3,4 and Enhancer Activation

Unlike Trx, Trr and its mammalian homologs MLL3,4 do not trimethylate H3K4 but mono- and di-methylate it. While MLL1 and 2 have partly redundant functions, MLL3 and 4 have entirely different functions that have more to do with enhancer accessibility and activation. A totally inactive enhancer is packaged into nucleosomes and generally not accessible to most DNA-binding proteins. When an enhancer is to be activated, it has to be made readily accessible to many enhancer factors and activating proteins. The process generally starts with a "pioneer" factor. Pioneer factors are a particular kind of DNA-binding protein that can find a toe-hold in nucleosomal DNA by a variety of strategies. Some bind through an HMG domain that bends DNA sharply, widening the minor groove and binding a reduced target sequence. Some use a winged helix DNA-binding domain that mimics the linker histone H1. By one or another strategy, pioneer factors serve as the initial entry into a nucleosome-packaged enhancer sequence and therefore as the prime activators to initiate new gene expression and cell-fate changes. The process continues when other factors interact with the pioneer factor and initiate chromatin changes. Typical is the recruitment of the CBP/p300 histone acetylase that acetylates histone H3K27. CBP and p300 contain domains that interact with an extraordinary variety of transcription factors (Figure 49). They can also recruit chromatin remodeling machines. This is facilitated by acetylation of H3K27. However, they are unable to acetylate previously inactive chromatin, which is dimethylated at H3K27 by the roaming PRC2 complex. Here is where Trr/MLL3,4 enter the picture. Poised enhancers bind Trr/MLL3,4 and are monomethylated at H3K4. It is not clear what recruits them but their involvement must begin after an initial partial opening of chromatin by pioneer factors or CBP/p300. Attention has been focused on the role of the H3K4me1 although it is not known what reads this mark. Loss of Trr or of MLL3,4 affects many features of enhancers. It causes loss of binding of CBP/p300 acetylases and therefore loss of H3K27ac,

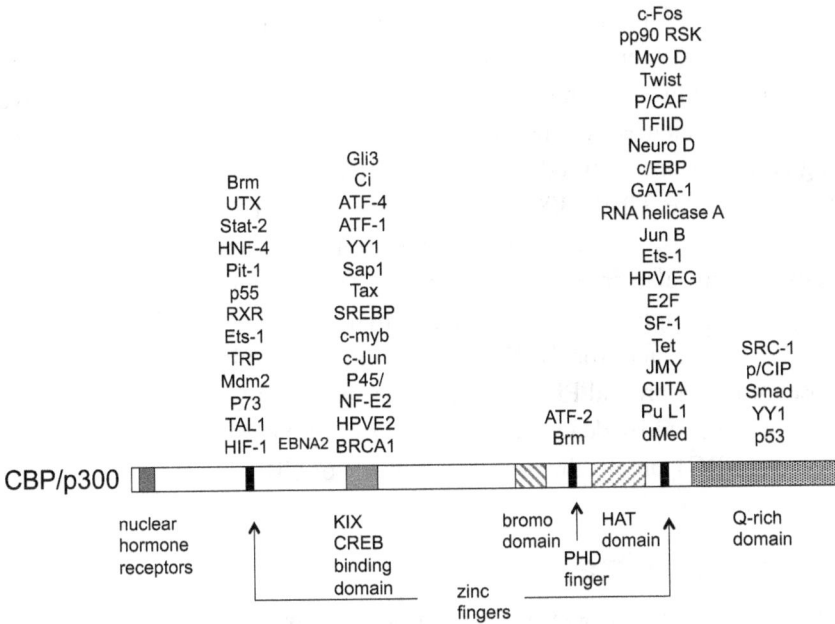

Figure 49.   Structure of the CBP/p300 acetylases. The binding sites of a large number of transcription factors are indicated.

loss of Mediator, loss of cohesin, and loss of enhancer transcription. There is also loss of contacts between enhancer and promoter, which could be attributed to the loss of cohesin and Mediator. Puzzling at first was the fact that mutations that only inactivated the catalytic activity of MLL3,4 did not have these drastic effects, provided the structural integrity of the protein and its ability to form the normal multiprotein complex were not affected. A partial explanation for this was suggested by the structure of the complex. In both flies and mammals, one important constituent of the complex is the UTX demethylase. This suggests that the H3K27 demethylation function of the complex is at least as important as the H3K4 methylation activity. This insight could also be turned around to account for the function of catalytically inactive UTY or UTX mutants that do not cause entire loss of MLL3,4 activities provided the UTX protein is still able to participate in the assembly of the MLL3,4 COMPASS complex.

   The combined action of K3K4me1 and the UTX demethylase activity, together with nucleosome removal by remodeling activities, results in loss of the H3K27 methylation, replacement by H3K27 acetylation, more active displacement of nucleosomes, and access to more DNA binding sites for additional enhancer factors. This is the state of the active enhancer. Enhancers are not the only places where these chromatin opening activities are required. A similar course of events takes place at promoters, where CBP/p300, Trr/MLL3,4, and UTX activities are also involved in promoter activation. Although it may seem paradoxical, these activities are also implicated in making *Drosophila* PREs accessible to Polycomb complexes. PREs are in fact major binding sites for *Drosophila* CBP, for Trr, and for H3K4me1. However, no histone acetylation is observed at or around PREs, possibly because it only occurs initially and is then removed by deacetylases brought in by Polycomb complexes and because PRC1 blocks the acetylase activity of CBP.

Further Reading

Blackledge NP, Farcas AM, Kondo T, King HW, McGouran JF, Hanssen LLP *et al.* (2014). Variant PRC1 complex-dependent H2A ubiquitylation drives PRC2 recruitment and Polycomb domain formation. *Cell.* **157**, 1445–1459.

Buchwald G, van der Stoop P, Weichenrieder O, Perrakis A, van Lohuizen M and Sixma TK (2006). Structure and E3-ligase activity of the Ring-Ring complex of Polycomb proteins Bmi1 and Ring1b. *EMBO J.* **25**, 2465–2474.

Davis AP, Witte DP, Hsieh-Li HM, Potter SS and Capecchi MR. (1995). Absence of radius and ulna in mice lacking *hoxa-11* and *hoxd-11. Nature.* **375**, 791–795.

Duboule D (2007). The rise and fall of Hox gene clusters. *Development.* **134**, 2549–2560.

Garcia-Fernandez J (2005). The genesis and evolution of homeobox gene clusters. *Nat Rev Genet.* **6**, 881–892.

Goodman RH and Smolik S (2000). CBP/p300 in cell growth, transformation, and development. *Genes Dev.* **14**, 1553–1577.

Lee H-G, Kahn TG, Simcox A, Schwartz YB and Pirrotta V (2015). Genome-wide activities of Polycomb complexes control pervasive transcription. *Genome Res.* **25**, 1170–1181.

Lemons D and McGinnis W (2006). Genomic evolution of Hox gene clusters. *Science.* **313**, 1918–1922.

Maeda RK and Karch F (2006). The ABC of the BX-C: The bithorax complex explained. *Development.* **133**, 11413–11422.

Margueron R, Justin N, Ohno K, Sharpe ML, Son J, Drury III WJ *et al.* (2009). Role of the polycomb protein EED in the propagation of repressive histone marks. *Nature.* **461**, 762–767.

Mohan M., Herz H-M, Smith ER, Zhang Y, Jackson J, Washburn MP *et al.* (2011). The COMPASS Family of H3K4 Methylases in *Drosophila. Mol Cell Biol.* **31**, 4310–4318.

Qin S, Li L and Min J (2017). The chromodomain of Polycomb: Methylation reader and beyond. In: *Polycomb Group Proteins*, V. Pirrotta, ed. Boston: Elsevier Inc., pp. 33–56.

Schuettengruber B, Bourbon H-M, Di Croce L and Cavalli G (2017). Genome regulation by Polycomb and Trithorax: 70 years and counting. *Cell.* **171**, 34–57.

Schwartz YB and Pirrotta V (2007). Polycomb silencing mechanisms and the management of genomic programmes. *Nat Rev Genet.* **8**, 9–22.

Smith ER, Lee MG, Winter B, Droz NM, Eissenberg JC, Shiekhattar R *et al.* (2008). *Drosophila* UTX is a histone H3 Lys27 demethylase that colocalizes with the elongating form of RNA polymerase II. *Mol Cell Biol.* **28**, 1041–1046.

Struhl G (1981). A gene product required for correct initiation of segmental determination in *Drosophila. Nature.* **293**, 36–41.

Chapter 8

Genome Architecture

Introduction

Classical views of the genome considered it to be a linear continuum with no region blocked off from other regions or closely apposed to other regions. The genome was clearly tightly folded in the nucleus but architectural considerations were not implicated in gene function. Widely accepted models for enhancer function began to require a degree of local looping, but this could be accounted for by local random movements. Soon, however, many observations began to indicate that where genes were located in the genome and, in particular, their topological relationship to other genes or genomic features made a difference in the way they were expressed. In the genome, genes are unevenly distributed. Certain regions are crowded with genes, while others are sparsely populated. We know that in many cases enhancers important for the function of certain genes can be located tens and even hundreds of kb away from the promoter they control. This means that enhancers can potentially act across fairly large distances. How does the genome prevent enhancers from acting inappropriately on the wrong gene just because it lies nearby?

As so often, many key observations were made in the study of gene expression in *Drosophila*. Salivary gland polytene chromosomes showed that the interphase genome consisted of condensed chromatin regions (bands) alternating with regions 10 times less condensed (interbands). Heat shock genes, located in band regions, and their sudden massive transcriptional activation upon a temperature increase, were discovered by the sudden appearance of local decondensation of the corresponding chromo-some band. The so-called puffs formed at the chromosomal site of heat shock genes (see Figure 16 of Chapter 4) correspond to their chromatin decondensation, transcriptional activation, and the accumulation of large amounts of RNA transcripts, associated RNA-binding proteins, and splic-ing factors. The sharp localization of the heat shock puffs and their boundaries raised the question in the mind of Paul Schedl at Princeton University whether some structural or functional boundary was present in the genome to prevent the local decondensation from spreading and the transcriptional activation from affecting flanking genes. Looking for such features in the genomic sequences flanking two heat shock genes, Schedl found unusual DNase hypersensitive chromatin regions on either side (Figure 1). These regions, which he called *Special Chromatin Sequences SCS* and *SCS'* appeared to delimit the region decondensed upon heat shock gene activation.

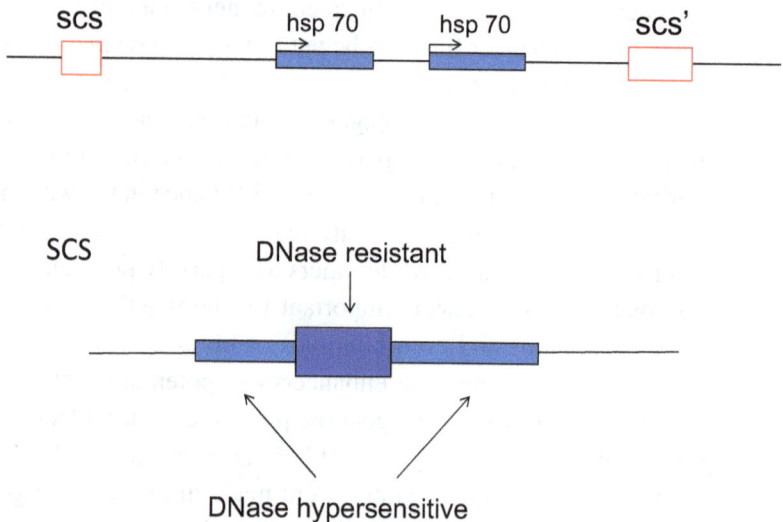

Figure 1.   Boundary or insulator elements at the heat shock genes. The heat shock genes are flanked by two chromatin sites that have an unusual structure consisting of a Dnase-resistant core between two DNase hypersensitive regions. They were called Special Chromatin Structures: scs and scs'.

Source: Udvardy *et al.* (1985).

In 1992, Kellum and Schedl went further and asked if these structures might also explain why heat shock activation did not also activate near-by non-heat shock genes. These structures might define boundaries separating chromatin regions that are independently regulated. To test this, they devised an enhancer-blocking assay. They constructed reporter genes expressed under control of specific enhancers, for example, an enhancer region from a *Drosophila* segmentation gene called *fushi tarazu (ftz)*. This gene is important for specifying the *Drosophila* segmentation and is expressed in a characteristic set of stripes in the early embryo. Kellum and Schedl inserted the *scs* sequence between the enhancer and the promoter and found that the striped expression was completely lost but only if the *scs* sequence is inserted between the enhancer and the promoter, not if it is on the other side of the enhancer (Figure 2). This topologically determined behavior indicated that *scs* elements constituted a new kind of

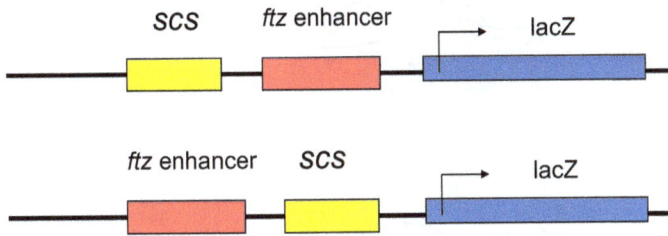

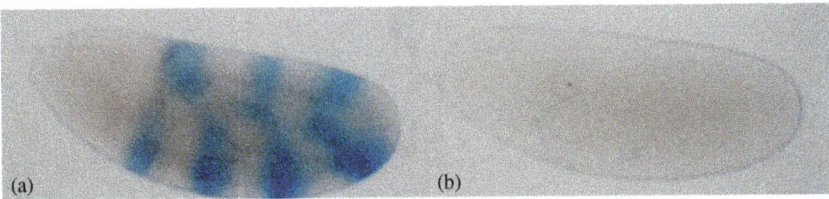

Figure 2.   Enhancer blocking. In a reporter transgene, the *ftz* enhancer drives expression in the *Drosophila* embryo in the form of seven stripes. (a) The insertion of an *scs* element upstream of the *ftz* enhancer does not prevent the enhancer action. (b) When the *scs* element is inserted between the *ftz* enhancer and the promoter, the enhancer is completely blocked and no expression takes place.

Source: Kellum and Schedl (1992).

regulatory element that acted as a boundary between two chromatin domains. Vazquez and Schedl proposed that looping contacts were possible within a domain but the insulator acted as a block preventing interactions between domains. In this model, the insulator was a self-standing element that behaved as a separatory element and could, by itself, create a boundary between two regions (Figure 3).

How exactly the boundary or insulator element separated two domains and what kinds of interactions it prevented between them were not very

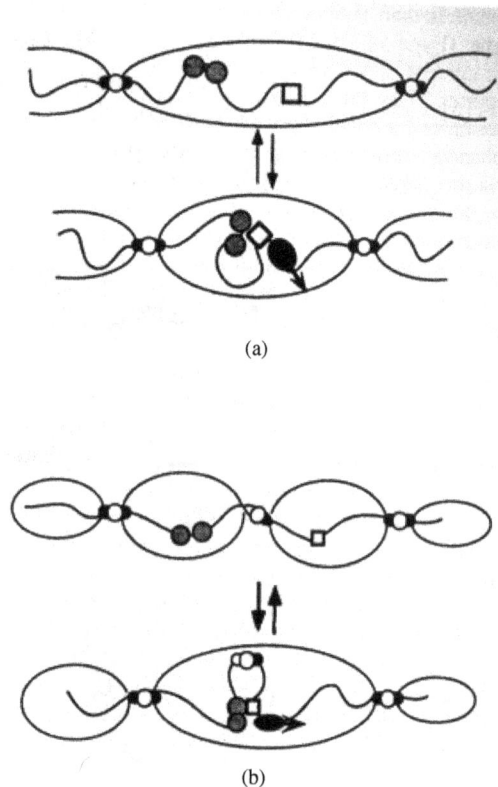

(a)

(b)

Figure 3.   Chromatin boundary model. (a) Vazquez and Schedl proposed that the scs element acted as the boundary of a chromatin domain within which folding and looping interactions are possible but which prevents such interactions with a domain on the other side of the boundary. (b) If a boundary element is introduced in the middle of such a chromatin domain, it separates it into two domains insulated from one another.

Source: Vazquez and Schedl (1994).

clear (Figure 4). Was there something transmitted from enhancer to promoter that could be blocked by the insulator? A prominent model for enhancer action was based on a predicated looping contact between the enhancer element and the promoter. Did the insulator capture the enhancer on its way to contact the promoter? Or did it in some way topologically prevent the looping that brought the two in contact? Tests to distinguish among these possibilities showed that the insulator was not a repressive element: it did not inactivate an enhancer or prevent it from acting on another promoter on the distal side (Figure 5). Furthermore, the insulator blocked both enhancers and silencing elements such as a Polycomb Response Element (Figure 6). It did not capture the enhancer by acting as a decoy or false promoter. A remarkable observation strengthened the idea that a topological explanation was required. It was found that, while an insulator element blocked the interaction of enhancer and a promoter, two insulator elements separated by a small segment not only failed to block

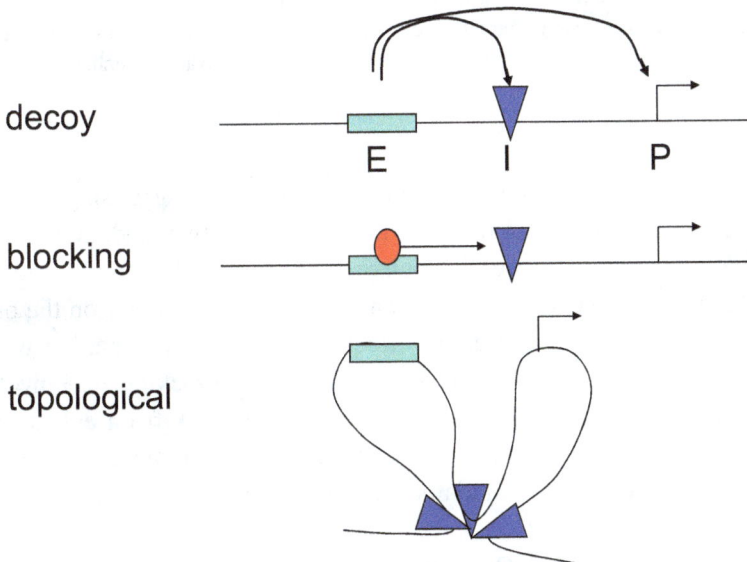

Figure 4.   Models of insulator action. In the decoy model, the insulator acts as a false promoter, a decoy distracting the enhancer from contacting the true promoter. In the blocking model, the insulator blocks the progress of a putative factor that moves along the DNA to contact the promoter. In the topological model, insulators interacting with one another fold chromatin into loops that may not be able to contact one another.

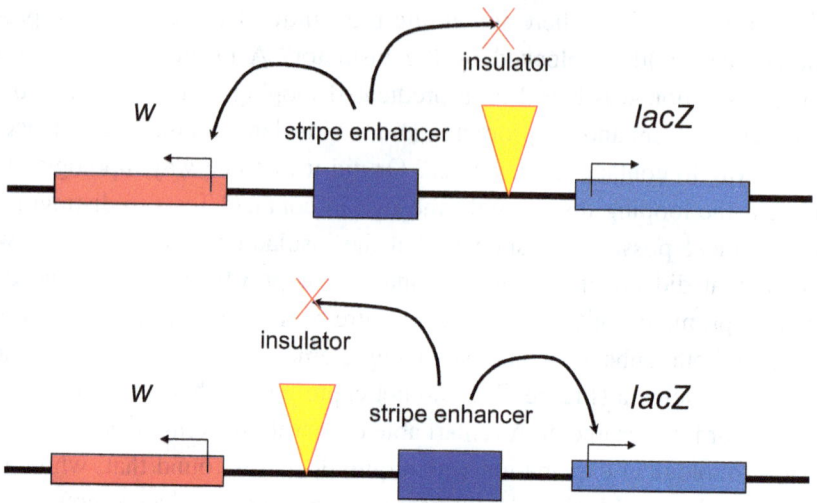

Figure 5.   Tests of insulator model. In reporter transgenes in which the enhancer is placed between two divergent reporter genes, an insulator blocking the gene to the right does not prevent the enhancer from acting on the gene to the left. Conversely, if the insulator is inserted to block the gene to the left, it does not prevent the enhancer from activating the gene to the right. This shows that the insulator does not inactivate the enhancer: it has a topological function.

but actually facilitated the interaction (Figure 7). This surprising observation suggested that, by interacting with one another, two tandem insulators canceled out by looping out the intervening segment and actually shortening the distance between enhancer on one side and promoter on the other (Figure 8). The double insulator effect is clearly not compatible with a tracking model of enhancer action and enhancer blocking that involves transmission of a substance or signal along the DNA from enhancer to promoter. It was one of the earliest observations that suggested that the role of insulators is not fundamentally to block but to form chromatin loops.

Further study of the *Drosophila* insulators showed that specific insulator-binding proteins were required for insulator action. The early studies quickly identified at least four different insulator families (Figure 9), each requiring a specific DNA binding protein (several more have been found more recently). One particularly powerful and consistent insulator

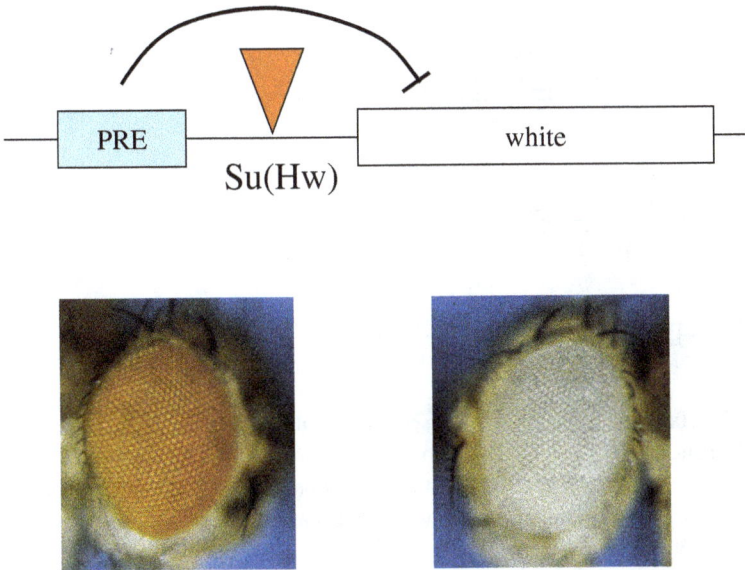

Figure 6. An insulator can block the repressive action of a **PRE**. A reporter gene construct containing the *white* gene and a Polycomb Response Element (PRE) with or without the insertion of a gypsy Su(Hw) insulator between them. The insulator blocks the repressive action of the PRE (bottom left). Without the insulator, the white gene is totally repressed (bottom right).

Source: Sigrist and Pirrotta (1997).

element was the *gypsy* insulator, so called because it resided within a retroviral transposable element called *gypsy* (Figure 10). Typically, in fact, insertion of the *gypsy* retrotransposon in the regulatory region of a gene prevented the action of regulatory elements more distal from the insertion site. The *gypsy* insulator contains 12 consensus binding sequences for the Suppressor of Hairy wing protein, the product of the *Drosophila Su(Hw)* gene (Figure 11). This gene in turn had been identified because a *gypsy* insertion in the regulatory region of the *Hairy wing* gene resulted in misregulation of the gene and formation of multiple wing hairs and the hairy wing phenotype that gave the gene its name. Mutations in the *Su(Hw)* gene rescued the hairy wing phenotype by restoring normal *Hairy wing* expression. Clearly, the discovery of the *gypsy* insulator provided the explanation that made everything clear: the *gypsy* insulator blocked the

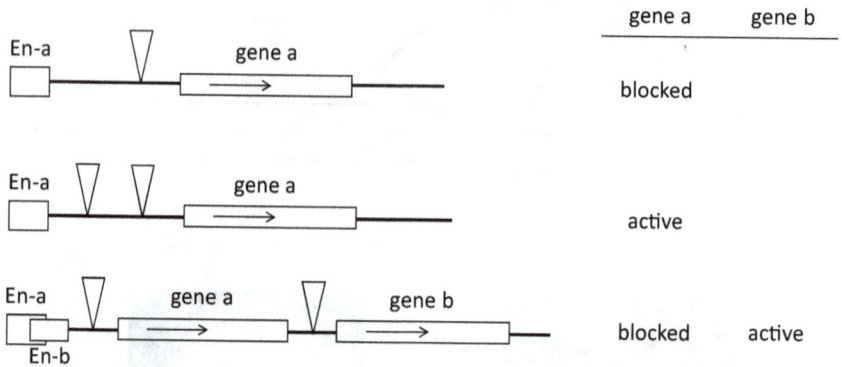

Figure 7.   Tandem insulators. While inserting an insulator between the enhancer and gene a blocks gene a activation, inserting two insulators, surprisingly, restores the ability of the enhancer to contact gene a. In the third configuration, activation of gene a is blocked by one insulator but activation of gene b, with two enhancers intervening between En-b and gene b, is not blocked.

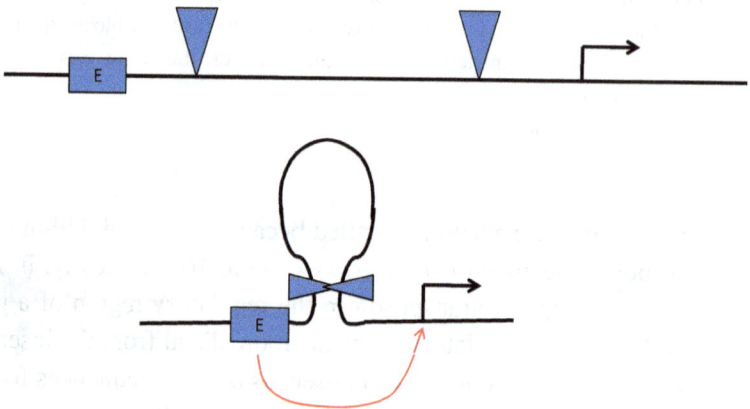

Figure 8.   Insulators and chromatin looping. The tandem insulator effect shows that insulators are not just enhancer blockers. By directing looping of the intervening chromatin fiber, two insulators can form a separate domain. This no longer prevents interactions between enhancer on one side of the loop and promoter on the other side. Instead, by bringing the two closer together, the looping can facilitate contact between enhancer and promoter.

Insulator binding proteins

Drosophila

Insulator type	Binding protein	Binding motif
scs	Zw5	8 zinc fingers
scs'	BEAF-32	1 zinc finger
gypsy	Su(Hw)	12 zinc finger
CTCF	dCTCF	11 zinc fingers
	CP190	2 zinc fingers + BTB domain
	Mod(mdg4)	BTB domain

Mammalian

CTCF (CCCTC Binding Factor) is the only known mammalian insulator protein

Figure 9.   Insulator types and binding proteins. The four best known types of insulators in *Drosophila* are listed, together with their corresponding binding protein. Two additional types of proteins do not bind to DNA directly but serve as auxiliary "glue" proteins linking insulators to form chromatin loops. In contrast to *Drosophila*, only one insulator protein has been so characterized in mammals.

interaction of a regulatory element of the *Hairy wing* gene but this insulator action required the binding of a protein, the product of the *Su(Hw)* gene. When the Su(Hw) protein was not available, the *gypsy* insulator lost its insulator action and restored normal regulation of the *Hairy wing* gene.

The insulator-binding proteins identified in *Drosophila* contained zinc finger DNA-binding domains, often multiple zinc fingers. Another kind of insulator-associated protein does not bind directly to DNA but rather to the DNA-binding protein that binds to the insulator. The two best-defined proteins of this type are the CP190 protein and the Mod(mdg4) protein (Figure 12). Both contain a powerful protein–protein interaction domain called BTB/POZ domain that mediates homo- and in some cases hetero-dimerization (Figure 13). These proteins might be thought of as "glue"

insulator

gypsy retrotransposon

680.   700.   720.   740.
ATTCGCAAAAACATTGCATATTTTCGGGAAAGTAAAATTTTGTTGCATACCTTATCAAAAAATAAGTG
       760.   780.   800.
CTGCATACTTTTTAGAGAAACCAAATAATTTTTATTGCATACCCGTTTTTAATAAAATACATTGCATA
     820.   840.   860.
CCCTCTTTTAATAAAAAATATTGCATACTTTGACGAAACAAATTTTCGTTGCATACCCAATAAAAGAT
.880   900.   920.   940.
TATTATATTGCATACCCGTTTTTAATAAAATACATTGCATACCCTCTTTTTAATAAAAAAATATTGCATA
       960.   980.   1000.
CGTTGACGAAACAAATTTTCGTTGCATACCCAATAAAAGATTATTATATTGCATACCTTTTCTTGCCA

Figure 10.   The *gypsy* transposable element and its insulator. *Gypsy* is a retrovirus-type transposable element with long terminal repeats that contain promoters. A powerful insulator element is located downstream of the 5′ repeat. The sequence of the insulator region is shown below, with the 12 binding sites for the Su(Hw) protein. The multiplicity of binding sites probably accounts for the gypsy's unusual insulator strength.

12 zinc fingers

N-ter   C-ter

Su(Hw) insulator protein

enhancer   Hairy wing

gypsy
transposon

Figure 11.   The structure of the Su(Hw) protein. Su(Hw) is the protein that binds to the gypsy insulator and hundreds of other genomic sites in *Drosophila*. If the gene encoding Su(Hw) is mutated, all these insulators lose their activity. The multiple zinc fingers allow Su(Hw) to bind flexibly to target sequences and interact with other proteins. Insertion of a gypsy transposon can inactivate a gene by blocking an enhancer. A mutation in the *Hairy wing* gene is produced by the insertion of a gypsy transposon between the enhancer and the promoter, producing a hairy wing phenotype. If the *Su(Hw)* gene is mutated, the insulator function is lost and the hairy wing phenotype is suppressed. This is what gained Su(Hw) its name.

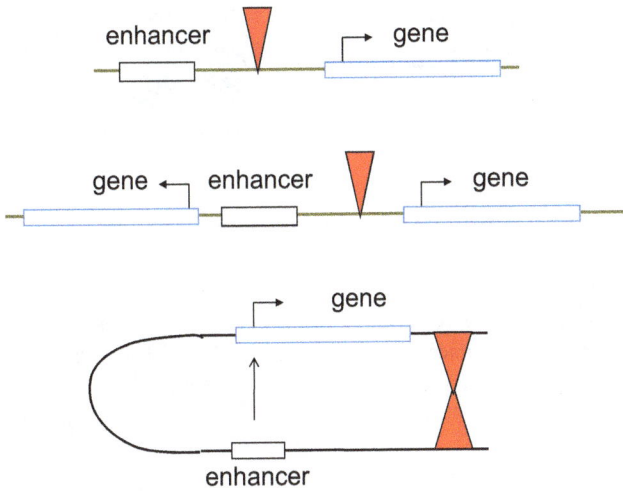

Figure 12.   Some roles played by insulators. In addition to the enhancer blocking function (top), which can be made to regulate gene activity, insulators can protect a gene from inappropriate action of a nearby enhancer, repressor, or heterochromatic region (middle). A vital role of enhancers is to bring distant enhancers close to their target gene (bottom). All these functions depend on the ability of insulators to form chromatin loops by interacting with other insulators.

proteins, necessary to cause association of insulator elements and the looping of the intervening chromatin region. In addition, multiple insulator proteins, as well as "glue" proteins, often bind in close vicinity to one another. It appears, in fact, that effective enhancer blocking activity requires the clustered binding of multiple insulator proteins. Most insulator protein binding sites, especially stand-alone binding sites for single insulator proteins, do not exhibit enhancer blocking activity and can be found not only in intergenic regions but also near the 5′ or 3′ ends of genes or in intronic regions. The most effective insulator site is the *gypsy* insulator, which contains 12 binding sites for the Su(Hw) insulator protein.

The efficacy of insulators as enhancer-blocking agents seems therefore to depend on the binding of multiple insulator-associated proteins forming an insulator body that brings together loops of chromatin and joins them by means of many protein–protein interactions (Figure 14). This may be further increased by interactions of the insulator body proteins with the nuclear lamina. It is not easy in this model to understand

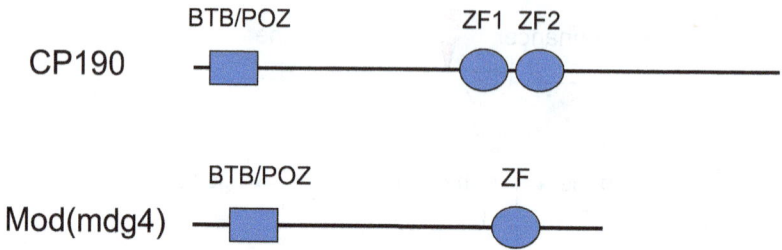

Figure 13.   Insulator-linking or looping proteins. In *Drosophila*, insulators interact with one another through the action of "glue" proteins. These are proteins that bind to insulator factors such as Su(Hw) and interact strongly with "glue" proteins bound to other insulator sites. Two such "glue" proteins are CP190 and Mod(mdg4), both of which have protein–protein interaction domain called BTB/POZ. This domain cross-links sites by dimerizing or heterodimerizing.

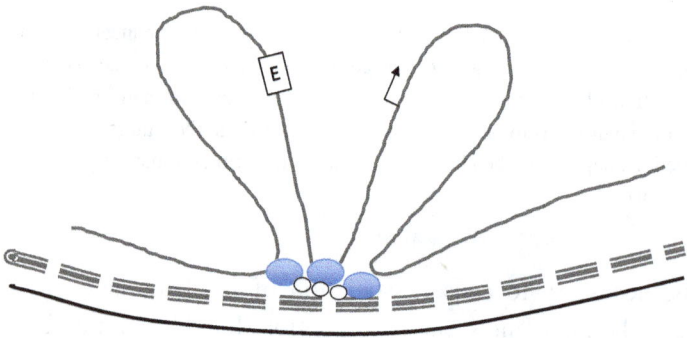

Figure 14.   Chromatin loops formed by insulator proteins. Proteins bound to insulator elements may come together, forming "insulator bodies". Some evidence suggests that these may bind to structures like the nuclear lamina. These assemblies organize a three-dimensional chromatin architecture that governs how different chromatin elements interact with one another.

how loop formation prevents the interaction between a site on one loop and a site on another loop. Greater insight into this question came only from technical advances in the study of chromatin architecture.

Mammalian Insulators

Instead of the multiplicity of insulator proteins found in *Drosophila*, only one insulator protein has been demonstrated in mammalian genomes. This is the CTCF protein, containing 11 zinc fingers, with significant homology to a *Drosophila* insulator protein, which is therefore called dCTCF. Insulator proteins are clearly major constituents of the genome: in *Drosophila*, there are hundreds of binding sites for each insulator protein; in mammalian genomes, there are 15–20,000 binding sites for CTCF. No homologs of the *Drosophila* "glue" proteins have been found in mammals. Instead, their role is taken over by the cohesin complex, which in mammals is closely associated with CTCF binding.

Cohesin is a multiprotein complex whose ring-like appearance is created by two long coiled-coil proteins of the Structural Maintenance of Chromosome (SMC) family called SMC1 and SMC3 (Figure 15). In each, the N-terminal and C-terminal come together to form an ATPase domain.

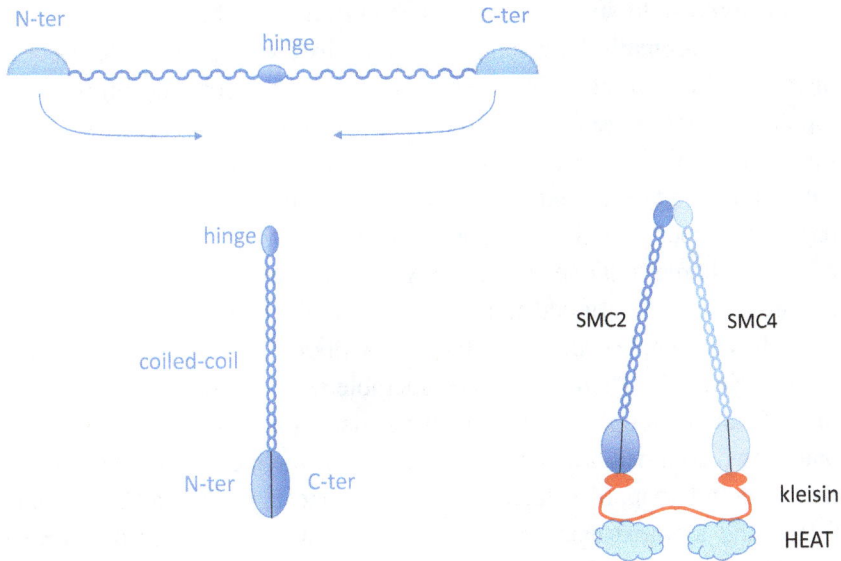

Figure 15. Structure of the condensin complex. The basic structure depends on the Structural Maintenance of Chromosomes (SMC) proteins, which consist of two long coil regions joined by a hinge domain and ending with a head domain. The coil regions fold together to form a long coiled-coil region with the hinge domain at one end and the two joined head domains at the other end. The joined head domains have ATP binding activity and ATP hydrolysis provides the energy for condensin movement along DNA. SMC2 and SMC4 proteins join at their hinge domains and their head domains are connected at the other end by a kleisin component and two HEAT repeat subunits. Cohesin has a very similar structure and related molecular activity.

A hinge domain in the middle of the protein separates two long arms that fold together forming antiparallel coiled-coil structures connecting the hinge domain and the ATPase domain. The hinge domain also mediates the hetero-dimerization of the SMC1 and SMC3 components while the third core component, kleisin SCC1, connects the ATPase domains of SMC1 and SMC3, forming a ring structure. Association with an additional complex NIPBL, thought to serve to load cohesin onto DNA, is required for cohesin action. Cohesin was known principally for its role in holding together the sister chromatids during metaphase by enclosing two chromatin fibers within the ring structure. This requires opening the ring for topological enclosure of the DNA fibers. The fact that, in addition, cohesin has a pervasive role in chromatin architecture during interphase has been revealed only in the years since 2000.

In contrast to its action in sister chromatid cohesion, the role of cohesin in chromatin loop formation arises by the loop extrusion mechanism where a loop of DNA is threaded through the cohesin ring without topological enclosure (Figure 16). Here, the ATPase domains operate by translocating DNA or moving along the DNA powered by ATP hydrolysis. According to the loop extrusion model, the cohesin complex can bind a chromatin fiber and then pull a loop into the ring. Movement of the ATPase subunits relative to the DNA pulls in more DNA, enlarging the chromatin loop. Continued action increases the size of the loop and moves the cohesin complex along the two DNA fibers forming the base of the loop (Figure 17). There is still considerable debate concerning the structural details of loop extrusion. In particular, opinions differ on whether one or two cohesins are needed at the base of the loop to pull both DNA fibers into the loop. Movement stops when cohesin reaches a DNA-bound CTCF and loop extrusion ends when two CTCF proteins in the correct orientation are met. The studies of mammalian CTCF suggested a much broader role for what had been called insulator proteins. The insulator effect is only one possible result of their activity as anchor points for the formation of chromatin loops and shapers of genomic architecture. Other factors can play similar roles. For example, the Mediator complex recruited to activate enhancers also brings in cohesin to help form the chromatin loop that brings together enhancer and promoter (Figure 18).

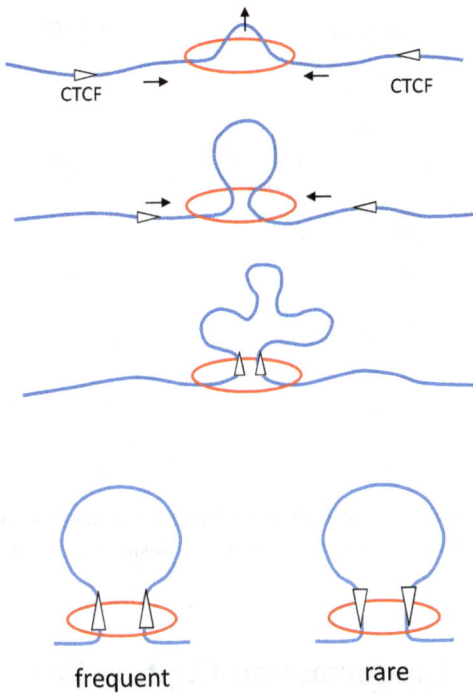

Figure 16.   Model of loop extrusion. Cohesin captures a loop of chromatin in its ring and pulls it along (using ATP hydrolysis) until it reaches a CTCF molecule. When two CTCF molecules in the correct orientation are pulled up, cohesin stops, forming a relatively stable loop. The CTCF binding sites must be not only aligned but pointing toward the loop. The inverse orientation is rarely observed.

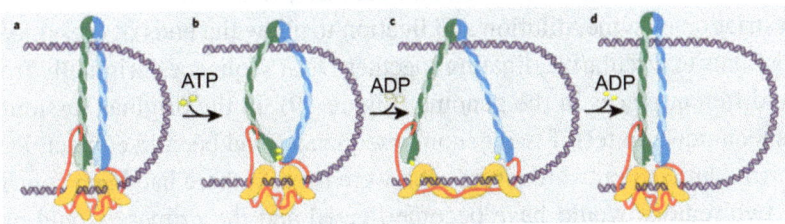

Figure 17.   One of many models of loop extrusion progression. The two head domains together bind two ATPs whose hydrolysis provides the energy for cohesin to pull DNA into a chromatin loop loosening or tightening it like a noose. In this model, cohesin pulls only one side of the loop. Studies of loop extrusion indicate that both sides are pulled, whether by a variant of this model or by two cohesin complexes working on each side of the loop.

Source: Nichols and Corces (2018).

enhancer   promoter

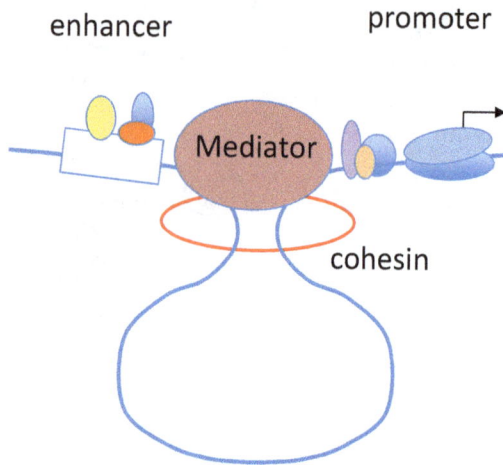

Figure 18.   Other factors can also recruit cohesin to produce looping. For example, Mediator bound to activate enhancers can recruit cohesin to facilitate looping to contact the promoter.

Chromosome Conformation Capture Techniques

Efforts to demonstrate directly looping interactions and the effect of insulators on chromatin folding spurred the application of a technique originally developed by Job Dekker to determine which part of a chromosome was near which other part of the genome in the yeast nucleus. The technique, called Chromosome Conformation Capture (3C), used chromatin crosslinking to freeze the chromatin contacts, followed by cleavage with a restriction enzyme, dilution and ligation to allow the ends of crosslinked fragments to circularize, ligating together DNA sequences originally from two different places in the genome (Figure 19). In the original version of this technique, to test if two genomic sequences had been in contact, PCR primers directed outwards from each were used. If there had been contact, the two regions would have become ligated and the primers would produce a PCR fragment spanning the ligation site. If no contact, no PCR primer would be produced. The frequency of contacts had some relationship to the quantity of the PCR product produced. Appropriate controls could be introduced to take into account ligation efficiencies, etc. This approach demonstrated that indeed an enhancer looped to contact a

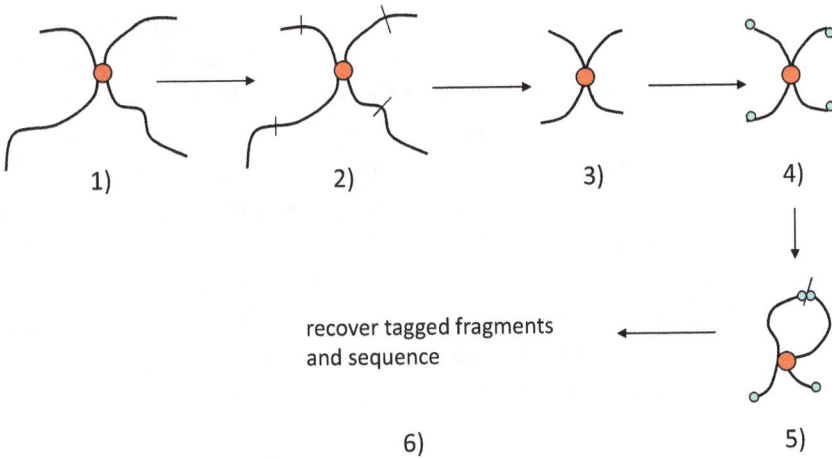

Figure 19. Chromatin Conformation Capture (3C) techniques. The core concept of this approach is to crosslink chromatin to freeze in place any chromatin–chromatin interaction (crosslink in red). The chromatin is then fragmented (2). In the Hi-C version, DNA ends are generally tagged to facilitate recovery (4). The free ends are ligated together (5). The tagged DNA is then recovered and sequenced. Extensive computer power is then applied to identify the genomic position of the sequences and of what other genomic sequence each has become ligated to. The result is a tabulation of the frequency with which each genomic sequence becomes ligated to any other sequence. This is taken to represent the contact frequency.

promoter and that, if an insulator was placed between them, this interaction was prevented.

The original 3C technique was marvelously informative but it required testing for each possible contact individually. The more sequences tested, the more detailed information could be obtained but this became very labor-intensive and inefficient if the spatial interactions over a larger genomic region were to be determined. A variety of modifications, called 4C, 5C, and variations on that theme, were soon developed to ask broader questions. The most general version of these, called Hi-C, could survey the frequency of contacts of any genomic region with any other genomic region (for more details on 3C, Hi-C, and related techniques, see Chromatin Contacts in Chapter 13). These genome-wide approaches were made possible by the growing number of genome sequences determined after the completion of the human genome sequence. It also depended on the increased affordability of large-scale sequencing resulting from commercial Next-Generation sequencing machines and the development of the computational, statistical, and hardware computer tools required to deal with billions of sequence fragments. The results of these experiments are typically reported as a matrix of contact frequencies (the higher the frequency, the more intense the color) of each site in a sequence against all other sites in that sequence (Figure 20). Self-contacts are along the diagonal and the two sides of the diagonal are mirror images.

The first conclusion derived from these studies was that contacts among genomic sequences were high within certain regions called Topologically Associating Domains or TADs but low between TADs. In

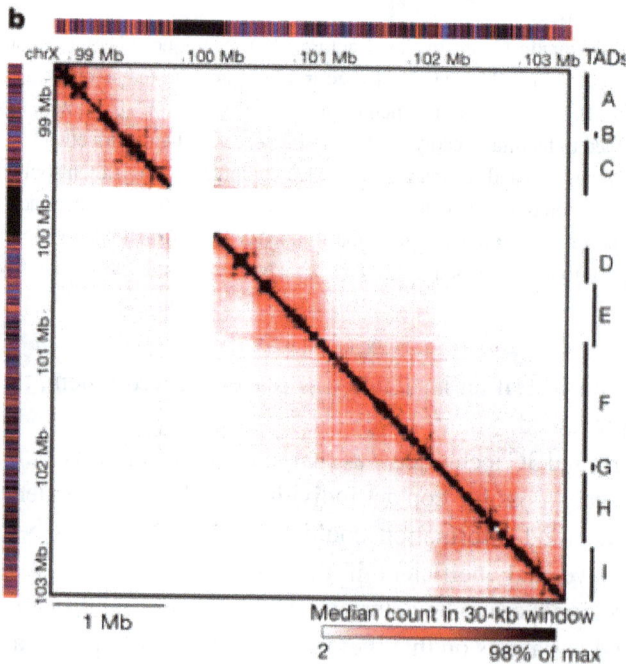

Figure 20.   Hi-C contact matrix. Long-distance interactions in chromatin are shown by the contact frequencies between any two positions in the chromosome interval represented here. The higher the frequency, the darker the color. The matrix plot shows regions in which every sequence interacts with nearly every other sequence (Topologically Associated Domains or TADs), separated by nodes across which interactions are greatly reduced.

Source: Nora *et al.* (2012).

the human genome, TADs range in size from 200 to 1000 kb. Two adjacent TADs are separated by a short region that acts as a node, a boundary decreasing or preventing contacts from occurring between sequences across the boundary (Figure 21). This situation is very similar to that proposed by Vazquez and Schedl in 1994 (Figure 3). Indeed, Hi-C analysis of *Drosophila* diploid and polytene chromosomes shows that the condensed chromatin in polytene band regions corresponds well to a TAD organization (Figure 22). However, a single insulator binding site, whether CTCF in the human genome or any of the insulator proteins in *Drosophila*, is not generally sufficient to create an architectural boundary and insulator protein-binding sites and local loops occur frequently within TADs. However, inter-TAD regions frequently contained multiple insulator binding sites, leading to the conclusion that a certain density of insulators may be needed to form a boundary separating TADs. Within a TAD, a high density of contacts prevails, not least between promoters and their enhancers. Many of these are guided by specific CTCF binding sites. Experiments in

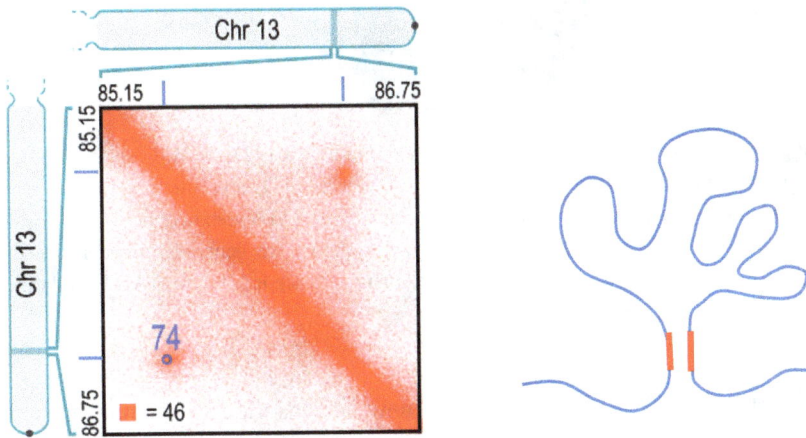

Figure 21.   Loop structures revealed by Hi-C. A configuration frequently seen in mammalian genomes reveals strong contacts at the two ends of a TAD (off-diagonal spots), corresponding to the stem or anchor point of a loop. The anchor may be due to CTCF binding sites, due to Polycomb complexes, and, in some cases, even due to gene regulatory sequences or other strongly interacting protein complexes.

Source: Rao *et al.* (2014).

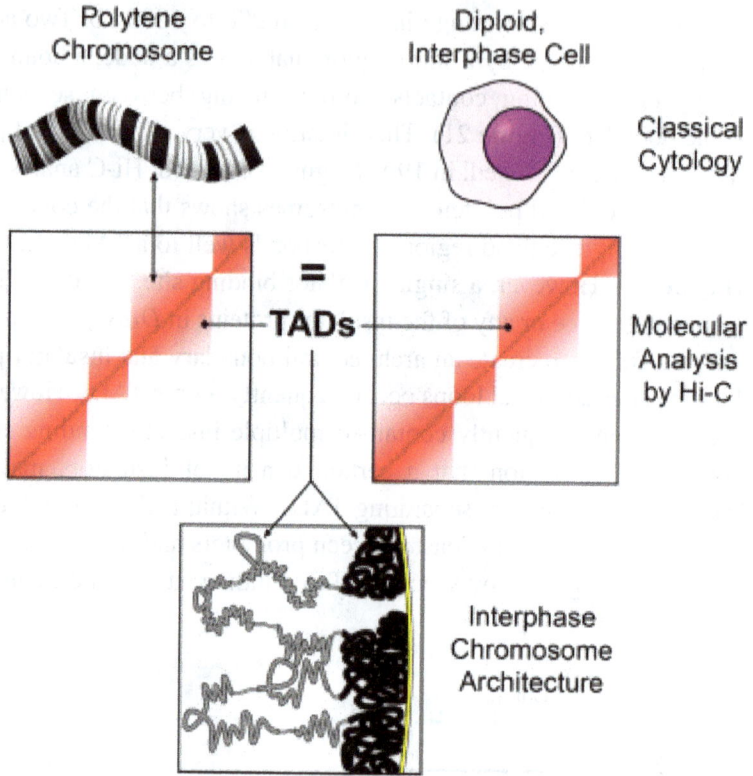

Figure 22.   Polytene chromosome bands correspond to TADs. A Hi-C study of polytene chromosomes showed that bands correspond well to TADs and interbands to the regions connecting TADs. Polytene TADs were identical to the TADs seen in diploid cells. Insulator sites are present within TADs but multiple insulators are generally found in interband regions, suggesting that several insulator elements are needed to form TAD boundaries.

Source: Eagen *et al.* (2015).

which a CTCF site is deleted or a new site inserted show that many promoters still depend on CTCF sites to create the local loop necessary for enhancer contact. A new view of CTCF binding sites now sees them not as boundaries or insulators but as means to bring together two chromatin sites and form a loop. They are as likely to bring enhancer and promoter together as to lock the enhancer in a configuration that prevents its contact with a promoter. According to this view, then, mammalian CTCF and other similar factors in *Drosophila* are better thought of as "architectural proteins" that contribute to the three-dimensional organization of chromatin than as insulator factors.

TADs Segregate into Compartments

The resolution of the Hi-C approach depends on many factors. Two of the most important are the size of the fragments into which the genome is cut up and the number of crosslinked fragments sequenced. Initially, restriction enzymes were used to fragment the genome into pieces of a few thousand kb. More frequently-cutting enzymes increased the resolution and recent experiments now use enzymes such as micrococcal nuclease to make fragments of a few hundred nucleotides. As sequencing technologies increased, it is now common to sequence billions of fragments per Hi-C experiment. Extending the computations for contacts farther from the diagonal in contact matrices showed that there are weaker but still significant contacts between sites farther distant from each other and revealed that some TADs have appreciable interactions with certain other TADs (Figure 23). These inter-TAD contacts are not random. If each TAD is given a score for the frequency of "active" chromatin marks (such as H3K4me3 or histone acetylation) versus "repressive" chromatin marks (such as H3K9me3 or H3K27me3), it is apparent that "active" TADs tend to contact other "active" TADs while "repressed" TADs contact other "repressed" TADs (Figure 24). In other words, chromatin domains segregate into a more "active" or A compartment and a more "repressed" or B compartment. The two compartments tend to physically separate from each other. This fits well with the finding that repressed chromatin regions tend to be attached to the nuclear envelope while active chromatin regions tend to be found in the nuclear interior. It was not a surprise, therefore, to find that B compartment TADs essentially correspond to Lamin Associated Domains or LADs (see Chapters 4 and 5).

The segregation of TADs into A and B compartments can be accounted for by interactions between heterochromatic TADs combined with their attachment to the nuclear envelope. This was made clear by the remarkable nuclear architecture of rod photoreceptor cells of nocturnal animals. In these cells, lamin A/C and Lamin B Receptor (LBR) are not expressed and heterochromatin does not attach to the nuclear lamina. The architecture of

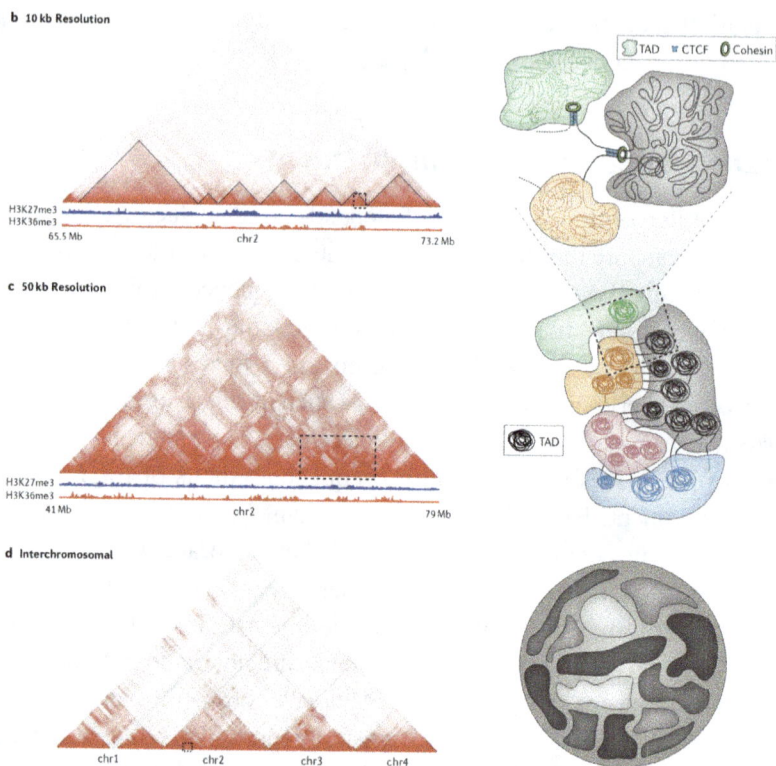

Figure 23.   Weaker interactions occur between TADs. While contacts are dense and abundant within TADs, significant contacts can be detected off the diagonal (towards the apex in this representation). The ability to see these less frequent contacts depends on the resolution of the Hi-C approach, which depends in part on the size of the chromatin fragments produced and on the number of fragments sequenced. Interactions among TAD segregate them into an active A compartment and a repressed B compartment and correspond to the density of active chromatin marks in A TADs and repressive marks in B TADs.

Source: Bonev and Cavalli (2016).

the genome in these cells is not a haphazard mix of active and repressed TADs. It is the inverse of that found in normal cells: heterochromatin forms in the inner nucleus in concentric shells with the densest innermost, while euchromatin occupies the periphery (Figure 25). This allows more light to reach the photosensory part of the rod cell and shows that heterochromatic regions tend to condense together even when not anchored to the nuclear envelope. This causes physical segregation of repressed TADs

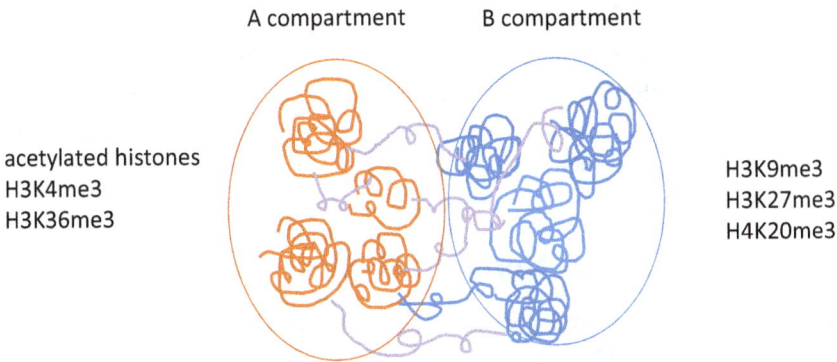

Figure 24.   Associations among TADs reveal chromatin compartments. Contacts among TADs are not random. TADs with high levels of active histone marks tend to contact one another, forming the A compartment. TADs with high levels of repressive histone marks tend to contact one another, forming the B compartment. Not surprisingly, the B compartment corresponds well with lamin-associated domains or LADs and tends to be found at the nuclear periphery.

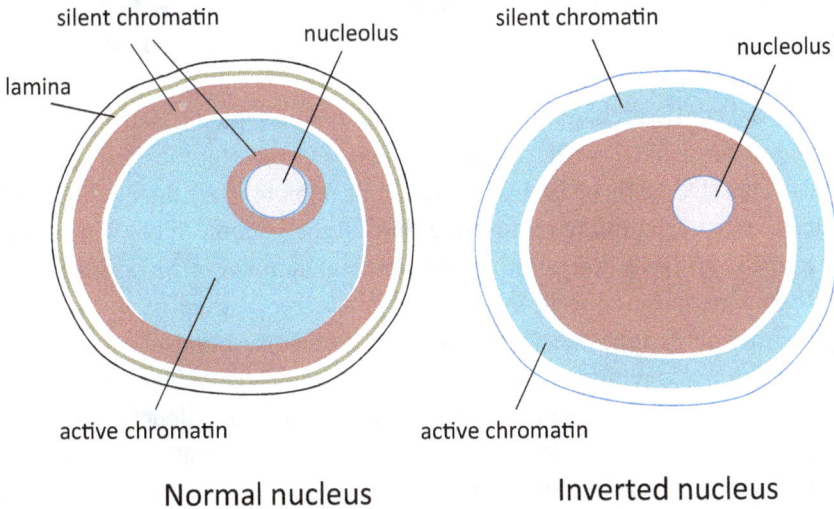

Figure 25.   Normal and inverted nuclear organization. In a normal nucleus, the nuclear lamina anchors silent chromatin and heterochromatin through lamin-associated proteins such as LBR. Some silent chromatin is also attached to the periphery of the nucleolus, while active chromatin fills the interior of the nucleus. In inverted nuclei such as those of rod photoreceptors in nocturnal mammals, LBR and lamin A/C are absent and attraction among silent chromatin domains accumulates them in the interior of the nucleus, while active chromatin is pushed to the periphery.

from active TADs. There does not seem to be an equally strong interaction among active TADs. As a result, repressed TADs cluster in the interior of the nucleus while active TADs are pushed to the nuclear periphery. A similar inverted nuclear architecture is observed in cells with a knockout mutation in lamin B (see also Chapter 12).

Lamin-Associated Domains (LADs)

To identify and map the genomic domains associated with the nuclear lamina, the classical technique of chromatin immunoprecipitation (ChIP) is not a convenient approach because the nuclear lamina itself is a large, insoluble structure. Modifications of this technique are possible to side-step this difficulty but the approach of choice used by van Steensel and collaborators is the DamID method (see Chapter 13), in which the lamin B1 protein was fused to a bacterial DNA adenine methyltransferase (Dam). The approach is based on the idea that the Dam domain will methylate any DNA that comes into sustained proximity to the lamina. The methylated DNA can then be visualized in the cell by antibody staining or identified by sequencing.

The DamID technique showed that genomic regions 10kb–10Mb in size are associated with the lamina and are therefore called Lamin-Associated Domains or LADs. Human cells contain more than a thousand such LADs, constituting almost one-third of the genome. They tend to be gene-poor, to have little or no transcriptional activity, to be enriched for H3K9 methylation, and to be depleted for active histone marks such as H3K4me3 or histone acetylation. In fact, they correspond to most of the heterochromatic regions of the genome but include also many regions that are facultative heterochromatin, that is, regions that are silent in some tissues but active in others. In fact, they include most chromatin marked with H3K27me2 and H3K27me3. Comparison of the genomic sequences shows that LADs correspond to a large extent to the B compartment TADs, confirming other evidence showing that genomic regions that are predominantly silent tend to be associated with the nuclear lamina (see Chapter 4). Analysis of LAD sequences indicates that multiple smaller sequence domains contribute to associate a LAD with the lamina. Given the chromatin features of LADs and the types of proteins known to bind to lamins, it seems clear that at least one important component of the interaction is heterochromatin, heterochromatin proteins such as HP1 and heterochromatic chromatin marks such as H3K9me2/3 and H4K20me3. It is likely that lamin A, whose farnesylated C-terminal is cleaved off and therefore is not directly associated with the nuclear membrane, is more internally located than lamin B and more likely to make contacts with chromatin. In agreement with this, the retinal rod cells of mice, which have an inverted genome architecture with heterochromatin internal and active chromatin peripheral, express neither lamin A/C nor the lamin B receptor LBR, which binds HP1. If these are ectopically expressed in retinal rod cells, the usual nuclear architecture is restored and heterochromatin relocates to the nuclear periphery. Conversely, in normal differentiated cells, knocking out both lamin A/C and LBR releases heterochromatin from the nuclear periphery and causes it to aggregate in the nuclear interior, as in the retinal rod cells. The evidence suggests then that LBR, which is anchored to both lamin B and the inner nuclear membrane, as well as lamin A/C bind to substantial, though probably not identical fractions of genomic heterochromatin. Other nuclear envelope proteins, such as emerin, have been proposed to interact with and help bind fractions of heterochromatin to the nuclear envelope and may be partly redundant with one another and with the lamins.

Inevitably, chromatin brought into proximity with the nuclear envelope is not uniformly heterochromatic. Some potentially active genes may be brought close to the envelope by genomic proximity with silenced heterochromatic regions. Such genes would find themselves in an environment rich in heterochromatin proteins, histone deacetylases, and methylases and may therefore be sensitive to becoming silenced through their environment. It remains unclear, however, to what extent recruitment to the nuclear lamina contributes to silencing and to what extent silencing contributes to lamina recruitment. It is interesting therefore that LAD edges tend to be enriched for CTCF binding sites and for active promoters. Both of these would tend to antagonize extension of heterochromatic regions and protect the activity of promoters, thus preventing their direct association with the lamina.

While LADs are reproducibly associated with the nuclear envelope, tracking individual LADs through cell cycles, and therefore through cycles of dissociation of the nuclear envelope and its re-assembly, shows that many LADs may alternatively be found associated with the nucleolus. A cloud of heterochromatin is in fact usually found surrounding the nucleolus. The relationship between nucleolus and heterochromatin is very interesting but not very clear. It may be related to the fact that specific mechanisms exist for silencing individual copies of the ribosomal RNA genes in the rRNA gene array and it has been proposed that the nucleolus is instrumental in the formation of heterochromatin in the very early embryo. It is clear, however, that part of but not all heterochromatin may alternatively associate with either nucleolar periphery or with the nuclear lamina.

Single-Cell Genome Architecture

High resolution Hi-C experiments were typically done with large numbers of cells and vast amounts of sequencing, with the idea that, for a given sequence, each cell could only give one possible interaction partner but multiple interactions might occur in fact, either because they might be dynamic or because several sequences might cluster together at the same time. Averaging over a large number of cells might then give an inadequate view of the real contacts in individual cells. Other questions arise: Is the TAD and compartment organization the result of averaging over large numbers of cells? How stable are these structures? How variable are they from cell to cell? Are the maternal and paternal genomes folded the same way? To answer these questions, it was necessary to develop single-cell Hi-C techniques. The drawback of such techniques is a loss in resolution for fine details but this does not prevent the analysis of TAD organization. The result of thousands of single-cell Hi-C shows that TADs exist at the single-cell level but chromatin conformation is not stable from one cell to another or across the cell cycle. Chromatin loops are absent during mitosis. After mitosis, chromatin decondensation continues until DNA replication starts and then chromatin starts to compact again. While chromatin loops appear to be stable, active TADs become looser, TAD boundaries start to fade after G1 phase, and contacts across TAD boundaries increase. Unlike the TAD structure, the compartment organization persists and increases in definition to a maximum at the end of S phase. This picture is consistent with other observations suggesting that chromatin loops, TADs, and compartments are distinct features. Chromatin compartments do not require the presence of TADs and the two are organized independently, while loops can exist without the high degree of intra-loop contacts that characterizes TADs.

A difficulty in single-cell Hi-C is that the two copies of the genome in diploid cells do not vary in conformation synchronously. Hi-C does not generally distinguish the two copies and therefore the results cannot build a consistent conformation model. To avoid this problem, the experiments were done using haploid cells, thus limiting the applications of this approach. A different approach that can distinguish the two copies of the genome is one based on high-resolution microscopy. To visualize a chromatin region, a series of fluorescently labeled oligonucleotides are sequentially hybridized and imaged to compute the 3D distance between each and map the configuration of a genomic region. This approach is limited to a small region of the genome at a time but it allows conformation mapping in real time, not only distinguishing one chromosome from its homolog but also visualizing changes as they occur. The microscopy approach confirmed the single-cell Hi-C results and demonstrated that decondensation within a TAD takes place as a gene becomes transcriptionally active. This probably explains the changes in TAD organization seen in single-cell Hi-C, as active genes undergo transcription bursts.

Intrinsically Disordered Proteins and Liquid Phase Transitions

It has been known for a long time from cytogenetics that heterochromatic chromosome regions tend to be "sticky". This is shown, for example, by the association of the pericentric regions of the four *Drosophila* chromosomes to form a chromocenter. More recently, some of the interactions driving heterochromatin associations have become clearer. Heterochromatin contains very high densities of certain proteins such as HP1, which bind essentially to every nucleosome. HP1 binds to nucleosomes as a dimer and can form multimers, cross-linking chromatin regions. HP1 also binds to many other chromatin proteins such as histone methyltransferases, DNA methyltransferases, histone deacetylases, methyl-binding proteins such as MeCP2, etc. Such large-scale interactions among heterochromatin proteins could account for the tendency of heterochromatic domains to cohere. Another kind of association has recently attracted much attention. This results from many weak and less-specific interactions between protein domains that lack a defined structure, remain highly flexible, and are called Intrinsically Disordered Regions or IDRs. Such domains cannot be mapped by X-ray crystallography or NMR structural methods because they do not assume a fixed conformation. Their sequences are often repetitious in amino acid content, with clusters or runs of repetitious amino acids. Charged or hydrophilic amino acids tend to promote disorder or lack of stable structure because they are stabilized by water molecules. They also favor weak associations with similarly disordered regions of other protein monomers or even different proteins. *In vitro*, IDR proteins can reach a critical concentration at which they separate from the aqueous phase and form a separate liquid phase. Interactions with RNA molecules, which are also charged and highly flexible, can promote the liquid phase transition. The result is the formation of liquid droplets that move, flow like droplets, and can fuse with other droplets. The HP1 N-terminal region and the hinge domain of HP1 contain IDRs and HP1 has been shown *in vitro* and *in vivo* to form foci with droplet-like appearance and behavior. These foci are dispersed by solvents such as dihydroxyhexane, which disrupt weak hydrophobic interactions. Protein diffusion rates in and out of these foci are consistent with the formation of a separate phase (Figure 26). Liquid phase formation can account for the ability of heterochromatic regions to condense with one another. It can also account for the exclusion of other proteins that have a well-defined and self-contained structure. HP1 droplets have been reported to permit the inclusion of nucleosomes and DNA but to deter the inclusion of some transcription factors. The assembly of proteins and RNAs to form condensed phase structures could also account for other membraneless nuclear or cytoplasmic structures such as nucleoli, nuclear speckles, splicing bodies, polar granules, and stress granules. Disordered regions are involved in allosteric

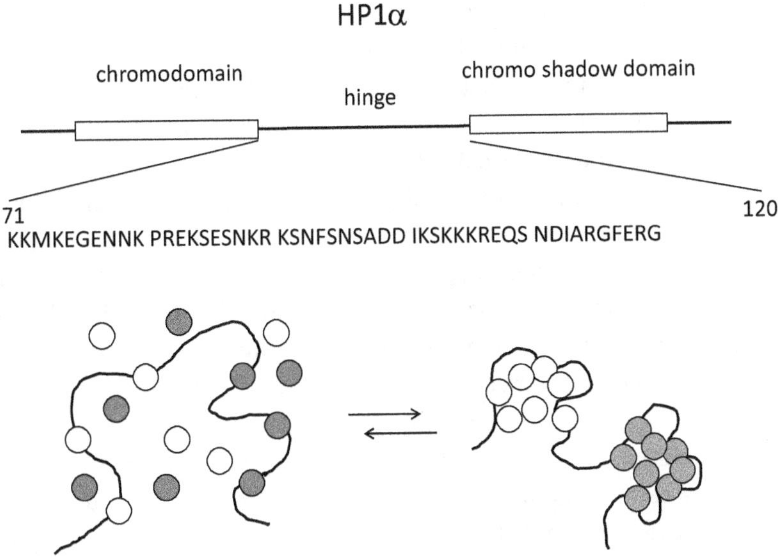

HP1α

chromodomain

hinge

chromo shadow domain

71

120

KKMKEGENNK PREKSESNKR KSNFSNSADD IKSKKKREQS NDIARGFERG

Figure 26.   HP1alpha hinge region. Amino acids 71–120 constitute a disordered domain that can result in liquid phase transition *in vitro* in the presence of DNA. Below is a representation of globules formed through IDR interactions between (for example) transcriptional activators (white) and heterochromatin proteins (gray). The evidence suggests that these interactions might reach a critical point at which they form separate liquid phases within an aqueous nuclear environment.

interactions; they can assume a definite conformation by induced-fit when they bind to globular proteins. They are particularly abundant among proteins involved in transcription and chromatin remodeling. Many transcription factors, repressors such as some Polycomb proteins, and even the RNA pol II CTD show behaviors typical of IDRs. Interactions mediated by such proteins in euchromatin may account for more local interactions but the proteins never reach the concentrations achieved by heterochromatin proteins like HP1 which bind essentially to every nucleosome. On a more local level, similar kinds of relatively non-specific interactions are thought to drive local euchromatin clustering interactions driven by weak affinities between transcription and other "active" factors on one hand and repressive factors on the other hand. Even nucleosomes have been reported to undergo liquid phase separation, driven by the histone tails, which are themselves typical IDRs and associate at ionic strengths and concentrations similar to those found in nuclei. Acetylation of the histones prevents droplet formation. These reports suggest that chromatin has an intrinsic tendency to associate and, promoted by the binding of many types of protein, can pass a critical point where it forms a separate liquid phase. Such liquid droplets have the effect of increasing the local concentration of participating components without preventing the diffusion of other proteins.

Despite the favorable reception that these concepts have found, they have also encountered criticism. The evidence for such liquid phase separations has often been vague and the criteria not very stringent. While the concept is appealing, it is not always clear that it produces qualitative or quantitative predictions that can be used to decide whether the liquid phase separation model is objectively more useful than earlier concepts. Weak interactions between macromolecules, favored by IDRs, may lead to local concentrations without necessarily causing a phase transition. Whether the IDR proteins and their interactions reach concentrations sufficient to produce phase separation is still debatable but there is no doubt that IDR domains interact and can support a degree of local condensation that can account for associative interactions between chromatin domains.

There are clearly interactions between chromatin sites, whether heterochromatic or euchromatic, that shape local chromatin configurations. Looping, which can be enhanced by cohesin loop extrusion, can occur between enhancers and promoters, between enhancers, stabilized by Mediator complexes or by interactions between enhancer and promoter binding factors. In some cases, large loops caused by the association of two chromatin regions give rise to the characteristic appearance of a TAD with foci off the diagonal of the contact profile corresponding to the interaction that forms the base of the loop (see Figure 21). Interactions between Polycomb complex binding sites have been detected through such structural effects as well as through biochemical experiments. In *Drosophila*, some TADs show the characteristic appearance of a loop with Polycomb binding sites at the base of the loop, such as shown in Figure 21. In conclusion, CTCF/cohesin is not the only way to form chromatin loops and this raises the question of how important they are for genome architecture and for regulated gene expression.

How Important Is CTCF or Cohesin?

We started the discussion of genomic architecture with the role of what were then called chromatin insulators. These are now better called architectural elements or architectural proteins since their primary role is in forming chromatin loops, whose functional consequence may be to separate an enhancer from inappropriate gene targets or it may be to bring together a regulatory element with the promoter it controls. We have also seen that cohesin plays an important role in generating loops, which may be locked in by CTCF or other proteins. But how important is CTCF or cohesin in constructing the larger architectural domains in which the genome is organized? And how important are they in determining the general features of gene activity? Many experiments have been done to answer these questions using loss of function CTCF mutants or inducing degradation of cohesin components. A particularly thorough study employed RAD21, a key component of cohesin, modified by the inclusion of a sequence that renders the protein rapidly degradable when an inducible ubiquitin ligase is expressed. The ubiquitin ligase TIR1 is induced from an auxin-activated transgene, ubiquitylates the modified RAD21, and induces rapid degradation by the proteasome machinery. Thus, Hi-C contact mapping can be done both before and after TIR1 induction to compare the results with and without functional cohesin. The loss of cohesin has a range of effects depending on the genomic region. In some situations, where cohesin forms the base of a loop containing a TAD, the loss of cohesin leads to the loss of the TAD: local interactions almost disappear (Figure 27). In many other situations, though loop structures disappear, the TADs become more diffuse but the condensed domains remain. Interestingly, contacts farther off the diagonal increase, indicating increased contacts between TADs. Another study prevented cohesin function with a mutation in NIPBL, a factor necessary to load cohesin on chromatin. This work reports similar results but also an increased fragmentation within TADs, as if each TAD broke up into smaller domains, separating regions of higher activity from those with lower activity. Each of these subdomains entered into more distant contacts with other domains with similar levels of transcriptional activity (Figure 28). These results indicate that, although cohesin-dependent loops promote interactions

A

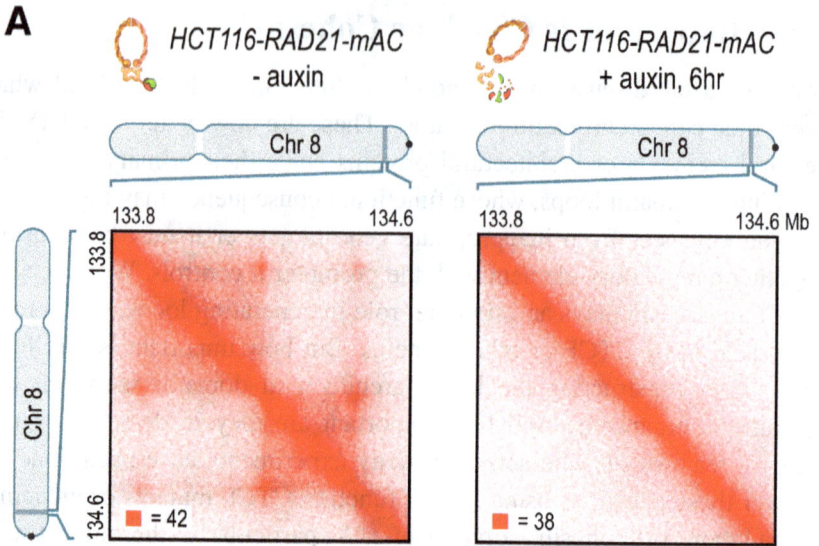

Figure 27A.   Effects of the loss of cohesin. If CTCF and cohesin are so important for chromatin architecture, what happens when they are missing or mutated? To see the results, Hi-C mapping has to be done at a very high resolution (billions of sequencing reads). In this experiment, auxin induced the degradation of RAD21, a core component of the cohesin complex. After auxin induction, this region loses TAD structure, and the bases of the TAD loops no longer interact (right).

Source: Rao *et al.* (2017).

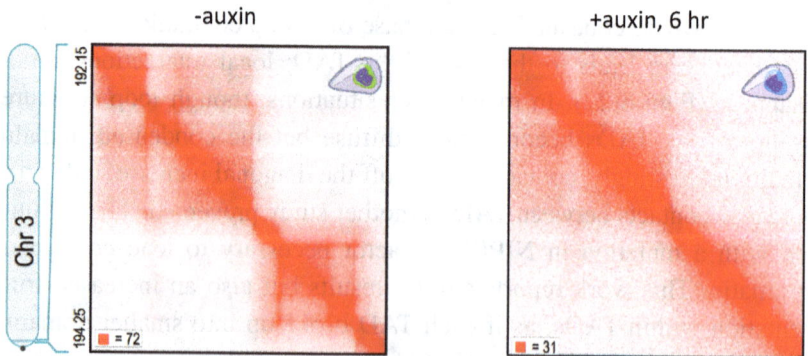

Figure 27B.   Effects of the loss of cohesin. In some regions, not all interactions are lost. Some TAD structure remains but more diffuse. Contacts off the diagonal increase indicating more interactions between domains.

Source: Rao *et al.* (2017).

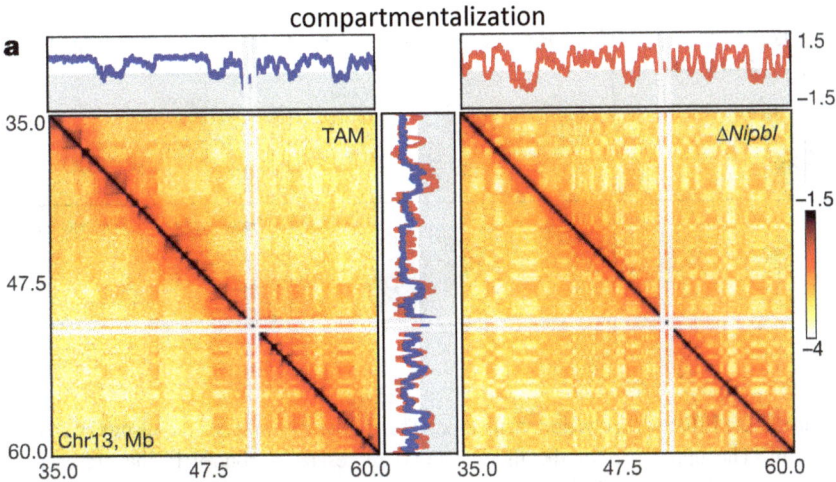

Figure 28. Effects of cohesin inactivation. This experiment induced the loss of NIPBL, a factor necessary to load cohesin on chromatin, to inactivate cohesin. When NIPBL is deleted (right), the results confirm the partial loss of TAD structure but also show a fragmentation of TADs into smaller domains and an increase in contacts among distant domains with similar compartment score. The blue and red tracings at the top indicate the compartment score: high is compartment A-like and low is compartment B-like.

Source: Schwarzer *et al.* (2017).

within the loop region, these interactions persist in the absence of cohesin and extend to other domains with similar chromatin states. The organization into active and repressed compartments is not affected. The role of cohesin seems to be to confine and focus the range of chromatin contacts within a TAD and minimize the interactions among subdomains with similar chromatin states that lie farther distant along the DNA sequence. This makes a TAD behave as a whole in associating with other TADs with a similar chromatin state. One could go further and speculate that the attachment of repressed or heterochromatic TADs to the nuclear lamina is an effective way to achieve a spatial separation between active domains and repressed domains, preventing the latter from getting too close to active domains where they might interfere with gene activity.

When the effects of transcriptional activity are examined, it appears that loss of cohesin has relatively mild consequences. Regulatory effects are less precise: the range of enhancer action is reduced; there may be ectopic activation of inappropriate promoters or transfer of enhancer

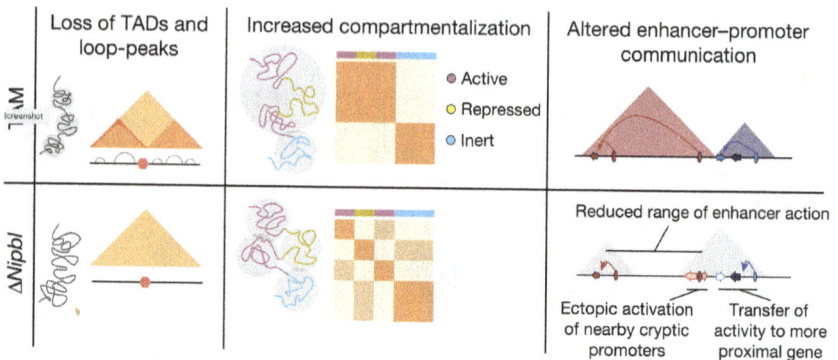

Figure 29. Effects of cohesin inactivation. This figure summarizes the results of loss of cohesin. The upper part of the figure (TAM) represents a control in the presence of cohesin. The lower part (Delta NIPBL) represents the effects of NIPBL deletion and loss of cohesin. In the absence of cohesin, TAD structure is partly lost and domains fragment into more numerous smaller interacting structures. Gene expression analysis shows a tendency to disorganize long-distance enhancer–promoter communication.

Source: Schwarzer *et al.* (2017).

action to a more proximal gene (Figure 29). These results show that CTCF/cohesin mechanisms are not the only source of looping interactions and contacts among chromatin regions. The associations among subdomains of similar chromatin states persist in the absence of cohesin, suggesting that "active" chromatin complexes can play a role in bringing together transcriptionally active regions. This may be the origin of what have been called "transcription factories", the tendency to find multiple transcriptionally active sites clustered together in the nucleus. Similarly, interactions among Polycomb repressive complexes bring together Polycomb-repressed regions and can form the base of a chromatin loop generating a TAD. Like transcription factories, multiple Polycomb-repressed domains tend to form clusters in the nucleus. We have already seen that heterochromatin complexes tend to interact and associate with each other. In both cases, the clustering enhances the transcription or repression, respectively.

In the absence of cohesin, then, the ability to form loop domains and organize genome architecture is not totally lost (Figure 30). In particular,

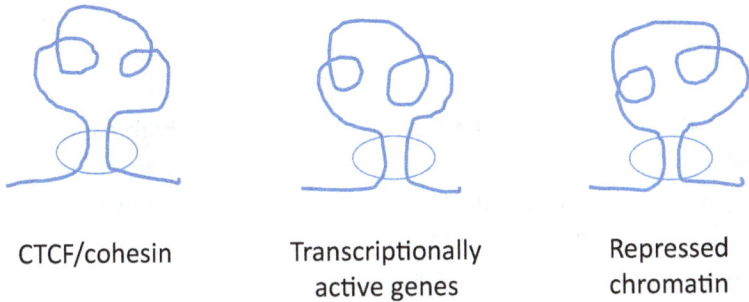

CTCF/cohesin   Transcriptionally   Repressed
                         active genes   chromatin

Figure 30.   Loop anchors. In addition to CTCF-anchored cohesin, other chromatin proteins can create loop anchors. Active promoters, particularly those that bind the same
activators tend to associate forming "transcription factories". Domains of repressed chromatin tend to associate and to bind to the nuclear lamina. Polycomb target regions tend to
associate. In embryonic stem cells, regions that bind pluripotency factors tend to associate.
The higher-order organization affects the stability of regulatory circuitry and the transcriptional potential of genes.

local domains rich in transcriptional activity can interact with similar
domains and generate a loop anchor. Domains binding Polycomb complexes can interact with one another, forming loops across large genomic
distances. Similarly, local domains rich in repressive marks can interact
with other similarly repressed domains and generate a loop anchor.
Cohesin-mediated looping adds to the precision of the loops and folding
domains that are formed. Local contact details require the presence and
correct positioning of CTCF binding sites and cohesin-mediated looping
also in the interior of TADs. Specific enhancer–promoter contacts may be
lost in the absence of CTCF or cohesion. Is genomic architecture structurally hardwired? Or is it a dynamic, stochastic assemblage of local states,
each with a short half-life and each independent of the others? Does architecture drive transcription or does transcription specify architecture? Or
are they mutually interacting to result in the dynamic architecture
observed in individual cells?

Chromatin architecture plays a particularly important role in the functioning of what are now called super-enhancers. These are genomic
regions containing multiple enhancers and multiple binding sites for
whole sets of transcription factors, particularly such as control major

decisions of cell fate and identity. A prototypic example is given by the regulatory regions that bind pluripotency factors and other factors coordinated with them in embryonic stem cells (see Chapter 9). A characteristic of super-enhancers is that they tend to cluster physically though they may be separated by large genomic distances. This clustering is thought to give them greater potency in activating transcription of their target genes. The clustering has been shown to result from the interactions of intrinsically disordered domains frequently found in transcriptional regulators, leading to liquid phase separation.

Further Reading

Bonev B and Cavalli G (2016). Organization and function of the 3D genome. *Nat Rev Genet.* **17**, 661–678.

Brodsky S, Jana T, Mittelman K, Chapal M, Kumar DK, Carmi M *et al.* (2020). Intrinsically disordered regions direct transcription factor *In vivo* binding specificity. *Mol Cell.* **79**, 459–471.e454.

Capelson M and Corces VG (2004). Boundary elements and nuclear organization. *Biol Cell.* **96**, 617–629.

Dekker J, Marti-Renom MA and Mirny LA (2013). Exploring the three-dimensional organization of genomes: Interpreting chromatin interaction data. *Nat Rev Genet.* **14**, 390–403.

Eagen KP, Hartl TA and Kornberg RD (2015). Stable chromosome condensation revealed by chromosome conformation capture. *Cell.* **163**, 934–946.

Hassler M, Shaltiel IA and Hearing CH (2018). Towards a unified model of SMC complex function. *Curr Biol.* **28**, R1266–R1281.

Kellum R and Schedl P (1992). A group of scs elements function as domain boundaries in an enhancer-blocking assay. *Mol Cell Biol.* **12**, 2424–2431.

Kubo N, Ishii H, Xiong X, Bianco S, Meitinger F, Hu R *et al.* (2021). Promoter-proximal CTCF binding promotes distal enhancer-dependent gene activation. *Nat Struct Mol Biol.* **28**, 152–161.

Lafontaine DLJ, Riback JA, Bascetin R and Brangwynne CP (2021). The nucleolus as a multiphase liquid condensate. *Nat Rev Mol Cell Biol.* **22**, 165–182.

Muravyova E, Golovnin A, Gracheva E, Parshikov A, Belenkaya T, Pirrotta V *et al.* (2001). Loss of insulator activity by paired su(Hw) chromatin insulators. *Science.* **291**, 495–498.

McCord RP, Kaplan N and Giorgetti L (2020). Chromosome conformation capture and beyond: Toward an integrative view of chromosome structure and function. *Mol Cell*. **77**, 688–708.

Nagano T, Lubling Y, Stevens TJ, Schoenfelder S, Yaffe E, Dean W *et al.* (2013). Single-cell Hi-C reveals cell-to-cell variability in chromosome structure. *Nature*. **502**, 59–64.

Nichols MH and Corces VG (2018). A tethered-inchworm model of SMC DNA translocation. *Nat Struct Mol Biol*. **25**, 906–910.

Nora EP, Lajoie BR, Schulz EG, Giorgetti L, Okamoto I, Servant N *et al.* (2012). Spatial partitioning of the regulatory landscape of the X-inactivation centre. *Nature*. **485**, 381–385.

Rao SSP, Huang S-C, Glenn St Hilaire B, Engreitz JM, Perez EM, Kieffer-Kwon K-R *et al.* (2017). Cohesin loss eliminates all loop domains. *Cell*. **171**, 305–320.e324.

Rao SSP, Huntley MH, Durand NC, Stamenova EK, Bochkov ID, Robinson JT *et al.* (2014). A 3D map of the human genome at kilobase resolution reveals principles of chromatin looping. *Cell*. **159**, 1665–1680.

Rowley MJ and Corces VG (2018). Organizational principles of 3D genome architecture. *Nat Rev Genet*. **19**, 789–800.

Sanborn AL, Rao SSP, Huang S-C, Durand NC, Huntley MH, Jewett AI *et al.* (2015). Chromatin extrusion explains key features of loop and domain formation in wild-type and engineered genomes. *Proc Natl Acad Sci USA*. **112**, E6456–E6465.

Schwarzer, W, Abdenur N, Golborodko A, Pekowska A, Fudenberg G, Loe-Mie Y *et al.* (2017). Two independent modes of chromatin organization revealed by cohesin removal. *Nature*. **551**, 51–56.

Shin Y and Brangwynne CP (2017). Liquid phase condensation in cell physiology and disease. *Science*. **357**, 1253.

Sigrist CJA and Pirrotta V (1997). Chromatin insulator elements block the silencing of a target gene by the Drosophila polycomb response element (PRE) but allow trans interactions between PREs on different chromosomes. *Genetics*. **147**, 209–221.

Strom AR, Emelyanov AV, Mir M, Fyodorov DV, Darzacq X and Karpen GH (2017). Phase separation drives heterochromatin domain formation. *Nature*. **547**, 241–245.

Udvardy A, Maine E and Schedl P (1985). The 87A7 chromomere: Identification of novel chromatin structures flanking the heat shock locus that may define the boundaries of higher order domains. *J Mol Biol*. **185**, 341–358.

van Steensel B and Belmont AS (2017). Lamina-associated domains: Links with chromosome architecture, heterochromatin, and gene repression. *Cell.* **169**, 780–791.

Vazquez J and Schedl P (1994). Sequences required for enhancer blocking activity of scs are located within two nuclease-hypersensitive regions. *EMBO J.* **13**, 5984–5993.

Yang J and Corces VG (2012). Insulators, long-range interactions, and genome function. *Curr Opin Genet Dev.* **22**, 86–92.

Zhang D, Huang P, Sharma M, Keller CA, Giardine B, Zhang H *et al.* (2020). Alteration of genome folding via contact domain boundary insertion. *Nat Genet.* **52**, 1076–1087.

Chapter 9

Stem Cells

Introduction

A nerve cell looks very different from a muscle cell or a skin cell; it expresses many genes that others do not and does not express certain genes that are active in other kinds of cells. Yet all the cells have the same DNA and exactly the same genes. What is different is the program of gene expression in the different kinds of cells and the epigenetic marks that are both the cause and the result of the different programs. One way to appreciate how genomic programming comes about is to look at a kind of cell in which previous programming has to be erased, set to zero in a sense, eliminating all or nearly all previous chromatin marks specific for previous patterns of differentiation. This is what happens in the fertilized egg, in which the genome has to be rewired to establish a state from which all possible types of cells in the body may be produced (Figure 1).

In the fertilized egg, the sperm and egg genomes start out in very different states. Each is the end product of a process of gametogenesis, a complex process of differentiation designed to result in an egg or a sperm cell. This involves the expression of genes specific to each process and the long-term inactivation of all other genes that are not needed for that process. Long-term gene silencing is done by DNA methylation of the promoter regions (see Chapter 3). The egg genome and the sperm genome have therefore different sets of epigenetic marks: patterns of DNA methylation and histone modifications specific for oogenesis or for spermatogenesis. These will have to be re-set to direct embryonic development.

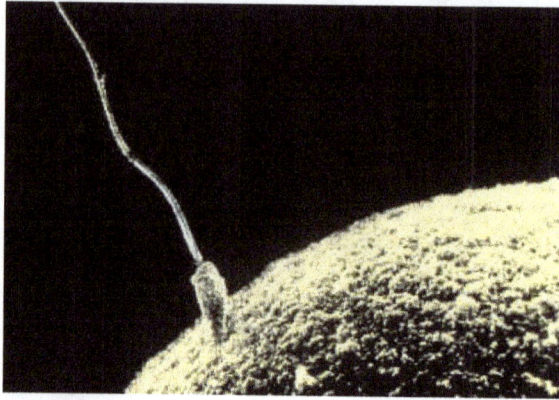

Figure 1.   Fertilization. A spermatozoon attempts entry into an oocyte. The image renders a realistic comparison of the relative sizes and of the extremely asymmetric products of egg and sperm differentiation. Source: unknown author. Public domain: http://www.pdimages.com/web9.htm.

In addition, both gametes have massive amounts of DNA methylation of repetitive sequences and transposable elements, designed to minimize transposon dynamics and prevent changes in the genome that is going to give rise to a new organism.

It is clear at first sight that the end products of oogenesis and of spermatogenesis are physically profoundly different (Figure 2): the egg is very large and full of yolk and other constituents that will go to help the growth of the future embryo. The sperm has a very small, dense head containing a highly compacted genome and a very long flexible tail. Spermatogenesis is designed to produce large numbers of these small and highly mobile spermatocytes for the large numbers and high mobility are essential in order for at least one sperm to find and fertilize the egg. Eggs, on the other hand, are produced one at the time or at best a few at the time during embryogenesis and are stored, waiting for sexual maturity and fertilization. They are large, full of yolk, RNA, histones, and other raw materials and gene products. They are primed to sustain the critical first few nuclear divisions after fertilization. Another important difference between sperm and egg genomes in all metazoans is that the sperm DNA has been largely (but not completely) stripped of nucleosomes, which are replaced by protamines and polyamines. Protamines are small proteins of about 50 amino

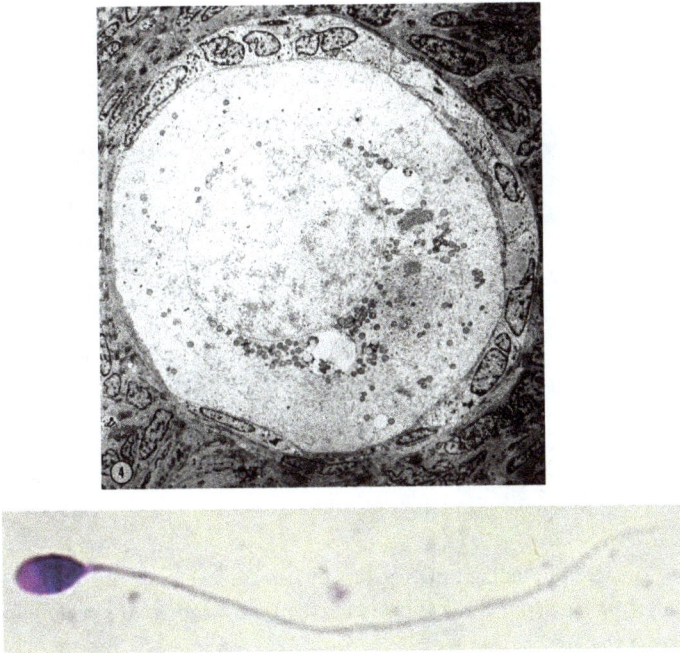

Figure 2.   Human oocyte and spermatozoon. The images are not to scale: the oocyte is far larger than the spermatozoon.

Source: Hertig and Adams (1967).

acids, very rich in arginine and therefore very basic (Figure 3). Protamines bind to the DNA major groove, neutralize the acidic phosphates of the DNA backbone, and promote its tight packaging into the sperm nucleus. Recent work has shown that not all histones are removed: in human sperm, about 10–15% of the histones remain bound to the sperm genome and are associated with early embryonic genes. These histones carry post-transcriptional marks that are important for the appropriate expression of those genes.

In the fertilized egg, the paternal and maternal pronuclei behave initially very differently. The sperm genome in the paternal pronucleus is decondensed, the DNA is released, and for a short period, it is potentially almost entirely accessible to DNA-binding proteins and needs to be rapidly reassembled into chromatin. Since it is not replicating, the normal replicative chromatin assembly machinery is not available and the reassembly

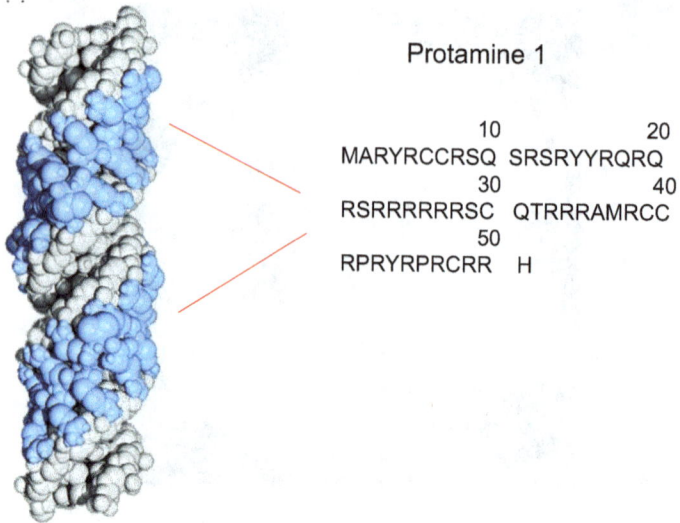

Protamine 1

```
         10              20
MARYRCCRSQ SRSRYYRQRQ
         30              40
RSRRRRRRSC QTRRRAMRCC
         50
RPRYRPRCRR  H
```

Figure 3.   Protamines binding to DNA. Protamines are small proteins ~50 amino acids long, rich in arginine, and highly basic, bind to the DNA major groove and fold it tightly. *Source*: Balhorn (2007).

involves non-replicative histone variants such as H3.3. Until it is reassembled into chromatin, the paternal genome remains more available to transcriptional activity than the maternal genome. It makes sense therefore that, during spermatogenesis, the sperm DNA becomes almost entirely methylated to prevent uncontrolled gene expression in the fertilized egg.

Erasing the DNA Methylation Marks

The fertilized egg is totipotent: it will make all the kinds of cells and tissues of the embryo as well as the extraembryonic tissues like the placenta and membranes surrounding the embryo itself. Therefore, it has to reset the programming of the maternal and the paternal genomes to zero. To do so, it must remove the previous DNA methylation marks and start with a clean slate. This is done by both active and passive demethylation. Passive demethylation is the simplest way: if CpG methylation is not maintained, every round of DNA replication without methylation would reduce the level of methylation by a half. Four rounds will reduce the level of 5mC to 1/16 of the original level. Passive demethylation occurs because DNMT1o, the oocyte-specific isoform of the maintenance DNA methylase, is exported out of the nucleus and into the cytoplasm of the fertilized egg by a maternal protein named STELLA or PGC7, which binds to its co-factor UHRF1. DNMT1 is unable to accumulate in the nucleus until the eight-cell stage (Figure 4). At this point, the original level of

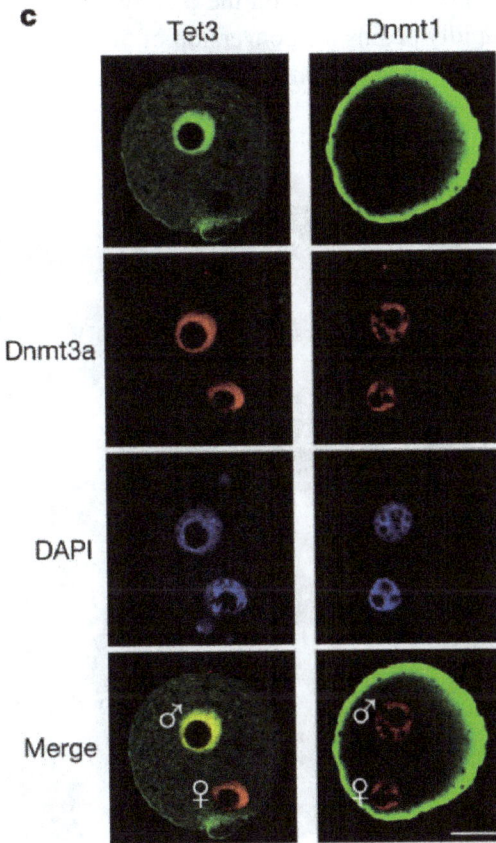

Figure 4.   Parental pronuclei in the fertilized egg. The fertilized egg on the left is stained with antibodies against TET3 (green) and DNMT3A (red), as well as with DAPI (blue) to identify the pronuclei. The antibodies show that TET3 enters only the paternal pronucleus but DNMT3A is available in both pronuclei. The fertilized egg on the right is stained with DNMT1 (green), showing that the maintenance methylase is segregated to the cytoplasm.

Source: Gu *et al.* (2011).

methylation would have dropped to 1/256 of the oocyte level. This is very effective but slow.

Active demethylation occurs through the action of the demethylating enzymes for which mammalian genomes have three closely related genes: Ten-Eleven Translocation (TET) 1, 2, and 3, so called after the genetic mutation through which the first TET gene was discovered (see DNA Methylation chapter). TET3 is the major demethylase present in the oocyte (Figure 5). It acts readily on the paternal pronucleus in the fertilized egg and rapidly begins the conversion of 5mC to 5hmC which leads to the loss of CpG methylation. In the maternal pronucleus, however,

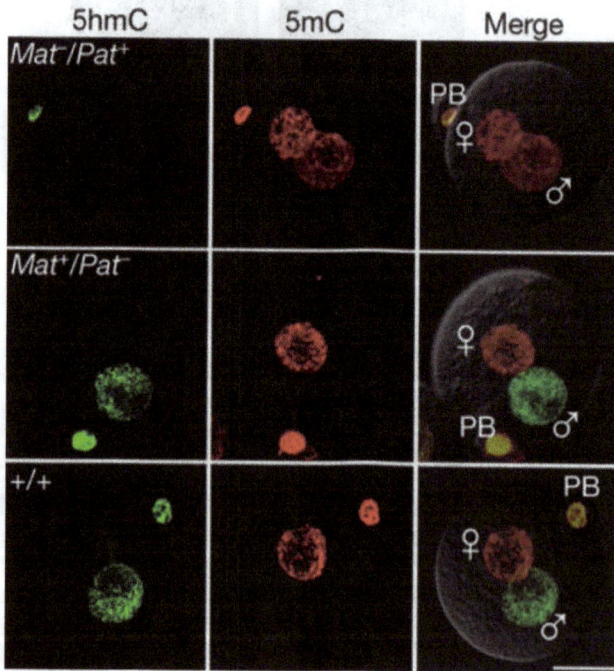

Figure 5.   The TET3 in the fertilized egg comes from the oocyte, not from the paternal genome. The fertilized egg is stained with antibody against 5hmC (green) and 5mC (red) to reveal the extent of demethylation. If the maternal TET3 gene is mutated, no demethylation is observed in the fertilized egg. If the paternal TET3 gene is mutated, maternal TET3 strongly demethylates the paternal but not the maternal genome.

Source: Gu *et al.* (2011).

STELLA binds to H3K9me2, which corresponds to DNA methylated site, and apparently prevents TET3 from binding to the maternal genome. STELLA is not present in the paternal pronucleus. As a result, although TET3 is maternally produced, it only acts on the paternal genome, resulting in its rapid demethylation. Note that this asymmetric activity would similarly occur if any somatic nucleus were introduced into the oocyte. This can be done by gentle manipulation to suck out the nucleus from a somatic cell and even more gently transplanting it into a mature oocyte (Figure 6). Using this technique, a somatic nucleus can be efficiently demethylated and reprogrammed, as discussed in the following.

The result of the active and passive DNA demethylation is that the paternal genome is demethylated rapidly, while in the maternal genome,

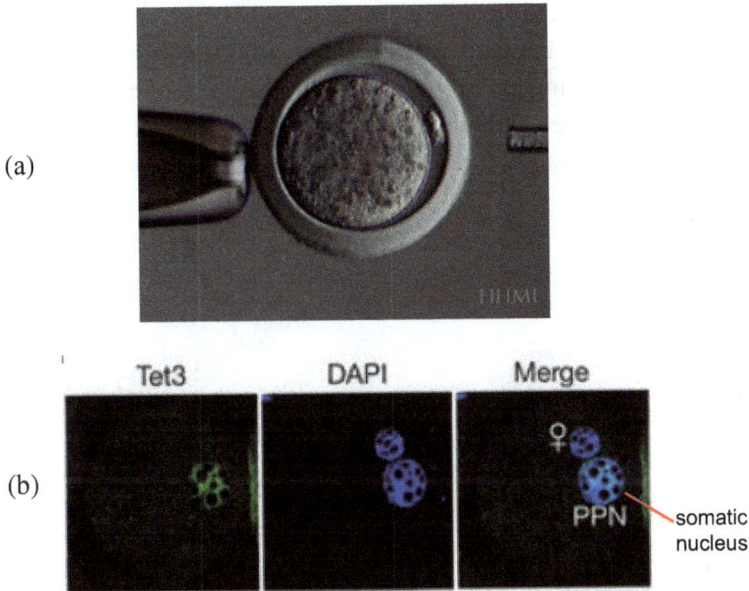

Figure 6. Oocyte TET3 acts on a transplanted nucleus. (a) Nuclear transplantation. The large, round-tipped pipette on the left holds the oocyte under gentle suction while a very fine pipette introduces a nucleus removed from a somatic cell. (b) A somatic cell nucleus was introduced into an oocyte as in (a). The oocyte was stained with an antibody against TET3 (green) to show that, while this enzyme is not visible in the oocyte nucleus, it can enter the somatic nucleus (PPN).

Source: Figure 6(a) Dietrich Egli, Figure 6(b) Gu *et al.* (2011).

demethylation is slower and not completed until the blastocyst stage, shortly before implantation of the developing embryo in the uterine wall (Figure 7). The rapid kinetics of demethylation and high early accessibility of the paternal genome cause incipient derepression of genes and transposable elements. This is a dangerous time for the paternal genome. However, it is also an important stage for the early expression of some key genes that will be important for the reprogramming of the zygotic genome. In particular, the paternal genome contributes early expression of pluripotency factors OCT4 and NANOG, essential for reprogramming and establishing the pluripotent state in embryonic stem cells (see the following). This is a situation in which maternal and paternal gene copies, though identical in sequence, are treated differently during development. We will see more situations in which the asymmetric expression of the two alleles is specifically produced (see Chapter 10).

Remethylation begins early through the maternally produced DNMT3A *de novo* methylase but does not gain the upper hand until the early blastocyst stage when the embryo consists of 64 cells. Until then, at the 16- and 32-cell stages, the embryo is at the morula stage, a ball of cells

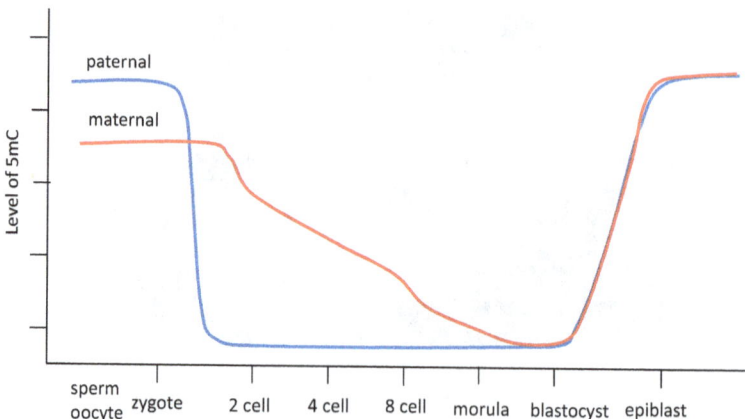

Figure 7.   Demethylation in zygote and early embryo. The paternal genome starts out higher because of hypermethylation in sperm DNA. Active demethylation by TET3 causes earlier loss of 5mC from the paternal genome, while the maternal genome depends on much slower passive demethylation. *De novo* methylation begins at the blastocyst stage and rapidly remethylates the genome.

thought to be in principle developmentally identical. By the 64-cell or early blastocyst stage, the ball of cells has become hollow, with an outer layer of cells that will give rise to extra-embryonic tissues and an inner lump of cells, called the Inner Cell Mass (ICM), that will become the embryo proper (Figure 8). Until now, the cells of the developing early embryo, known as blastomeres, are thought to be identical. Although they might start to do different things, they are as yet uncommitted and equally able to take up any role. This can be tested by embryonic manipulation and cell transplantation. An individual blastomere cell can be isolated from a morula-stage embryo and introduced into a different morula-stage embryo. If the first embryo is marked in a readily detectable way, for

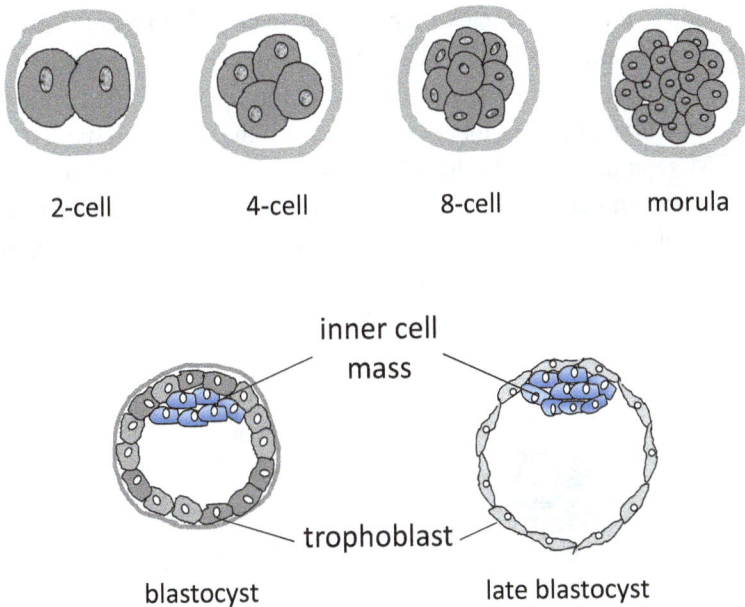

2-cell   4-cell   8-cell   morula

inner cell
mass

trophoblast

blastocyst   late blastocyst

Figure 8.   Pre-implantation embryo. As the fertilized egg divides several times, the cells (blastomeres) are interchangeable and totipotent. By the 32 cell stage, the cells form a hollow sphere, the blastocyst. However, a group of cells remains in the cavity. The first important developmental decision differentiates the trophoblasts from the inner cell mass. The trophoblasts are specialized cells that will not be part of the embryo proper but will form the trophectoderm, a layer of cells that surrounds the early embryo and eventually will form a connection with the uterine wall: the placenta.

example, with a marker gene or a mutant allele so that its cells can be easily identifiable, after the transplant, we can ask how the progeny of the transplanted cell behaves when the chimeric embryo grows and differentiates. The result is that progeny cells can be found in any tissue and any differentiated state, showing that the morula blastomeres are still totipotent.

In the morula, the blastomere cells occupy equivalent positions. Each has a polarity: the outer surface is different from the inner surface, which contacts the other blastomere cells. Beyond the eight-cell stage, the cleavage plane is oriented so that the cell division produces an outer cell and an inner cell. The different signals received by the inner and outer cells specify different cell fates and produce the first developmental decision. The outer cells will become trophoblasts, constituting the trophectoderm. These cells will produce the extraembryonic tissues that form the placenta and the membranes protecting the embryo proper. The outer cells pump water into the morula, which swells, becoming a hollow ball called the blastocyst with a clump of inner cells that form the inner cell mass (ICM). The ICM separates into the hypoblast, which produces the extraembryonic yolk sac and chorion, and the epiblast from which the future embryo will develop (Figure 9). The cells of the epiblast remain transiently undifferentiated but acquire the capacity to develop into any kind of cell in the embryo proper and are now said to be pluripotent, no longer totipotent

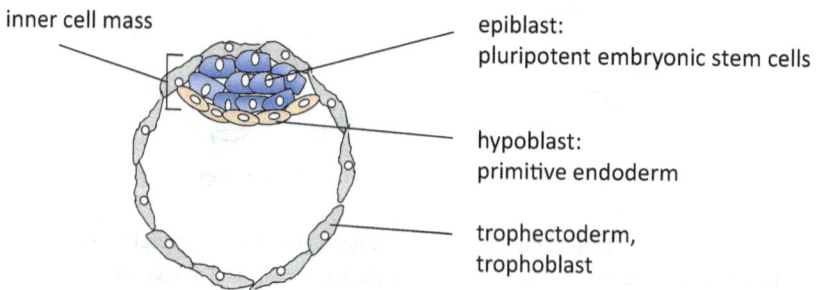

inner cell mass

epiblast:
pluripotent embryonic stem cells

hypoblast:
primitive endoderm

trophectoderm,
trophoblast

Figure 9.   Late blastocyst stage. The inner cell mass separates into the primitive endoderm, which will form the yolk sac and chorion, and the epiblast, which will form the embryo proper. Epiblast cells are pluripotent embryonic stem cells. They will give rise to all tissues of the embryo.

because they will no longer have the opportunity to become trophecto-derm or epiblast. For a brief moment then, these cells are the pluripotent embryonic stem cells (ESCs). They still have the ability to differentiate into any type of cell of the embryo itself but are held briefly in this pluri-potent state until appropriate signals are received to drive them into one or another differentiation pathway.

The fate of the ICM cells is strongly determined by the signals they receive from their surroundings. If these cells are transplanted into an adult, they will grow and start differentiating haphazardly into different kinds of cells forming a mass of mixed cell types, including pluripotent stem cells. This is called a teratoma. Similar teratoma tumors can also occur naturally due to errors during oogenesis or spermatogenesis. They are normally slow growing and non-malignant but may turn into rapidly growing malignant teratocarcinomas. Pluripotent stem cells derived from teratocarcinomas provided the first such *in vitro* cell cultures for early stem cell studies.

Embryonic Stem Cells

It was a major achievement of the 1990s and early 2000s that culture sys-tems were devised allowing the growth of mouse and later human embry-onic stem cells in culture while carefully suppressing their differentiation to maintain their pluripotent state. Mouse embryonic stem cell lines were first obtained in the early 1980s by Martin Evans and Matthew Kaufman at Cambridge and by Gail Martin in San Francisco. Early procedures involved growing cells from the inner cell mass in serum over a feeder layer of fibroblast cells treated to prevent their own growth (Figure 10). Key to success in establishing many mouse ESC lines was the realization that the feeder layer could be eliminated by supplying two ingredients: Leukemia Inhibitory Factor (LIF), which induces the JAK/STAT signaling pathway, and Bone Morphogenetic Protein (BMP) that effectively inhibit differentiation by partly opposing differentiation cues. Together, these fac-tors allow maintaining ESCs in culture for an indefinite number of cell divisions. Withdrawing these factors or supplying specific hormones or growth factors initiates their differentiation. The fact remains that ES cells grown in LIF plus serum (to supply BMP) do not completely block

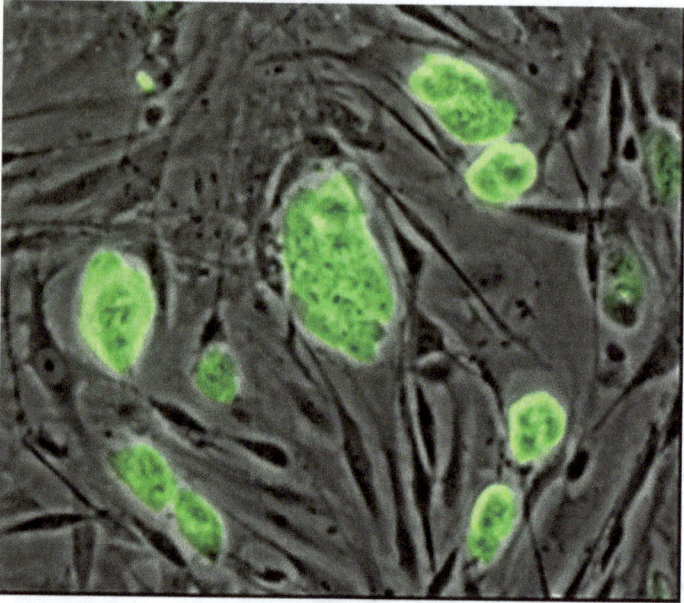

Figure 10.   Mouse embryonic stem cells. Epiblast cells, the embryonic stem cells, carrying a fluorescent marker, can be grown on a fibroblast feeder layer. The fibroblast cells themselves are prevented from growing by irradiation.

Source: https://kids.kiddle.co/Image:Mouse_embryonic_stem_cells.jpg. Public domain.

differentiation signals. They are in a state of partially conflicting and opposing signals. For this reason, human ESC lines proved to be more difficult to establish and it was not until some 15 years later, in 1998, that the team of James Thomson in Madison, Wisconsin, established the first human ESC lines. The cells in the human lines are in a somewhat different state from the mouse lines and the LIF-BMP factors are not sufficient to suppress differentiation. Early success was obtained using bFGF growth factor combined with growth on a layer of feeder fibroblast cells to supply other needed factors, often under conditions in which the feeder cells themselves are unable to grow. Conditions have now been developed to support growth of human ESCs without the use of feeder cells. Nevertheless, human ESC lines have different properties from mouse ESC lines. Most significantly, human ESCs introduced into a blastocyst embryo cannot give rise to chimeric embryos: they have lost some degree of potency compared to mouse ESCs.

It is important to realize that, *in vivo*, ESCs are a transient state not intrinsically organized for self-renewal. Different stem cell lines isolated by these procedures may represent somewhat different states of a pluripotent equilibrium and different solutions to achieve self-renewal. The presence and abundance of different factors in the blastocysts of different mammalian species and the details of the transitions from one stage to another greatly affect the stability of the epiblast-stage pluripotent cells. These differences may underlie the facility with which ESC lines can be established from different species. It is now thought that, at implantation in the uterine wall, mouse epiblast cells progress to a stage that has different culture requirements and in which some differentiation has begun. Post-implantation epiblast cell lines have been obtained and are called EpiESC lines. These cells are still largely pluripotent but have begun to express new genes and can no longer produce all adult tissues, particularly germ cells, if transplanted back into a blastocyst. It is thought that cells of the inner cell mass represent a ground state of pluripotency now called the naïve state while the post-implantation epiblast cells are at a more advanced state predisposed for differentiation into early lineages, now called the primed state. Human ESC lines correspond more to mouse EpiESC lines than to mouse ESCs in many features and are thought to be in a primed state, probably because in the process of establishing the lines *in vitro*, the naïve state advances to the primed state. More recently, the use of small-molecule inhibitors of two early acting protein kinases that promote differentiation (glycogen synthase kinase 3, GSK3, and mitogen-activated protein kinase, MEK) plus LIF has proved to be more effective in suppressing signaling and preventing the heterogeneity of mouse ESCs grown in serum/LIF. The new growth regime, developed by the group of Austin Smith, is now known as 2i/LIF, referring to the two small molecule inhibitors. It produces a more open overall chromatin structure, with lower levels of *de novo* DNA methylases and higher levels of TET demethylases, and higher and more homogeneous levels of pluripotency factors. ESCs grown in 2i/LIF are considered to be in a ground state, naïve pluripotency (Figure 11).

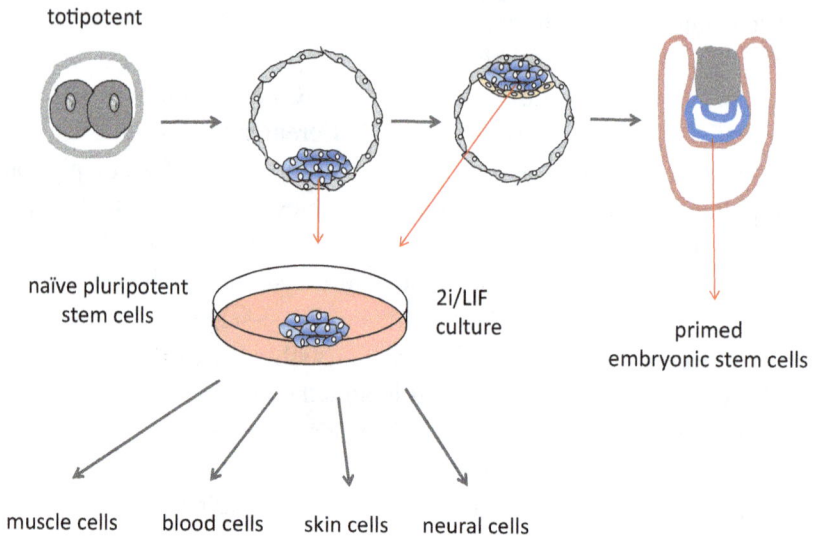

Figure 11.   Mouse pluripotent stem cells. The fertilized egg and early cleavage-stage embryonic cells are totipotent. In the mouse blastocyst stage, the inner cell mass cells are pluripotent: they can no longer give rise to trophectoderm but they can produce all cells in the fetus. They can be grown in culture without losing their pluripotency and can still differentiate into all body tissues.

The isolation of human naïve ESCs has proved to be more difficult. The 2i/LIF conditions are not sufficient to maintain the naïve state in culture. Addition of other inhibitors proved to be necessary but different researchers used different combinations, some including histone deacetylase inhibitors, growth factors, transcription factors, and inhibitors (Figure 12). These various conditions yielded cells that approach more closely the state of human inner cell mass cells, which is somewhat different from and more heterogeneous than that of mouse inner cell mass naïve ESCs (Figure 13). Unlike the sequential, unidirectional initial differentiation of mouse cells into inner cell mass and trophectoderm, human inner cell mass cells can still be reverted to the trophectoderm state. The model of sequential specification and lineage restriction seen in the mouse blastocyst does not apply to the human blastocyst and epiblast, whose cells remain plastic and capable to regenerate the blastocyst until implantation.

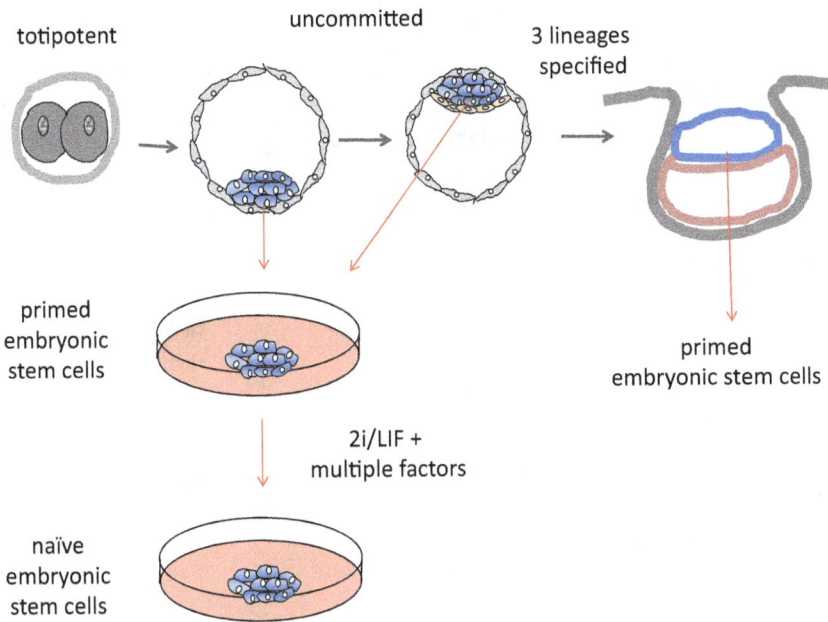

Figure 12. Human pluripotent stem cells. The fertilized egg and early cleavage-stage embryonic cells are totipotent. In the human blastocyst stage, the trophectoderm lineage has not been established. The inner cell mass cells are still uncommitted and can still give rise to trophectoderm. The three lineages trophectoderm, epiblast, and hypoblast are specified at the implantation stage. Inner cell mass cells are in principle naïve pluripotent but, if put into culture, they progress to the primed state. Culture conditions have been found to return to the naïve pluripotent state, for example, in a medium containing 2i/LIF, protein kinase C inhibitor (PKCi), ROCKi, ACTIVIN, and FGF2.

The 2010s years have seen intense interest in and efforts to characterize pluripotent human embryonic stem cells and to derive pluripotent stem cell lines that reflect the naïve state of inner cell mass cells. Embryonic stem cells can, in principle, be made to differentiate into any type of cell in the adult body. They are therefore of extreme interest today both for basic science: they allow us to probe the questions of how the genome can be programmed and reprogrammed, and at the same time, they are extremely powerful tools for regenerative medicine and cell replacement therapeutic approaches.

FGF2 + Activin A

naïve hPSCs   ⟶
              ⟵   primed hPSCs

2i/LIF +
a variety of cocktails

Features

naïve	Features	primed
Rounded	Shape	Flat
High	E-Cadherin	Low
Low	DNA methylation	High
Low	H3K27me3	High
X_aX_a	X chromosome	X_aX_i
Oxidative phosphorylation	Metabolism	Glycolysis
Good	Primordial germ cell differentiation	Poor
Aberrant	Genomic imprinting	Maintained
frequent	Chromosomal aberrations	Less frequent

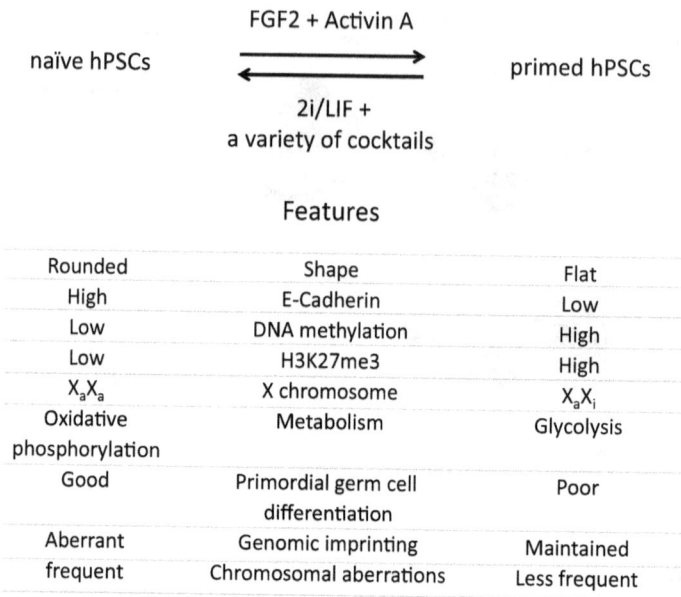

Figure 13.   Comparison of naïve and primed hPSCs. Human PSCs isolated from the blastocyst inner cell mass shift to a primed state when cultured in medium containing FGF2+Activin or on a fibroblast feeder layer. They can be made to recover a naïve state by culturing in 2i/LIF plus a variety of additional factors in different protocols. Some of the principal differences between the two states are listed. X chromosome inactivation status is discussed in the X Inactivation chapter and genomic imprinting is discussed in Chapter 10.

Source: Yilmaz and Benvenisty (2019).

Tests of Pluripotency

What does it mean to say that ES cells are pluripotent? The simplest test is to ask whether they can be induced to differentiate to produce different types of cells *in vitro*. This is not a very stringent criterion because it does not tell us what the cells can do *in vivo*. Another test that was often used in the past is to graft them into an adult mouse to see if they produce teratomas. Teratomas are growths containing different types of differentiated cells. A more stringent test is to see if, when they are introduced into an early mouse embryo at the blastocyst stage, they can contribute to all different kinds of tissues of the adult. Such an adult is called chimeric because it has some cells from the original embryo and some from the grafted ES cells. This shows that the cells can contribute to all different somatic tissues. A still more stringent test is to ask if they can also contribute to a functional germ line: if they can produce gametes that give rise to viable progeny. The most stringent test is to introduce the cells into the blastocyst produced by tetraploid cells. Tetraploid cells are obtained by fusing the two cells at the two-cell stage of a normal embryo. Tetraploid embryos develop to the blastocyst and early implantation stage but will die afterwards. If cells grafted into the tetraploid blastocyst are truly pluripotent, they will take over from the tetraploid cells and proceed to make an embryo that will survive and which will be entirely derived from the grafted cells (Figure 14). The ability of cultured mouse embryonic stem cells to give rise to viable mouse embryos is of fundamental importance. It means that they can be manipulated *in vitro*, modified genetically by introducing transgenes, expanded by growth *in vitro*, selected for mutations, and still generate live mice. The situation is much more complicated for human pluripotent stem cells, partly because of the more heterogeneous nature of human inner cell mass and epiblast cells and partly because of the moral limitations involved in working with human embryos. Only the first two of the criteria for pluripotency listed in Figure 12 can be applied to human ESCs, so the true pluripotency of human stem cells cannot be established.

Differentiation of cultured cells	Does not test for in vivo functionality
Formation of teratomas	Shows ability to generate multiple lineages but does not test developmental functions
Formation of chimeric embryos	Shows ability to contribute to normal development of a blastocyst
Formation of functional germ line	Shows ability to contribute to the germ line
Complementation of tetraploid embryos	Shows ability to provide all functions to a tetraploid blastocyst and develop all cells of a normal embryo

Figure 14.   Evaluation of developmental potency. The tests are listed in order of increasing stringency. The ability to fully complement a tetraploid blastocyst is the most stringent.

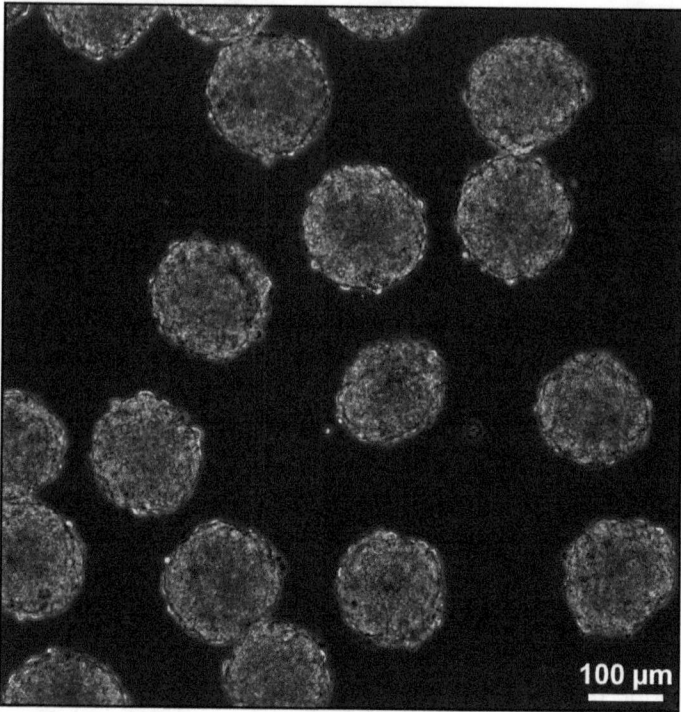

Figure 15.   Embryoid bodies. These embryoid bodies were produced from mouse embryonic stem cells in suspension culture. The suspension conditions and absence of factors
that suppress differentiation allow the cells to aggregate into spheroids that start to differentiate. All three germ lineages are produced: ectoderm, endoderm, and mesoderm.

Source: Stemcellscientist, Creative Commons https://commons.wikimedia.org/wiki/File:MESC_
EBs.jpg.

Embryonic stem cells will start to differentiate spontaneously if the
differentiation-suppressing factors are withdrawn. In this case, they will
produce clumps of cells called embryoid bodies (Figure 15). Cells in
embryoid bodies differentiate heterogeneously, producing muscle cells,
neural cells, bone cells, skin cells, etc. that assemble to form tissues and
organ-like structures. More orderly and specific patterns of differentiation
can be obtained by adding specific factors to induce, for example, neural
differentiation or muscle differentiation, or epidermal differentiation.
With the appropriate factors and culture methods, embryonic stem cells

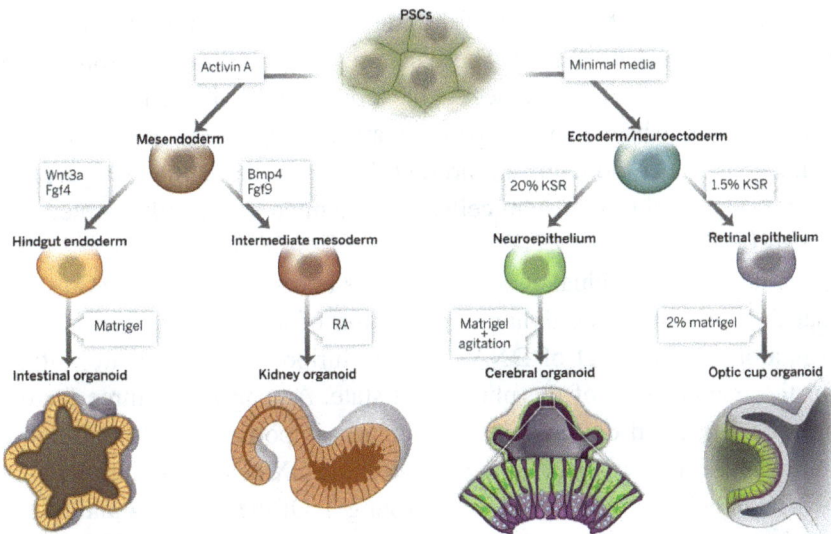

Figure 16. Production of organoids. In the presence of the appropriate factors in the medium and in the appropriate environment (hanging drops, etc.), pluripotent embryonic stem cells (PSCs) can not only enter particular pathways of differentiation but can also self-organize to produce patterned assemblies of different cell types, producing **organoids**. It may soon be possible to control this process well enough to produce functional organs.

Source: Lancaster and Knoblich (2014).

can not only initiate specific pathways of differentiation but can also produce patterned assemblies of cell types called organoids that resemble the way specific organs are generated in the developing embryo (Figure 16). Research is advancing rapidly in this field and it may be possible soon to control this process well enough to produce functional organs.

The Pluripotent State

What is the pluripotent state and how is it achieved? In other words, how can embryonic stem cells have the potential to express any gene and enter any differentiation pathway but at the same time be held back from doing so? The differentiation genes are kept in a state that is not permanently silenced but is nevertheless not active. Embryonic stem cells have low levels of DNA methylation, lack extensive heterochromatin, their nucleus is large relative to the nucleus of differentiated cells, and the chromatin is in a fairly decondensed state. These features suggest that the chromatin of ESCs is relatively open and accessible, compared to the genome of most somatic cells. Chromosome territories are already established and some lamina-associated domains are present. However, the lamins A/C are not expressed in embryonic stem cells, so the lamina is not fully formed nor are all LADs.

Studies of individual genes and factors bound to them in ESCs show that they are under the dynamic regulation of a remarkable network of regulators. A small set of DNA-binding pluripotency factors are critical for the maintenance of the pluripotent state. Among these, three factors have been singled out as being particularly important: Octamer-binding transcription factor 4 (OCT4), SRY-box 2 (SOX2), and NANOG (from "Tir na nÓg", Irish for "Land of the Young"). Of these, OCT4 and SOX2 can form a heterodimer and are critical for pluripotency and self-renewal, while NANOG is necessary to establish pluripotency in the inner cell mass, stabilizes and protects it from drifting into differentiation pathways. These three factors bind together to the regulatory regions of many other genes as well as to control elements of the three pluripotency genes themselves (Figure 17). The first thing to notice is that these three factors stimulate one another, creating a circuit that maintains the pluripotent state. In the second place, they also stimulate a number of other genes needed to support pluripotency and proliferation by recruiting both specific and generalized co-activators. Some of these factors, such as KLF4, are characteristic of the naïve state. KLF4 is turned off upon transition to the primed state and is therefore thought to be an important contributor to maintain the naïve state. A general co-activator of major importance is c-Myc, which binds to many core promoter sites and recruits P-TEFB, therefore stimulating the release of paused RNA Pol II. C-Myc acts as a volume control, increasing the level of expression of the genes activated by the pluripotency factors and promoting the release of paused RNA polymerase.

The pluripotency trio also bind to a large number of genes known to control lineage differentiation. These genes are kept silent in ESCs in part through the action of the pluripotency factors, which recruit the SETDB1 H3K9 methylase, in part with help from Polycomb repressive complexes.

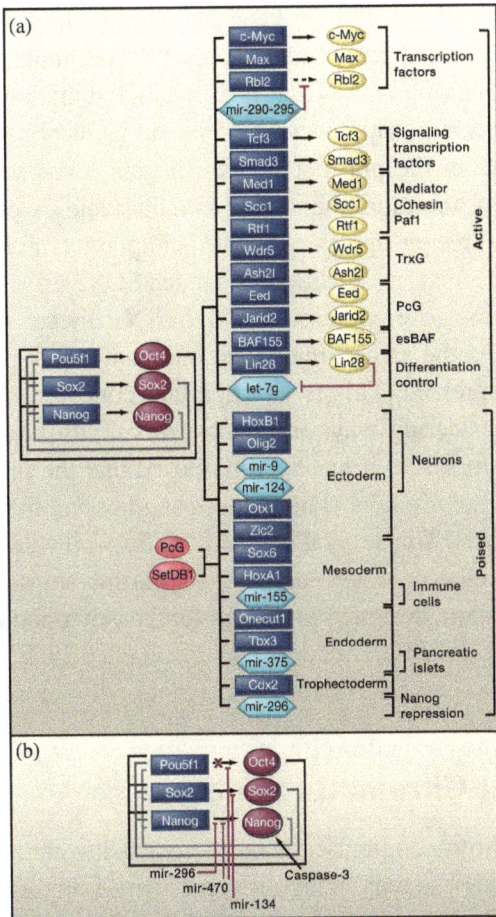

Figure 17. The pluripotency circuitry. The core circuit is that which links the three pluripotency factors: Oct4, Sox2, and NANOG. These three factors also regulate one another
(b), forming an autoregulatory loop, which is further modulated by miRNAs. The three
factors bind, usually together, and regulate a large number of other genes. One set of the
target genes is necessary for self-renewal and pluripotency of the stem cells. Note that this
set includes components of the Polycomb Repressive Complexes. Another set of target
genes consists of key activators of differentiation genes that would specify the main cell
lineages. These genes are kept repressed by the pluripotency factors and repressive activities that they recruit.

Source: Young (2011).

The PcG proteins therefore help keep the undifferentiated state. Here, a distinction has become clear: while variant PRC1 complexes are required to maintain the repression, PRC2 is not essential: mutations in PRC2 proteins do not prevent pluripotency but result in gross abnormalities when differentiation from the pluripotent state begins. Even with the help of PRC1 repression, the pluripotent state is metastable. A precise relationship among the three pluripotency factors is important: an excess of OCT4 promotes mesodermal specification; too much SOX2 drives neuroectodermal differentiation; overexpression of NANOG directs mesendodermal differentiation. At the same time, when one pathway is promoted, other pathways are repressed. This is an important concept to which we will return when considering ways in which genomic differentiation can be reprogrammed. In ESCs, it has been proposed that the pluripotency factors maintain the pluripotent state by each suppressing the pathways promoted by the others. This mutual competition fits well with the impression that, in normal embryonic development, the pluripotent state of ESCs is a precarious condition, designed to be transient, easily tilted towards one or another pathway of differentiation and maintained in ESC lines established *in vitro* by providing factors that suppress differentiation.

The Bivalent Chromatin State

Studies of the chromatin landscape in ES cells using chromatin immunoprecipitation (ChIP) to map many different histone modifications and the distribution of many proteins such as RNA polymerase and PcG complexes have shown that several hundred genes bind the pluripotency factors. Many of these bind also the Polycomb complexes PRC1 and PRC2. These genes also contain H3K27me3 and are not actively expressed. However, surprisingly, they also bind RNA polymerase and contain H3K4me3 in their promoter region. These are marks of transcriptionally active chromatin. Are these genes active and repressed at the same time? Or are they repressed for a while and then weakly transcribed for a little while and then repressed again? CpG island promoters that have both H3K4me3 and H3K27me3 marks are called **bivalent** (Figure 18). The discovery of the bivalent state generated much surprise and was thought for a time to represent a special class of promoters poised for activation in

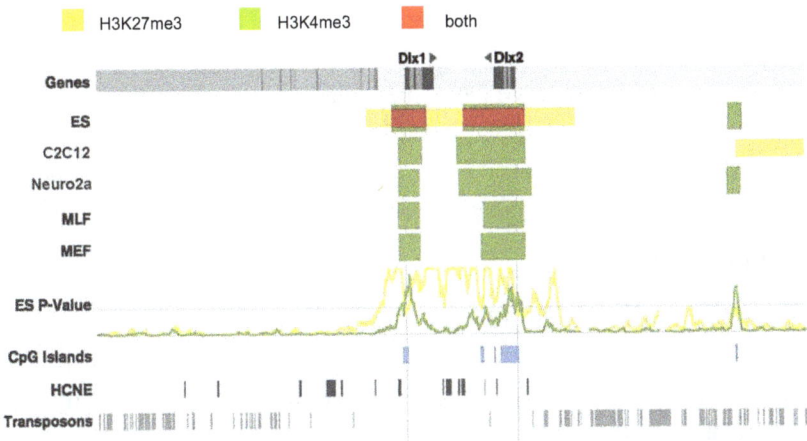

Figure 18. Bivalent domains. The two genes Dlx1 and Dlx2 have both active and repressed histone marks in embryonic stem cells. They lose the H3K27me3 mark and become completely active in all four differentiated cell types tested. The figure also shows the CpG islands and the abundance of transposon-derived sequences typical of mammalian genomes. HCNEs are Highly Conserved Non-coding Elements, which were thought to contain regulatory sequences.

Source: Bernstein *et al.* (2006).

pluripotent cells. In fact, H3K4 methylases are recruited to CpG islands because they contain a cofactor with a CXXC zinc finger domain. Therefore, most CpG islands acquire H3K4me3 at this stage. H3K4me3 in turn inhibits *de novo* DNA methylation. If a gene is not specifically activated at this stage, it will meet the two important conditions for recruitment of PcG complexes: a CpG island with no DNA methylation and no transcriptional activity. In this state, the promoter is kept free of DNA methylation and can bind RNA pol II but cannot carry out effective transcription because the RNA polymerase is paused near the promoter region and unable to elongate effectively in the absence of a specific activator. The block in transcription automatically results in the recruitment of PRC2 by the CXXC zinc finger protein KMD2B and is accompanied by H3K27 methylation (see Chapter 7). However, this is a consequence, not a cause of the block in transcription, which is caused by the pluripotency circuitry and the absence of specific activators. In fact, loss of PRC2 function at this stage does not derepress bivalent promoters. In sum, at

CpG promoters, CXXC zinc finger proteins are responsible for H3K4 methylation, which antagonizes DNA methylation, and for the binding of TET proteins, which remove DNA methylation. Therefore, these bivalent genes seem both repressed and poised to become active when transcriptional activators become available.

Differentiation

In vitro, ES cells can be readily induced to start differentiating. For example, simply adding retinoic acid (a powerful signaling substance important in the differentiation of many tissues) to a culture of ES cells initiates differentiation towards a neural type of pathway. Changing the balance of growth factors in the growth medium can also trigger differentiation in different directions and a fascinating series of studies now suggest that it may soon be possible to define cocktails of factors to induce any desired differentiation lineage. *In vivo*, of course, the pluripotent state in the early embryo is short-lived and cells begin almost immediately to become committed to different differentiation pathways.

What happens when ESCs begin to differentiate? The first thing that happens is that *Oct4* is turned off, first by the induction of repressive factors that bind to the *oct4* gene and recruit histone deacetylases and a histone methyltransferase called G9a that methylates H3K9. In addition, G9a also recruits the *de novo* DNA methylase Dnmt3B. As a result, the *Oct4* gene becomes soon targeted by multiple layers of repression and is epigenetically silenced. The stable silencing of *Oct4* is the pre-condition for further development. In the absence of Oct4, the other two pluripotency factors are also turned off. It is clear that it is undesirable for differentiated cells to start de-differentiating, resume proliferating, and generate different kinds of cells. The pluripotency factors are therefore strongly silenced and DNA methylation ensures that they remain stably silenced. One of the functions of differentiation genes is to ensure that this stable repression takes place. Ectopic expression of Oct4 in mouse causes rapid de-differentiation and powerful proliferation of cells, particularly in tissues that have populations of tissue-specific stem cells (the lining of the gut; the spleen and bone marrow; etc.). You will not be far off if you think that this looks like massive carcinogenesis.

Other changes in gene activity follow the repression of the pluripotency factors, depending on which differentiation pathway is activated. The selection of one pathway generally results in the repression of the factors controlling alternative differentiation pathways in a progressive fashion. What happens to those key regulatory genes that were maintained in a bivalent state? Upon entering a differentiation pathway, transcription factors specific for that pathway fully activate the corresponding bivalent, while the genes that promote alternative pathways now become fully repressed, lose H3K4me3 and RNA polymerase, and eventually also acquire DNA methylation. Polycomb repression and DNA methylation are the two basic mechanisms that switch off unwanted genes during differentiation. In general, Polycomb mechanisms are used for dynamic, short-term repression, for example, of genes that might be needed again later for further differentiation. DNA methylation is used for long-term silencing.

The preceding account should make it clear that, during early development, the activities of a cell depend on the history of that cell and the kinds of inputs it has received. Furthermore, that history may modify the genomic chromatin in ways that are inherited by the cellular progeny. Here we have the clearest example of what epigenetic information is. The chromatin modifications preserve the information of the regulatory decisions that have been made and transmit it in subsequent cell divisions. Normally, this occurs through the roughly equal distribution of nucleosomal histones to the two daughter DNA molecules during DNA replication. This ensures that each of the two daughter cells receives half of the old histones carrying the histone modifications present in the mother cell. The histone-modifying complexes, such as the Polycomb complexes or the heterochromatin complexes, are recruited by the pre-existing histone modifications to extend the modifications to the histones that are newly deposited to restore a full complement. DNA methylation has its own way of ensuring the inheritance of the methyl mark. Since the preferred target of DNA methylation is at CpGs, the fully methylated DNA produces hemimethylated CpGs in the newly replicated daughter DNA molecules. Hemimethylated CpGs are the target of the maintenance DNMT1 that accompanies the DNA replication fork and rapidly restores full methylation (see the DNA Methylation chapter). Daughter cells therefore rapidly restore the DNA methylation status as well as the key histone marks present in the mother cell and with them also the pattern of gene expression. That these marks are instructive and determine the state of differentiation in the daughter cells is shown by a case in which they are specifically not equally transmitted to the daughter cells. Such an extreme case of asymmetric inheritance occurs in *Drosophila* spermatogenesis, where germ line stem cell division produces one stem cell that inherits the old histones with their histone marks and remains a stem cell. The other daughter cell recruits all new histones, with no marks, and initiates differentiation to produce spermatogonia. If the remarkable mechanisms that produce this asymmetry are interfered with, restoring a more equal partitioning of the old histones, the result is a failure to differentiate.

PcG Mechanisms and Epidermal Differentiation

PcG repression helps stabilize ES cells but is not absolutely essential for ES cell or pluripotency. However, it is essential for differentiation. ES cells that are defective for PcG mechanisms differentiate abnormally, cannot completely shut down the pluripotency genes, start expressing terminal differentiation genes prematurely, and result in abnormal tissues. To understand why this is so, a recent paper (Ezhkova *et al.*, 2009) described the process of differentiation of epidermis: skin.

The epidermis is not just a simple layer of leathery cells that covers the muscles and nerves. To function properly, the active layer of cells that generate the skin, the epidermal stem cells called basal keratinocytes, must continuously grow and produce successive layers of cells that become progressively differentiated to produce the proteins that make the horny outer layer of skin, cease proliferating and eventually die, and are sloughed off the skin (Figure 19). When the basal keratinocytes first appear in the embryo, they are already committed to the epidermal fate. The pluripotency genes are silenced and DNA-methylated, as are the key genes controlling alternative differentiation pathways. If the PcG mechanisms are turned off at this point, those genes do not become reactivated. However, the PcG complexes are still needed to keep repressed the genes for terminal epidermal differentiation. Without PcG repression, the basal keratinocytes

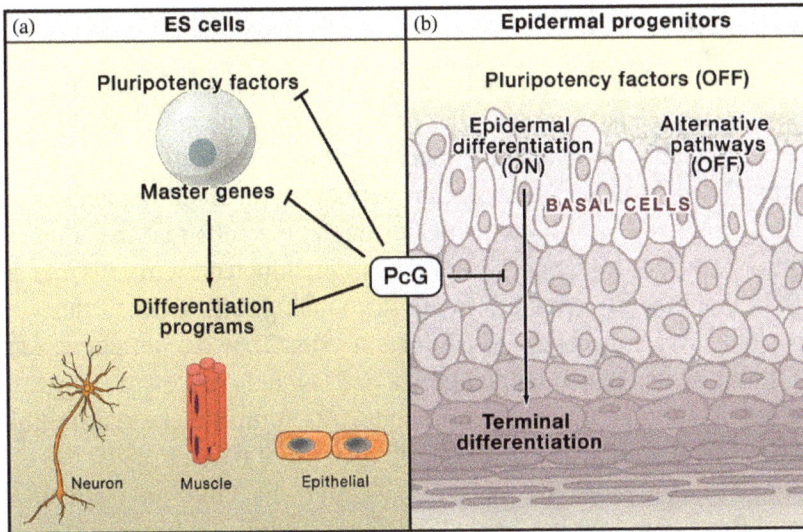

Figure 19.   Epidermal differentiation. As differentiation begins, pluripotency factors and alternative differentiation pathways are shut off first by H3K9 methylation and then by DNA methylation. Epidermal-specific bivalent genes move to being either wholly Polycomb-repressed (all H3K27me3) or wholly transcriptionally active (all H3K4me3). Polycomb mechanisms become essential to control differentiation genes, which become gradually derepressed as differentiation proceeds to terminal differentiation. In the case of epidermis, this ends with the death of terminally differentiated cells, which form the outer layer of the skin.

Source: Pirrotta (2009).

just immediately stop dividing, produce the horny layer, and die without building up the intermediate layers of cells that are critical to form functional skin. Why do they stop dividing and die? One of the things PcG complexes repress is genes that block cell cycle progression, particularly two related genes called *Ink4a/ARF* and *Ink4b* (see Chapter 7). When these are repressed by PcG, cells can still divide. When *Ink4a* and *Ink4b* are derepressed, the cells stop dividing. In normal skin, the expression of PRC2 components gradually decreases as differentiation progresses, allowing the gradual derepression of the epidermal genes as cell division slows down. Terminal differentiation and exit from the cell cycle occur only after the intermediate layers of cells have been produced.

Adult Stem Cells

Differentiation is a process, not a simple event. It generally goes through many stages, depending on the pathway, corresponding to different degrees of commitment and intermediate proliferation before reaching the terminally differentiated state. Many tissues retain small populations of cells that are still **multipotent**. For example, the cells that make up the lining of the gut include pockets that house multipotent stem cells that are kept in this state by signals from the surrounding cells. Cells of this kind are also known collectively as adult stem cells. They are not pluripotent: the stem cells in the gut are committed and can only make gut epithelium and gut-specific cells. The surrounding cells form a niche that inhibits further differentiation and supports cell division of the stem cells. As soon as they leave the protective niche or pocket in which they are maintained, they differentiate into gut epithelium (see Chapter 12, Figures 7–9). In some situations, the alignment of the mitotic spindle in the dividing stem cell is such that one daughter cell remains in the niche while the other is pushed out of the niche. This is a characteristic asymmetric division in which the cell that remains in the niche continues to be a stem cell, while the cell that exits the niche begins to differentiate.

A particularly multipotent kind of adult stem cell is the hematopoietic stem cell (HSC). HSCs are stem cells that can produce a large variety of blood cells (Figure 20). In adult mammals, these cells reside in an appropriate niche in the bone marrow and express factors that promote their self-renewal and regulate differentiation. In particular, they target Polycomb complexes to repress the INK4A locus, which would otherwise produce inhibitors of cell cycle progression, and therefore allow cell proliferation. Insufficient Polycomb repression would result in too few HSCs and consequently insufficient blood cells. HSCs that move out of the niche begin differentiating and, through a series of choices, can produce the many different kinds of blood cells as well as the B and T cells of the immune system.

De-Differentiation and the Reprogramming of Somatic Cells

As embryonic development proceeds, ESCs must differentiate to produce a vast variety of very different cells and tissues. As developmental

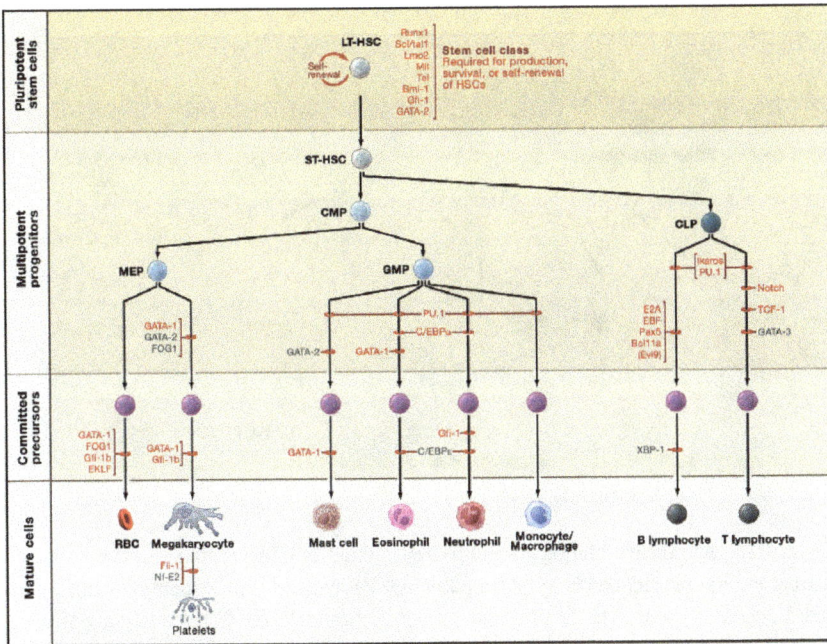

Figure 20. Hematopoietic stem cells. These multipotent cells reside in the bone marrow and thymus. The expression of different transcription factors indicated is required to proceed in the various differentiation pathways. LT-HSC/ST-HSC, long-term/short-term hematopoietic stem cell; CMP, common myeloid progenitor; CLP, common lymphoid progenitor; MEP, megakaryocyte/erythroid progenitor; GMP, granulocyte/macrophage progenitor; RBCs, red blood cells.

Source: Orkin and Zon (2008).

biologists have noted from the very early days, it looks like many alternative differentiation pathways are closed off and differentiating cells progressively narrow down their potential. Many biologists wondered how the decisions are made, whether any genetic information was progressively lost or if it might be possible to reverse the differentiation process (Figure 21).

In recent years, the enormous potential for the application of stem cells to regenerative medicine has become evident. For this to be therapeutically useful, the stem cells need to be generated from the patient's own cells. How can we take adult cells and reprogram them to become again pluripotent? Work over the past 60 years, beginning with John Gurdon's

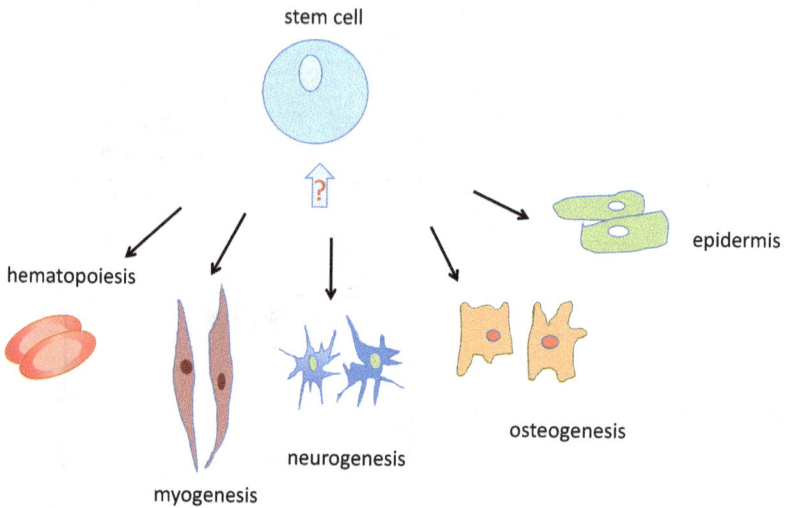

Figure 21.   Are differentiation programs reversible? It is beginning to be possible to instruct embryonic stem cells to take a particular pathway of differentiation, using appropriate cocktails of growth factors and growth conditions. As differentiation proceeds, alternative choices and pathways are closed off. Is something physically lost or irreversibly altered in differentiation? Or is it possible to reprogram differentiated cells to return to a pluripotent state?

experiments in the 1960s with nuclear transplantation and frog eggs, has shown that if somatic cell nuclei, even from terminally differentiated cells, are introduced into an egg from which the egg nucleus has been removed, it is possible to obtain a viable embryo that develops into an adult (Figure 22). This process, called somatic cell nuclear transplantation (SCNT), is rapid: somatic nuclei become reprogrammed in a matter of hours. But it is terribly inefficient in terms of success in generating viable and normal development. Even in frogs, the success rate is low. In mammals, it is even lower. Most of the resulting embryos die during development with various kinds of abnormalities: the genes of the transplanted nucleus have been incompletely reprogrammed. Nevertheless, these experiments, culminating with the production of Dolly the sheep, cloned by the team of Keith Campbell and Ian Wilmut from the nucleus of a mammary cell, showed that even terminally differentiated cells have not lost any genetic information and it is possible to reprogram the genome to

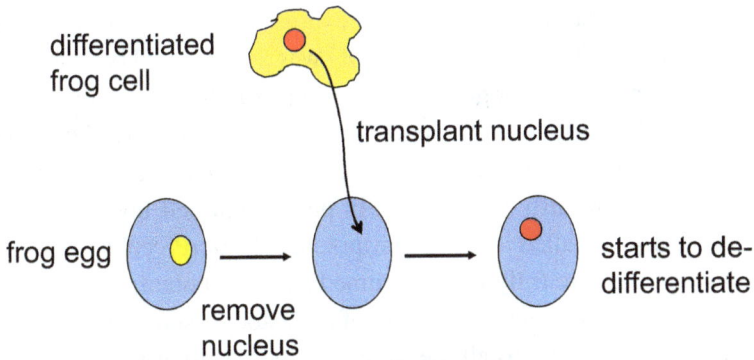

Figure 22. John Gurdon's nuclear transplantation experiment (1958). Has the nucleus of a differentiated somatic cell lost any essential information, compared to a fertilized egg? John Gurdon removed the nucleus from a frog oocyte and replaced it with the nucleus from a differentiated cell. The somatic nucleus starts to dedifferentiate but can it direct development into a frog?

the state of the embryonic stem cells from which all cells of the body can be produced.

Why is it so difficult? We begin now to understand what needs to happen. Silenced genes governing all differentiation pathways have to be reactivated by removing DNA methylation (remember, in the fertilized egg, this happens in the first two days). In nuclear transplantation, this happens because the TET3 DNA demethylase present in the egg can act on the transplanted nucleus, though it cannot act on the oocyte nucleus itself (see Figure 6). But differentiation genes must not become active: they must be effectively repressed by the pluripotency circuitry. Therefore, the critical events are the reactivation of genes, including the pluripotency factors but also the establishment of the pluripotency circuit before the differentiation genes start being expressed. Many experiments in the 1980s and 1990s had shown that differentiated cells could be reprogrammed by fusion with other kinds of cells. Fusion with embryonic stem cells could reactivate genes that had been silenced much earlier in development. Something in the cytoplasm of the embryonic stem cells was able to activate earlier programs of differentiation. In 2006, Shinya Yamanaka published a path-breaking article showing that somatic differentiated cells could be converted to something that behaved very much like ES cells by introducing into them four transgenes expressing OCT4, SOX2, cMYC, and KLF4 (OSKM). Exogenous NANOG was not essential because OCT4 and SOX2 turn on the endogenous *Nanog* gene (as well as the endogenous *Oct4* and *Sox2* genes). The efficiency was still very low, around one in 105 cells became reprogrammed, and it took several weeks, but it could all be done in the culture dish and resulted in pluripotent cell lines. The reprogrammed cells are called induced pluripotent cells or iPS cells (Figure 23). To show that they are fully reprogrammed and pluripotent, these cells can be introduced into the inner cell mass of a blastocyst stage mouse embryo and they will contribute to all the tissues of the resulting mouse.

The procedures have been repeated and improved by many other researchers in the subsequent years. It is clear that differentiation is not a one-way process but much more plastic than previously thought. Yamanaka's original work used retroviral vectors to introduce the genes into the cell culture, and the mice produced from these iPS cells developed tumors at high frequency, a major drawback. Intense work since 2006 has improved the procedures to generate iPSCs from mouse, human, and many other mammalian species without the use of retroviral vectors. Alternative cocktails of pluripotency factors have been explored and the process of reprogramming has been clarified. Successful reprogramming involves the reactivation of the endogenous *Oct4, Sox2,* and *Nanog* genes before the transgenic copies are lost or are shut down. Thus, the transgenes

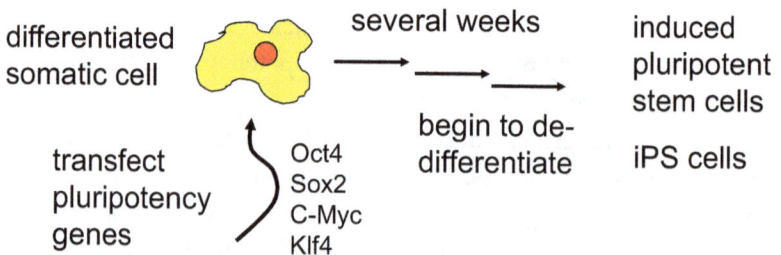

Figure 23.   Yamanaka's reprogramming experiment (2006). Yamanaka introduced pluripotency transgenes into the nucleus of a differentiated somatic cell. After several weeks, a very small fraction of the somatic cells show signs of having been reprogrammed to self-renewing pluripotent cells, now called induced pluripotent cells or iPSCs.

kickstart the pluripotency circuitry. To do this, it is important to keep the cells alive and dividing. cMyc is not specific for pluripotency but it is needed to promote cell proliferation, to increase gene expression, and to release paused RNA polymerase. KLF4 is specific for the naïve state of embryonic stem cells and helps direct the reprogramming to the pluripotent state. This is the role of the other two factors often used in the OSKM cocktail. However, the key factors are OCT4 and SOX2. OCT4 is irreducibly essential for the process. It has even been possible in some cases to obtain iPS cells just with exogenous OCT4 although at a much lower frequency. SOX2 and KLF4 can be replaced by related proteins SOX1 or SOX3 and KLF2 or KLF5, respectively. All MYC family members are equally effective. Substitutions of KLF and MYC factors are also possible and additional factors, based on the analysis of pluripotency networks, can sometimes improve efficiencies by replacing a factor with its downstream targets.

In agreement with the idea that endogenous pluripotency genes and other early genes need to be reactivated, DNA demethylation is important and *Tet2*, but not *Tet1*, is upregulated early in reprogramming. Inhibition of DNA methylation increases the efficiency of the process by helping reactivate endogenous *Oct4*, *Klf4*, and *Nanog*. This has been done by treating the cells with azacytidine, which does increase the frequency but at the risk of activating transposable elements and producing DNA damage. Surprisingly, significant DNA remethylation, which was thought to be needed to repress differentiated functions, occurs only in the late stages of reprogramming and is, in fact, not essential. Reprogramming has been achieved even with cells lacking the *de novo* DNA methylases DNMT3A and B. The pluripotency circuitry seems to be sufficient to turn off most unwanted gene expressions. PcG repression needs to be lifted from some genes and restored to others, particularly in the "bivalent" state. A variety of factors that promote cell proliferation and bypass the many safeguards that normally prevent cell proliferation can improve the efficiency of reprogramming to pluripotency. These are not just factors that act directly on gene expression. A remarkable effect is obtained not by a regulatory protein but by vitamin C, ascorbic acid, which stimulates the activity of histone demethylases KDM2A and KDM2B.

Reprogramming Intermediates

What happens during the lengthy process of reprogramming to pluripotency?

First of all, why is the efficiency of reprogramming so low? Are only a few cells in a large population susceptible to reprogramming? This is unlikely as lineage tracing shows that terminally differentiated cells of various types can be reprogrammed. The evidence shows instead that reprogramming is a process that traverses many stages and which most cells never complete.

An important step is a mesenchymal to epithelial cell transition. This is a transition that occurs in both directions during normal embryonic development in which motile, spindle-shaped cells with little cell adhesion (mesenchymal) convert to planar, polarized cells that adhere tightly and form cohesive and interacting structures (epithelial). A metabolic transition from oxidative phosphorylation to glycolysis is also an early step in reprogramming. In fact, primed ESCs utilize principally glycolysis rather than oxidative phosphorylation to drive their metabolism and have a correspondingly lower level of mitochondria. While this is consistent with the lower levels of oxygen available during embryogenesis, pre-implantation naïve ESCs have higher levels of mitochondrial aerobic utilization of pyruvate to generate acetyl CoA and have higher levels of oxidative phosphorylation than primed pluripotent cells. These metabolic shifts are not just changes in energy production but affect the potential for epigenetic chromatin changes. Acetyl CoA is, after all, necessary for histone acetylation and for the synthesis of S-adenosyl methionine, in turn required for histone and DNA methylation. During reprogramming, differentiation-specific genes must be turned off and silenced and chromatin needs to become more plastic and less condensed. A large number of genes and events are involved. Do these events occur in a defined progression towards pluripotency or is the process more haphazard and stochastic?

The OSKM proteins act as pioneer factors, binding to many sites not accessible to most transcription factors. Initially, through their high levels, they bind to a wide variety of genomic sites, including differentiation-specific genes. Some of this may be necessary but much is likely to regulate irrelevant genes, detracting from efficient reprogramming. Differentiation-specific genes tend to be shut off, as they are in ESCs, by the pluripotency factors. The process is haphazard and inefficient at first and involves turning off as well as activating genes to change metabolism, cell proliferation, cytoskeletal structures, and differentiated functions. This early stage involves principally c-MYC but KLF4 is also involved in repressing differentiated genes. Many partially reprogrammed cells enter dead-end pathways that cannot progress to pluripotency (Figure 24). A fraction retains the possibility to reach pluripotency with increasing frequency if exposure to OSKM is continued. As differentiated functions are silenced, a second stage involves the derepression of silenced functions associated with embryonic development and pluripotency. In contrast to the first stage, this involves gene reactivation and is promoted by DNA demethylases, by inhibitors of histone deacetylases, and by demethylation of repressive histone marks. This second phase is better defined, with reference to the pluripotency circuitry, and more predictable. Only at this stage is the expression of endogenous pluripotency genes reactivated. All these events occur much more efficiently when nuclei are introduced into eggs (SCNT), indicating that factors present in the egg cytoplasm or nucleus are much better at carrying out the reprogramming in the scope of a few days. In both iPS cells and nuclear transplantation, intermediate

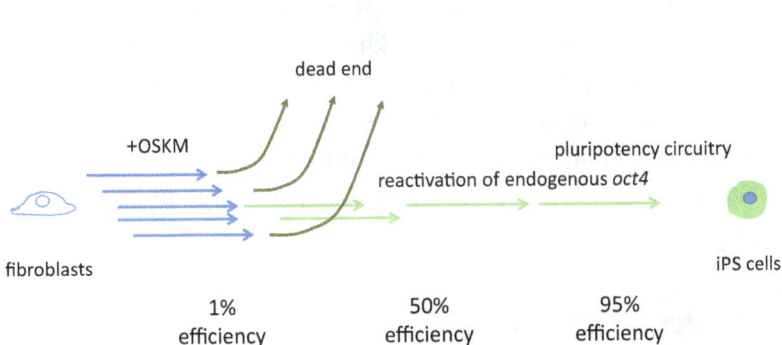

Figure 24.   Reprogramming intermediates. Analysis of intermediate stages in OSKM-induced reprogramming shows that initially many cells enter non-productive pathways that do not lead to pluripotency. Some cells, often those displaying certain surface marks, enter more promising pathways. Some of these reactivate endogenous oct4 gene expression and are very likely to re-establish the pluripotency circuitry and reach iPSC status.

states give a glimpse of the complex processes that have to take place. When we learn how to reproduce the oocyte environment *in vitro*, it might be possible to reactivate the endogenous pluripotency circuits in cultured cells without the need for transgenes.

An important advance for the therapeutic use of iPSCs was the development of efficient, non-retroviral vectors that do not integrate into the genome to introduce the OSKM genes into the cells. Instead of retroviral vectors, well-tested modified adenovirus vectors or lentiviral vectors were used. This avoided the possibility of generating insertional mutations as well as the risk of continued expression of an integrated c-MYC gene, which would be tumor-inducing. The use of defined inducible cassettes expressing the OSKM factors increased the efficiency of reprogramming to the level of several percent and showed that continued expression of these factors throughout the process was required. Cells from different somatic tissues required different OSKM levels and had different efficiencies of reprogramming. Generally, a higher ratio of OCT4 to SOX2 was more effective because it promotes transient mesendoderm-like gene expression, while higher SOX2 levels promote an ectoderm-like pattern. For research purposes, the introduction in the genome of cassettes expressing pluripotency factors under control of an inducible promoter has been the most useful and effective. An alternative that bypasses transgenes or OSKM entirely is the use of small molecules to inhibit or activate signaling pathways. A cocktail of small molecules has been reported to induce pluripotency in mouse somatic cells with a 0.2% frequency. The large variety of treatments that have been shown to be effective in reprogramming differentiated cells to pluripotency and the types of intermediate stages indicate that alternative pathways can reconstruct the pluripotency circuitry.

Properties of iPSCs

iPS cells derived from a patient's own tissues have a vast potential for applications in research, regenerative medicine, and therapeutic treatments. Cells of almost any desired genetic background can be used to generate iPS cell lines. For therapeutic applications, autologous stem cells (generated from the patient's own cells) are compatible genetically and immunologically. The principal feature of iPSCs is, of course, that they are pluripotent.

They are selected for this purpose, and the reprogramming process, though inefficient, reaches a steady state at pluripotency. iPS cells expanded in the culture conditions used for naïve embryonic stem cells express the typical markers of the naïve state and in chimeric embryos can produce every type of embryonic cell. For mouse iPSCs, this was conclusively shown by their ability to complement tetraploid blastocysts and produce normal live animals entirely derived from iPSCs. The ability of iPSCs to undergo extended self-renewal means that it is possible to generate large numbers of cells that can in principle be differentiated to any state in the body. For most clinical applications in regenerative medicine, iPSCs need to be differentiated to produce the type of cells and tissues required. This can be done by removing inhibitors and allowing them to differentiate freely and then selecting the desired type of cell. Directed differentiation would be more desirable and exploit the potential of iPSCs to produce large numbers of cells. For this purpose, specific and safe differentiation protocols suitable for clinical use need to be developed and applied.

While iPSCs are clearly pluripotent, there remain nevertheless differences among pluripotent lines produced from the same reprogramming procedure, even from the same type of somatic cells, confirming the idea that there is a good deal of randomness in the process. Clearly, the reprogramming process is variable not only in the path taken to pluripotency but also in the degree of reprogramming in different parts of the genome. Mutations, both point mutations and larger-scale genomic rearrangements have been reported in many studies of hiPSCs. The first clinical trial using hiPSCs of patient origin was suspended because of alterations and copy number variations detected in the cells that were not present in the original fibroblasts (Garber, 2015; Blair and Barker, 2016). These mutations might be due to the process of reprogramming itself, to the selection of rare mutations present in the original cell population, or to the expansion of the hiPSCs in extended culture. Studies indicate that some alterations can arise from all three sources.

A similar concern involves inappropriate epigenetic changes. An important example is DNA methylation. Reprogramming requires removal of DNA methylation from the promoters of pluripotency genes while the promoters of differentiated functions need to be methylated and shut down. This re-methylation is often incomplete so that some differentiated functions are not entirely silenced or just easier to reactivate. This results in a predisposition to differentiate to the type of cell originally used to derive the iPSCs. This is not necessarily a problem, depending on the use for which iPSCs are intended, but it is a concern that needs to be kept in mind. A related problem is the methylation of imprinted genes (see Genetic imprinting chapter). Some imprinted genes may lose their methylation imprint, others may gain an inappropriate methylation imprint, resulting in over- or under-expression of some critical functions. X chromosome inactivation is a process triggered when naïve embryonic stem cells begin to differentiate and involves DNA methylation as well as histone marks (see X Inactivation chapter). The reprogramming process should reverse inactivation and iPSCs should have both X chromosomes active. The control of X inactivation is often defective so that, when iPSCs are induced to differentiate and inactivate one of the two X chromosomes, the inactivation is incomplete or unstable, resulting in the expression of a double dose of some or all X chromosome genes.

To summarize the difficulties associated with reprogramming to iPSCs:

- it is slow, laborious, and inefficient
- there are risks from the use of oncogenes such as c-Myc
- there is induction or selection of genomic alterations
- iPS cells may not be fully reprogrammed
- residual DNA methylation patterns resembling the tissue of origin
- partial loss of imprinting and of X inactivation

Alternative Reprogramming Methods

Improvements in the reprogramming methods to produce and maintain human iPSCs have been made and are progressing. These improvements may reduce the disadvantages of human iPSCs, but for many purposes, there are now alternatives to reprogram cells for use in regenerative medicine.

Somatic cell nuclear transfer, SCNT, is the use of enucleated oocytes into which are introduced the nuclei of somatic cells from an individual patient for reprogramming. This method, similar to the John Gurdon type of experiment, is much more rapid than the iPS method as a means of reprogramming the somatic nucleus. Reprogramming to pluripotency in the oocyte cytoplasm takes hours rather than weeks. The reprogrammed cell may need further tweaking and growth in culture to expand the number of cells and does not escape the possibility of incomplete reprogramming. The main disadvantage of SCNT is that it is a laborious process that can only be done one cell at a time.

A very promising approach is that of direct lineage conversion. It has been known for a long time from studies in *Drosophila* and mammalian development that entire programs of differentiation are controlled by key regulatory factors. Strong expression of such lineage-determining key factors in an already differentiated cell has been shown to reprogram the genome to the alternative lineage. For example, ectopic expression of MyoD, a DNA-binding transcription factor, in fibroblasts is sufficient to convert them into myogenic cells. Lineage-specific transcription factors such as MyoD not only activate the necessary downstream differentiation genes but also suppress the expression of alternative lineage factors. As a result, a terminally differentiated cell is converted into a different type of terminally differentiated cell (Figure 25, upper row). A particularly striking

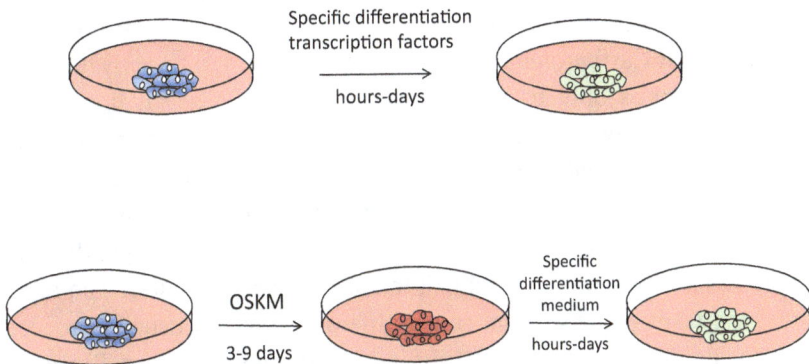

Figure 25.   Direct and indirect lineage conversion. Direct lineage conversion uses differentiated cells and induces expression of master differentiation factors that activate a gene expression program for specific differentiation while suppressing alternative pathways. It is fast and efficient but does not allow cell proliferation. Indirect lineage conversion uses the forced expression of the OSKM pluripotency cocktail (OCT4, SOX2, KLF4, and cMYC) for a brief period of culture to induce de-differentiation before inducing specific differentiation through the culture medium or expression of differentiation factors. This approach allows cell proliferation and expansion.

example is the direct conversion of mouse embryonic fibroblasts into neuronal cells. The introduction of three transgenes, *Brn2*, *Ascl1*, and *Mytl1* (the BAM factors) reprogrammed the fibroblasts within 24 hours to assume a neuronal morphology, form functional synapses, and express the typical electrophysiological features of excitatory neurons. A similar conversion could be obtained starting from primary hepatocytes, showing that even distantly related cells, of endodermal as well as mesodermal origin, could be converted to neurons (normally derived from ectoderm). Different combinations of factors successfully produced different neuronal subtypes. Direct conversion, usually of fibroblasts, has successfully produced not only neurons but hepatocytes and cardiomyocytes, using appropriate factors.

Direct conversion is much faster and more efficient than reprogramming to pluripotency. This approach has been used to convert differentiated cells, usually fibroblasts, to different types of differentiated cells. This includes not only different types of neurons but hepatocytes, cardiomyocytes, or other kinds of differentiated cells, limited only by the current state of knowledge about the appropriate factors necessary. Current approaches use CRISPR/Cas technology to activate or silence endogenous genes instead of introducing exogenous genes. The CRISPR/Cas methods (see Methods chapter) use small guide RNAs to target an activator fused to the bacterial Cas9 protein to the endogenous genes to be activated. This approach requires only transient expression of the Cas9 fusion protein because, once activated, the endogenous genes remain active and affect the program of lineage conversion. The direct conversion approach requires high levels of expression of the key reprogramming factors to overcome the previous epigenetic states, to silence the corresponding differentiation factors, and to establish the new epigenetic states. The reprogramming takes place without cell proliferation since it usually proceeds from one post-mitotic terminally differentiated state to another. Therefore, only relatively small numbers of cells are involved and there is usually no possibility of cell expansion.

An intermediate reprogramming strategy is the indirect conversion. Starting from differentiated cells, this approach is to first loosen the epigenetic state by a transient expression of some or all four OSKM factors. This brief treatment is not intended to achieve pluripotency but to remove differentiated marks and revert to a more plastic state that has the ability to

Reprogramming strategy	Time frame	Efficiencies	Differentiation potential	Requirement for cell proliferation	Expandability	Risk for teratoma	Mechanism
SCNT	Hours–days	Moderate	Pluripotent	None	Yes	High	De-differentiation
iPSC	Weeks–months	Very low	Pluripotent	Yes	Yes	High	De-differentiation
Direct lineage conversion	Hours–days	High	Unipotent	None	No	Low	Transdifferentiation
Lineage conversion by plastic induction	Days–weeks	High	Multipotent/unipotent	Yes	Yes	Moderate*	De-differentiation

Figure 26.   Comparison of the reprogramming approaches.

Note: *The extent of de-differentiation in the plastic induction process is heterogeneous. It is possible, therefore, that some of the cells reach pluripotency and are more subject to the risks attendant with pluripotent cells, including mutations, genomic rearrangements, and risk for teratoma formation.
Source: Sancho-Martinez Baek and Izpisua Belmonte (2012).

proliferate. After a few days of this preliminary treatment, the cells are cultured in a medium conducive to the desired differentiation of the new lineage (Figure 25, lower row). Alternatively, specific differentiation factors can be introduced or activated to achieve the desired terminal differentiation. This approach allows expansion of the cells before terminal differentiation. It also may allow a wider range of lineage conversion than is currently possible by direct conversion. Figure 26 summarizes the advantages and disadvantages of these different reprogramming approaches.

Further Reading

Bao S, Tang F, Li X, Hayashi K, Gillich A, Lao K and Surani A (2009). Epigenetic reversion of post-implantation epiblast to pluripotent embryonic stem cells. *Nature*. **461**, 1292–1295.

Balhorn R (2007). The protamine family of sperm nuclear proteins. *Genome Biol*. **8**, 227.

Bayerl J, Ayyash M, Shani T, Manor YS, Gafni O, Massarwa R *et al.* (2021). Principles of signaling pathway modulation for enhancing human naive pluripotency induction. *Cell Stem Cell*. **28**, 1549–1565.

Bernstein BE, Mikkelsen TS, Xie X, Kamal M, Huebert DJ, Cuff J *et al.* (2006). A bivalent chromatin structure marks key developmental genes in embryonic stem cells. *Cell*. **125**, 315–326.

Bizzotto S, Dou Y, Ganz J, Doan RN, Kwon M, Bohrson CL *et al.* (2021). Landmarks of human embryonic development inscribed in somatic mutations. *Science.* **371**, 1249–1253.

Black JB, Adler A, Wang H-G, D'Ippolito A, Hutchinson H, Reddy T *et al.* (2016). Targeted epigenetic remodeling of endogenous loci by CRISPR/Cas9-based transcriptional activators directly converts fibroblasts to neuronal cells. *Cell Stem Cell.* **19**, 406–414.

Blair NF and Barker RA (2016). Making it personal: The prospects for autologous pluripotent stem cell-derived therapies. *Regen Med.* **11**, 423–425.

Caldwell BA, Liu MY, Prasasya RD, Wang T, DeNizio JE, Leu, NA *et al.* (2021). Functionally distinct roles for TET-oxidized 5-methylcytosine bases in somatic reprogramming to pluripotency. *Mol Cell.* **81**, 859–869.e858.

Fasching L, Jang Y, Tomasi S, Schreiner J, Tomasini L, Brady MV *et al.* (2021). Early developmental asymmetries in cell lineage trees in living individuals. *Science.* **371**, 1245–1248.

Garber K (2015). RIKEN suspends first clinical trial involving induced pluripotent stem cells. *Nat Biotechnol.* **33**, 890–891.

Gu T-P, Guo F, Yang H-F, Wu H-P Xu G-F, Liu W *et al.* (2011). The role of Tet3 DNA dioxygenase in epigenetic reprogramming by oocytes. *Nature.* **477**, 606–610.

Hertig AT and Adams EC (1967). Studies on the human oocyte and its follicle: I. Ultrastructural and histochemical observations on the primordial follicle stage. *J. Cell Biol.* **34**, 647–675.

Ladstätter S and Tachibana K (2019). Genomic insights into chromatin reprogramming to totipotency in embryos. *J Cell Biol.* **218**, 70–82.

Li D, Shu X, Zhu P and Pei D (2021). Chromatin accessibility dynamics during cell fate reprogramming. *EMBO Rep.* **22**, e51644.

Lancaster MA and Knoblich JA (2014). Organogenesis in a dish: Modeling development and disease using organoid technologies. *Science.* **345**, 1247125.

Li M and Izpisua Belmonte JC (2017). Ground rules of the pluripotency gene regulatory network. *Nat Rev Genet.* **18**, 180–191.

Li Y, Zhang Z, Chen J, Liu W, Lai W, Liu B *et al.* (2018). Stella safeguards the oocyte methylome by preventing *de novo* methylation mediated by DNMT1. *Nature.* **564**, 136–140.

Loh KM and Lim B (2011). A precarious balance: Pluripotency factors as lineage specifiers. *Cell Stem Cell.* **8**, 363–369.

Michael AK, Grand RS, Isbel L, Cavadini S, Kozicka Z, Kempf G *et al.* (2020). Mechanisms of OCT4-SOX2 motif readout on nucleosomes. *Science.* **368**, 1460–1465.

Orkin SH and Zon LI (2008). Hematopoiesis: An evolving paradigm for stem cell biology. *Cell.* **132**, 631–644.

Perrera V and Martello G (2019). How does reprogramming to pluripotency affect genomic imprinting? *Front Cell Dev Biol.* **7**, article 76.

Pirrotta V (2009). Polycomb repression under the skin. *Cell.* **136**, 992–994.

Sancho-Martinez I, Baek SH and Izpisua Belmonte JC (2012). Lineage conversion methodologies meet the reprogramming toolbox. *Nat Cell Biol.* **14**, 892–899.

Schlesinger S and Meshorer E (2019). Open chromatin, epigenetic plasticity, and nuclear organization in pluripotency. *Dev Cell.* **48**, 135–150.

Shahbazi MN, Siggia ED and Zernicka-Goetz M (2019). Self-organization of stem cells into embryos: A window on early mammalian development. *Science.* **364**, 948–951.

Soldner F and Jaenisch R (2018). Stem cells, genome editing, and the path to translational medicine. *Cell.* **175**, 615–632.

Szabo E, Rampalli S, Risueno R, Schnerch A, Mitchell R, Fiebig-Comyn M and Bhatia M (2010). Direct conversion of human fibroblasts to multilineage blood progenitors. *Nature.* **468**, 521–526.

Theunissen TW and Jaenisch R (2017). Mechanisms of gene regulation in human embryos and pluripotent stem cells. *Development.* **144**, 4496–4509.

Thomson M, Li SJ, Zou L-N, Smith Z, Meissner A and Ramanathan S (2011). Pluripotency factors in embryonic stem cells regulate differentiation into germ layers. *Cell.* **145**, 875–889.

Wang X, Qu J, Li J, He H, Liu Z, Huan Y (2020). Epigenetic reprogramming during somatic cell nuclear transfer: Recent progress and future directions. *Fron Genet.* **11**, article 205.

Wu J, Ocampo A and Izpisua Belmonte JC (2016). Cellular metabolism and induced pluripotency. *Cell.* **166**, 1371–1385.

Yilmaz A and Benvenisty N (2019). Defining human pluripotency. *Cell Stem Cell.* **25**, 9–22.

Young RA (2011). Control of the embryonic stem cell state. *Cell.* **144**, 940–954.

Chapter 10

Allele-Specific Expression

Introduction

Sexually reproducing organisms have two copies of every gene: one coming from the mother and one from the father. In principle, the two should be treated the same way, be regulated the same way, and it should not matter whether a gene copy comes from the mother or from the father. This is true for the vast majority of genes but there are a few exceptions and special cases. X chromosome genes are a large exception that we will discuss separately. Another type of exception is a number of genes that have a parental "imprint", that is, they have an epigenetic mark that distinguishes the maternal from the paternal allele. Imprinted genes are expressed differently depending on whether a gene copy is paternally or maternally derived. This is quite different from sex-specific genes, for example, genes that are expressed only or mainly in females in response to female-specific hormone or developmental signals. Both alleles of sex-specific genes are expressed the same way independently of the parental provenance. In the case of imprinted genes, it is not the sex of the individual that determines which allele is expressed but whether it is derived from the mother or from the father. Only one of the two alleles is expressed. A number of such monoallelically expressed genes were discovered in the 1990s and we now know of about 150 genes in mouse (and about the same number in humans) whose expression is regulated by imprinting. In some cases, the maternal copy is turned off and only the paternal copy is active. In other cases, it is the paternal copy that is silenced and the maternal copy is active. Genetic imprinting was originally discovered in 1984 by Davor Solter and James McGrath and, independently, by Azim Surani and Sheila Barton, who found that mouse uniparental embryos died during embryogenesis. We know now that an embryo that gets both copies of an imprinted gene from the mother or from the father (a uniparental embryo) will be either dead (both copies of many imprinted genes are inactive) or very abnormal (both copies of other imprinted genes are active).

Although some examples of imprinting have been found in flowering plants, imprinting is a characteristically mammalian phenomenon. Imprinting essentially makes the organism haploid for some important genes. If the active allele carries a deleterious mutation, that gene's function is entirely lost. Much discussion has resulted from the need to explain how such a perilous mechanism could have evolved. Several theories have been proposed and the debate is still ongoing. I will present here the model that appears to me most straightforwardly explained and probably best supported by the available evidence. This is called **the parental conflict model**. It was observed early on that imprinted genes and their imprinting are generally conserved among mammals and are very often genes important for the growth rate of the embryo or its regulation or for control of behavior after birth. Some imprinted genes remain imprinted in all tissues while others lose the imprint in certain tissues or at certain developmental stages. An important class is imprinted specifically in the placenta.

The Parental Conflict Model

In cases when an imprinted gene stimulates growth, for example, if it is a growth factor gene, it is the maternal copy that is silenced while the paternal copy is active. In cases where an imprinted gene downregulates fetal growth, it is the maternal copy that tends to be active while the paternal copy is silenced. Evolutionary geneticists pointed out that this could be interpreted as the result of evolutionary selection resulting from the different selective advantages for the mother and for the father of placental mammals. Fetal growth is very demanding, maternal resources are limited and the best maternal strategy is to distribute them equally among all the

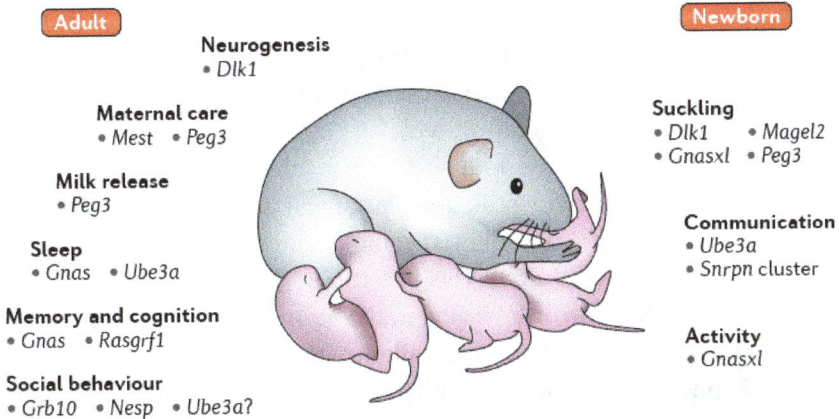

Adult

Neurogenesis
• *Dlk1*

Maternal care
• *Mest*   • *Peg3*

Milk release
• *Peg3*

Sleep
• *Gnas*   • *Ube3a*

Memory and cognition
• *Gnas*   • *Rasgrf1*

Social behaviour
• *Grb10*   • *Nesp*   • *Ube3a?*

Newborn

Suckling
• *Dlk1*   • *Magel2*
• *Gnasxl*   • *Peg3*

Communication
• *Ube3a*
• *Snrpn* cluster

Activity
• *Gnasxl*

Figure 1.   Imprinted genes affecting behavior in mice. In adult mice, imprinted genes affect milk release, maternal care of offspring, sleep and other behaviors. In infants, imprinted genes act on feeding behavior by regulating nipple attachment, suckling ability, locomotor activity and communication with the mother.

Source: Peters (2014).

offspring. In contrast, in promiscuous species, the paternal strategy is to maximize the growth of the father's own progeny and outcompete the progeny of other fathers. The result is a **parental conflict of interest** and an evolutionary selection pressure that, on the maternal side, favors turning off growth-promoting genes and turning on genes that control growth, while, on the paternal side, it tends to maximize the expression of growth genes and to minimize genes that control growth. Many imprinted genes affect the nervous system and some have clear behavioral phenotypes (Figure 1). A similar parental conflict argument can be made for a gene that promotes aggressive feeding behavior among a progeny litter. Competitive and aggressive behavior is advantageous for paternal genes but maternal interests promote a more equitable deployment of resources.

The Methylation Imprint

Whatever the evolutionary theory, imprinting requires an epigenetic molecular mark that distinguishes the paternal from the maternal allele.

To mark the parental origin of an imprinted allele, epigenetic modifications must be introduced during gametogenesis so they will control the expression of the imprinted genes during fetal growth. In the germ line of the fetus, the epigenetic modifications (the imprint) must be erased during gametogenesis and replaced with new modifications specific to the sex of the fetus. It was soon evident that maternal and paternal alleles differ in the DNA methylation of certain specific regions, called Differentially Methylated Regions (DMRs). The difference is already present in the gametes and is therefore established in the germ line. For a given DMR, all sperm will have the same mark and all eggs will have the opposite. More complicated is distinguishing the paternal from the maternal allele in the somatic tissues. This is generally done by using parents from different strains of mice that have sequence polymorphisms at or near the region of interest. As a result, the maternal allele will have some sequence differences relative to the paternal allele, usually **Single Nucleotide Polymorphisms** (SNPs), which allow the parental identification of the methylation mark and the molecular and genetic analysis (Figure 2).

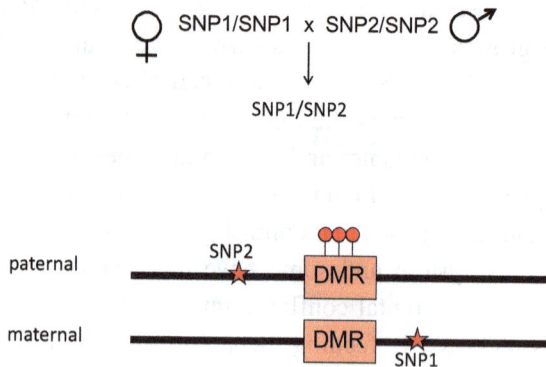

Figure 2.   Use of sequence polymorphisms to identify a parental allele. In a cross between two mice, each with known single nucleotide polymorphisms (SNPs), the mother is homozygous for SNP1 and the father for SNP2. In this example, the methylation marks linked with SNP2 will come from the paternal allele.

Genetic analysis made clear that monoallelically expressed genes are generally clustered. Though the cluster may involve several DMRs, one of them is generally the key site that governs the differential methylation of the other DMRs in the cluster. This key DMR site is the Imprinting Control Region (ICR).

DNA methylation is a fairly stable epigenetic mark. In principle, once it is created, it is reproduced by the maintenance of DNA methylase DNMT1 in every round of cell division. However, problems immediately arise. As we have seen (in the Stem Cells and Genome Programming chapter), a massive process of demethylation occurs in the early embryo, beginning with the fertilized egg. It proceeds faster in the paternal genome (active demethylation) and more slowly in the maternal genome (passive demethylation) but both genome copies are demethylated by the blastocyst stage. In principle, this would erase any methylation mark distinguishing a paternal from a maternal allele. Are DMRs specifically protected against demethylation? While some protective protein binding might be imagined to prevent active demethylation, it would not prevent passive demethylation. This puzzle has been solved only recently. ICRs are associated with several specific sequence motifs. It is these sites that protect the local methylation status by binding a zinc finger protein called ZFP57, which is a constituent of a heterochromatic complex that recruits the DNA methylases DNMT1, DNMT3A and B. The complex includes a repressor protein called KAP and other factors that recruit the SETDB1 H3K9 methylase and generates a locally repressed state that binds HP1 and other heterochromatin proteins (Figure 3). The ZFP57 complex only binds to a methylated target sequence and specifically restores the methylation and heterochromatic status surrounding the ICR in embryonic stem cells. Mutation of ZFP57 causes loss of the parental methylation marks in the early embryo at all the ICRs tested. In mouse, ZFP57 cooperates with another zinc finger protein, ZFP445, which, in some cases, can have the same function as ZFP57. Human imprinted ICRs bind principally ZFP445 and ZFP57 has a much reduced role.

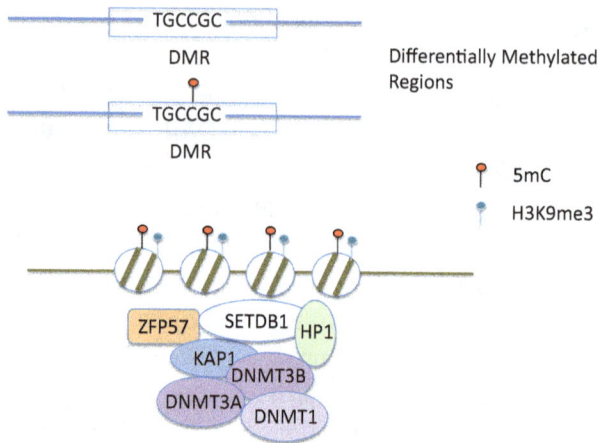

Figure 3.   Maintenance of methylation at DMRs. Global genome demethylation occurs in the early embryo. The methylation mark is preserved in Differentially Methylated Regions through the presence of specific sequence motifs. When these are methylated, they bind ZFP57, a zinc finger protein that recruits KAP1, *de novo* DNA methylases, as well as histone H3K9 methylase SETDB1 and HP1. This complex selectively restores and protects DNA methylation at previously methylated DMRs.

Creating the Parent-Specific Methylation Imprint

A second problem arises in the germ line, where the old parent-specific marks must be erased and new sex-specific marks (the imprints) need to be created. During embryogenesis, a second genome-wide wave of DNA demethylation occurs in the progenitor germ line cells (PGCs). This second wave of demethylation is very thorough and removes all CpG methylation prior to the differentiation of the male or female germ line cells. No ZFP57 is present to protect the ICRs. DNA remethylation takes place as the germ line cells differentiate, as it does when embryonic stem cells begin their differentiation in the somatic tissues of the embryo. Is there a sex-specific mechanism that recognizes and methylates specific ICRs? It has now become clear that the germ line methylation of ICRs does not work that way but rather depends on the different methylation patterns of the male and female germ lines. Sperm DNA methylation is very abundant but targets particularly repetitive sequences, transposons and intergenic regions. Oocyte methylation is more like that of other transcriptionally

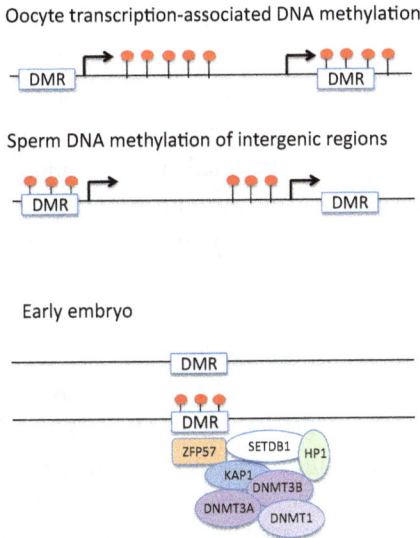

Figure 4.   Parent-specific methylation imprint. Maternal methylation imprints are produced non-specifically by transcription-associated DNA methylation in the oocyte. Paternal methylation imprints are also produced non-specifically when sperm DNA is abundantly methylated in intergenic regions. In both cases, the specificity arises after fertilization, when both paternal and maternal genomes are globally demethylated but DNA methylation is specifically maintained at ICRs by the ZFP57 complex.

active tissues: it targets the body of transcriptionally active genes, both introns and exons. This matches the distribution of known ICRs. Paternally methylated ICRs are found in intergenic regions, while maternally methylated ICRs are located generally in intronic CpG islands of genes that were actively transcribed during oogenesis. The resulting methylation pattern is not specific for ICRs: there is no ICR-specific methylation mechanism. The specificity arises after fertilization when the entire genome is demethylated but at the ICRs methylation is restored by the ZFP57 mechanism (Figure 4).

The *Igf2-H19* Imprinted Locus

Once the target genes are marked with ICR methylation, the monoallelic expression can result from different mechanisms. The first imprinted locus to be accounted for mechanistically was the *Igf2-H19* locus. This locus contains at least three genes: *Ins2* and *Ifg2* produce insulin and insulin-like growth factor, respectively. Both promote growth. *H19* is a gene that produces an RNA with no significant open coding region. Its sequence is well conserved in mammals at the nucleotide level but not at the codon level. *H19* can be deleted with little detectable growth effect, suggesting that it may not have any essential function, but ectopically driving H19 expression causes embryonic lethality. This and other evidence show that the RNA is in fact processed to produce a microRNA that downregulates growth. As might be expected from the parental conflict theory, *Ins2* and *Igf2* are expressed from the paternal allele only and the maternal alleles are silent. *H19* is actively transcribed from the maternal allele while the paternal allele is silenced (Figure 5). The monoallelic expression of this locus is important. Mutations deleting the Imprinting Control Region result in biallelic expression: both the maternal and

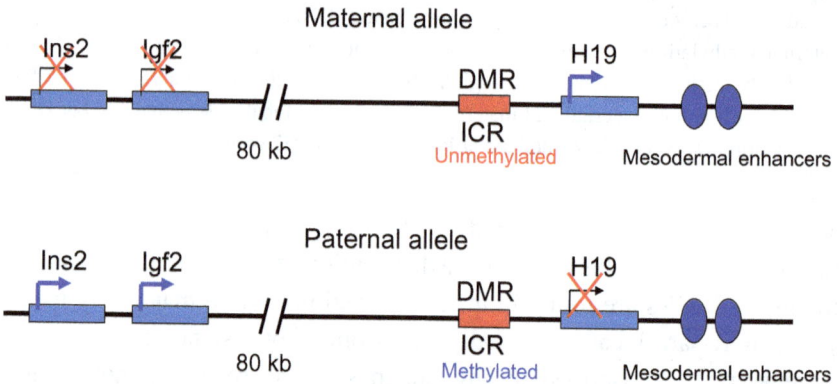

Figure 5. The imprinted *Igf2/H19* locus. The locus contains three principal genes governed by the same enhancers and several Differentially Methylated Regions. One of these DMRs is critical for imprinted expression: if deleted, imprinting is lost and expression is biallelic. This is the Imprinting Control Region or ICR. The ICR of this locus is methylated in the paternal allele. The methylation spreads to the promoter of the *H19* gene and silences it. In contrast, the *Ins2* and *Igf2* genes are active on the paternal allele. On the maternal allele, the ICR is unmethylated, *H19* is active and the *Ins2* and *Igf2* genes are turned off.

paternal alleles of the genes are expressed with serious developmental consequences known as the Beckwith–Wiedemann Syndrome (BWS). Patients with BWS display fetal and postnatal overgrowth, physical malformations, and tendency to develop tumors.

The Imprinting Control Region is situated a few kb upstream of the *H19* promoter, while the *Igf2* and *Ins2* genes are some 80 kb further upstream. The ICR is methylated in the paternal allele, which expresses *Igf2* and *Ins2* but not in the maternal allele in which these genes are silent. The *H19* gene is active in the maternal allele but is silenced in the paternal allele in which the ICR is methylated and methylation spreads to affect the *H19* promoter. The mechanism involved began to be clarified when the enhancers needed to activate the expression of all three genes were mapped downstream of the *H19* gene. These enhancers therefore need to make a short loop to contact the *H19* promoter but a rather long loop to contact *Igf2* and *Ins2*. Two groups came up with an account of the mechanism resulting in monoallelic expression. The laboratories of Gary Felsenfeld at NIH (Bell and Felsenfeld, 2000) and of Shirley Tilghman at Princeton (Hark *et al.*, 2000) independently found that the ICR contains multiple binding sites for the insulator protein CTCF. These CpG-rich sites are methylated in the paternal allele, preventing the binding of CTCF, but not methylated in the maternal allele, where CTCF can bind. Both groups also demonstrated that when CTCF binds it blocks the ability of the enhancers downstream of *H19* to loop and contact the *Igf2* and *Ins2* genes far upstream. Methylation of the ICR, extending to the *H19* promoter, prevents activation of *H19* transcription (Figure 6). These observations accounted for the monoallelic expression and fit well with the insulator mechanisms that had been demonstrated first in *Drosophila* and then at other CTCF sites in mammals.

As so often happens, a more detailed analysis of the region complicated this simple picture. The normal functioning of the locus depends on the correct folding of the chromatin, bringing together the regulatory regions that need to interact and pushing out of the action those that should not play a part. Other CTCF binding sites are involved in creating the configuration in the active allele and its alternative in the inactive

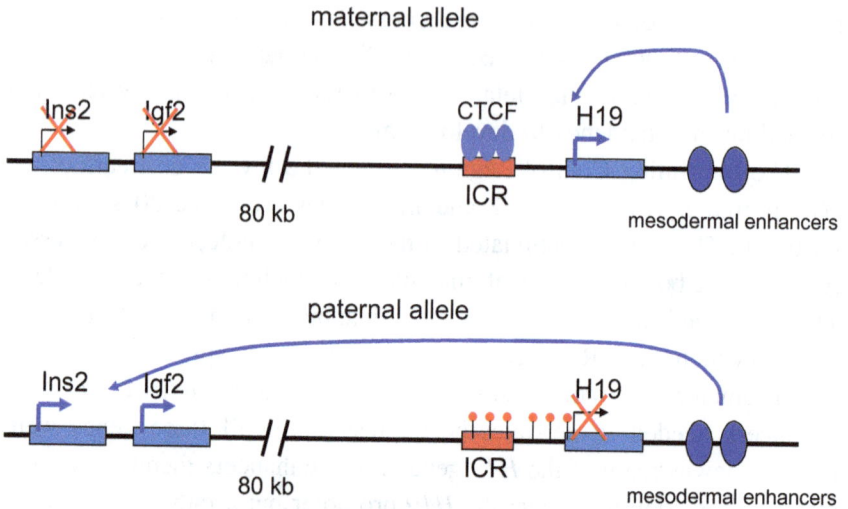

Figure 6.   Imprinted expression of the *Igf2/H19 locus*. The ICR contains multiple CTCF binding sites. The insulator protein CTCF binds to the ICR and prevents the mesodermal enhancers from looping to contact the *Igf2* and *Ins2* promoters. Only the *H19* promoter is activated. In the paternal allele, methylation of the ICR prevents the binding of CTCF but spreads to silence the *H19* promoter. The mesodermal enhancers are free to loop and contact the *Igf2* and *Ins2* promoters.

allele. A study based on the older, PCR-based 3C assays showed that the region encompassing *Igf2*, *H19* and the mesodermal enhancers is folded in a combination of loops held together by CTCF binding sites (Figure 7). In the maternal allele, in which the ICR is not methylated, the binding of CTCF holds together multiple loops, one of which secludes the *Igf2* gene and its promoters. In the paternal allele, *Igf2* is not locked away from the mesodermal enhancers. The *H19* promoter is still not distant from the enhancers but its DNA is methylated and silenced. The specificity of the enhancer contacts is not necessarily obvious from the two-dimensional representation in the figure but the 3C analysis shows clearly that in the paternal allele the enhancers contact the *Igf2* promoter region while in the maternal allele they do not but contact instead the *H19* promoter.

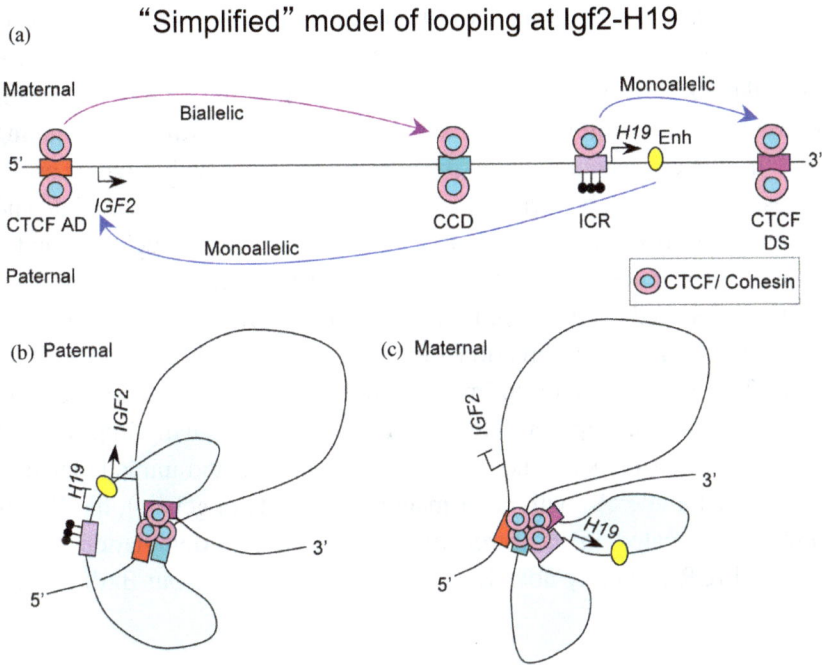

Figure 7. Chromatin looping at the *Igf2/H19* locus. Shown is a "simplified" model of the role of CTCF in the looping interactions that control the expression of this locus. Four CTCF binding sites are reported. One of these, at the ICR, is methylated in the paternal allele, preventing CTCF binding. Interactions between CTCFs, demonstrated by 3C mapping, suggest that, in the paternal allele, the enhancer region is brought close to the *Igf2* promoter, while, in the maternal allele, the enhancer and the *H19* promoter form a loop apart and cannot activate *Igf2*. The blue-tinged loops indicate transcriptionally active loops.

Source: Nativio *et al.* (2009).

The *Igf2r* Gene and lncRNA-Mediated Silencing

The analysis of the *Igf2-H19* imprinted locus seemed very satisfying but it provided no understanding for many other imprinted loci, and particularly for the *Igfr2* locus, which was being studied at the same time by the group of Denise Barlow. *Igf2r*, not to be confused with *Igf2*, produces the

IGF2 receptor. This is a mannose-6-phosphate receptor that binds many proteins tagged with this sugar, including IGF2. Its role is to remove proteins like IGF2 from the cell surface and convey them to the lysosome for destruction. It therefore has an anti-IGF2 effect in terms of promoting growth. It is consistent with the parental conflict theory that *Igf2r* has the opposite imprinting behavior: it is expressed from the maternal allele and repressed from the paternal allele (Figure 8). The *Igf2r* region includes several other genes that are coordinately imprinted, as well as some that are not imprinted. The difficulty arises from the fact that these genes are interspersed and their direction of transcription is also mixed (Pauler *et al.*, 2012). It is difficult to imagine an insulator-type model to account for imprinted transcription. Furthermore, *Igf2r* is maternally imprinted: it has an ICR that is methylated in the maternal allele and unmethylated in the paternal allele. As with other maternal imprints in general, the ICR is intragenic, located in an intron of the *Igf2r* gene. Methylation of the maternal ICR is clearly not silencing the maternal allele but Barlow soon

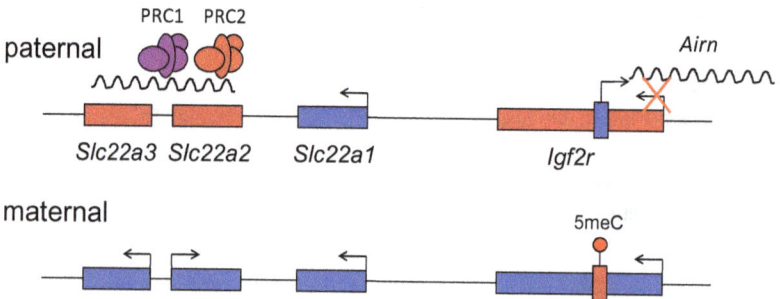

Figure 8.   The *Igf2r* locus. Many imprinted genes use a kind of mechanism that involves no insulator. Igf2r inhibits the utilization of Igf2 and its imprinting pattern is the opposite of that of Igf2: the maternal allele is active and the paternal allele is silenced. The ICR is in an intron of the *Igf2r* gene. It is methylated in the maternal allele, in which the *Igf2r* promoter is active. In the paternal allele, the ICR is not methylated but the *Igf2r* gene as well as *Slc22a2* and *Slc22a3* are silent. The *Slc22a1* gene, in the middle of the cluster, is active in both paternal and maternal alleles. The ICR contains the promoter of a lncRNA called Airn, transcribed antisense relative to the *Igf2r* promoter. Airn transcription through the *Igf2r* promoter blocks its activity. Airn also forms a cloud around the *Slc22a2,3* genes, recruits repressive Polycomb complexes and silences the paternal allele of those genes.

realized that it regulates a different transcript that initiates at the ICR and extends upstream in the antisense direction relative to the *Igf2r* promoter. It is also a very long transcript, over 100 kb, that seems to escape splicing, lacks significant coding capacity, and was called *Antisense imprinted RNA non-coding (Airn)*. Could this long non-coding RNA (lncRNA) produce a kind of antisense-based silencing? Or perhaps by transcribing across the *Igf2r* promoter it might prevent proper *Igf2r* promoter initiation. Neither of these models would account for the coordinate regulation of the two downstream genes *Slc22a2* and *Slc22a3* nor would they account for the biallelic expression of the intervening *Slc22a1* gene. Some three-dimensional folding is likely to occur in this locus but it does not suffice to explain the monoallelic expression.

The answer for *Igf2r* and for a number of other imprinted genes eventually showed that at least two distinct mechanisms are involved: one for the *Igf2r* promoter itself and one for the *Slc22a2,3* genes. The ICR contains the promoter for *Airn*, which is silenced when the ICR is methylated in the maternal allele. When no *Airn* is produced, the *Igf2r* gene is active and its transcription is not impeded by the methylation of the ICR; when *Airn* is produced, it has a silencing effect. *Airn* is highly unstable and probably remains associated with the DNA from which it is transcribed, so acts only in *cis* and not on the paternal allele. Detailed mapping experiments showed that the *Igf2r* promoter itself is primarily blocked by the antisense transcriptional activity that produces the Airn. This could result from the collision of the two convergent RNA polymerases initiating from the *Airn* promoter and from the *Igf2r* promoter or from the interference of the Airn transcript with the assembly of the *Igf2r* promoter complex. In such cases, the stronger promoter overcomes the weaker. In the case of Airn, the occlusion of the *Igf2r* promoter would be particularly effective if the Airn product remains associated with the DNA. A second, independent mechanism is required to account for the silencing of the *Slc22a2,3* genes, which do not overlap with the Airn transcript. Airn itself was shown to interact with the histone H3K9 methylase G9a and to recruit H3K9 methylation to the promoters of the silenced genes. In addition, Airn was found to form a cloud associated with the *Slc22a2.3* genes and with Polycomb complexes PRC1 and PRC2. The paternal allele of these genes is in fact marked by H3K27me3 and H2AK119ub, the products of

PRC2 and PRC1 complexes. The Air RNA acts as a scaffold that associates with the *Slc22a2,3* genes and recruits the repressive complexes. This specific repression clearly involves a correct local folding of the chromatin that leaves out *Slc22a1*, the *Airn* and the *Igf2r* promoters but this has not been analyzed in detail. Neither G9a nor the Polycomb complexes or their chromatin marks are found at the paternal *Igf2r* promoter itself, whose silencing is entirely due to transcriptional antagonism with the *Airn* transcript.

Another case of lncRNA-dependent imprinted silencing is that of the *Kcnq1* gene cluster (Figure 9), located not far from the *Igf2-H19* locus. Here again, multiple genes in both orientations are coordinately imprinted with *Kcnq1*, which contains the ICR within an intron. The ICR is DNA methylated in the maternal allele and *Kcnq1* is maternally expressed and paternally silent. A 91 kb lncRNA called *Kcnq1ot1* is expressed from the ICR in the paternal allele and runs antisense to the *Kcnq1* promoter. Here too, it is clear that the lncRNA is responsible for the silencing not only of *Kcnq1* but also for several other genes both upstream and downstream of

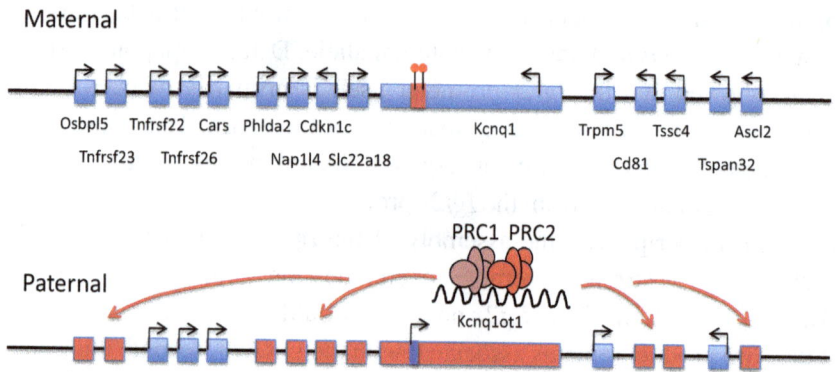

Figure 9.   The *Kcnq1* locus. The ICR is located in an intron of the *Kcnq1* gene and is methylated in the maternal allele. This silences the promoter of a lncRNA called Kcnq1ot1. In the paternal allele, the ICR is not methylated, and the Kcnq1ot1 promoter is active, producing a lncRNA antisense to the *Kcnq1* promoter. The Kcnq1ot1 lncRNA recruits Polycomb silencing complexes and, through looping interactions, silences several genes both upstream and downstream of *Kcnq1*.

Source: Ferguson-Smith (2011).

Kcnq1. Though, like *Airn*, *Kcnq1ot1* is transcribed antisense, a promoter blocking effect by the antisense transcription was excluded in this case by showing that, if a degradation inducing sequence is included at its 3′ end, it abolishes silencing. This shows that it is not the act of transcription but the lncRNA itself that produces the silencing. In this case, it was shown that the *Kcnq1ot1* lncRNA recruits not only G9a to methylate H3K9 but also the Polycomb Repressive Complex 2 (PRC2) and PRC1 to trimethyl-ate H3K27 and to ubiquitylate H2AK119. Like the *Airn* lncRNA, *Kcnq1ot1* lncRNA is highly unstable and probably remains associated with the chromatin from which it is transcribed. The contacts with the several coordinately regulated genes clearly demand a complex three-dimensional folding of the whole region to bring the RNA and its associated silencing complexes together with the genes to be silenced but not with the interspersed genes that are not monoallelically expressed. The details of the folding differ in the placenta from those in embryonic tissues since, while most of the genes in the cluster are paternally silent in the placenta, only some are paternally silent in embryonic tissues. If this model is correct, it raises the interesting question of how the *Kcnq1ot1* promoter itself is able to remain active when silencing complexes are recruited to the surrounding region, including the *Kcnq1* promoter close by. This clearly requires precise control of what the lncRNA contacts and what it can silence.

Evolution of Imprinting

Studies of the *Igf2r*, *Kcnq1*, and *Igf2* imprinting mechanisms and comparisons with other imprinted genes have shown that there is not a single canonical mechanism for imprinted gene regulation. The details vary not only among different imprinted gene clusters but also among the genes of a single cluster and even for the same genes in different tissues. It appears that the detailed workings have become adjusted under powerful selection for whatever produces the most advantageous results for each particular gene. Like other biological phenomena based on conflicting interests and advantages, imprinting mechanisms appear to evolve very rapidly and can change very fast, probably reflecting the strong selection for countermeasures to escape imprinting control and counter-countermeasures to regain control.

None of the genes known to be imprinted in placental mammals are imprinted in monotremes, non-placental relatives of mammals that include the duck-billed platypus and lay eggs instead of giving birth to live young. But some imprinted genes are already found in marsupials. Most strikingly, the *Igf2/H19* genes are imprinted in mouse and man, as well as in the marsupial wallaby but they have lost imprinting in a species of deer mouse that has life-long monogamous mating habits. This is consistent with the parental conflict model. Much of the imprinting-driving conflict of interests is based on the offspring of different fathers competing for maternal resources in the womb or in newborn litters. Much of the selective pressure for imprinting would be lost in a staunchly monogamous lifestyle. Not entirely, however. Overgrowth of a single embryo, straining the maternal resources, could still require control, as in the case of *Igf2/H19* in man. While many imprinted genes have to do with placental and embryonic growth, many affect postnatal growth and, in particular, several affect behavior in mouse and in man. Competition for maternal attention can still be an issue even among offspring of different ages, not born in a single litter.

It is not hard to see how the parental conflict could be generalized to apply to adult behavior as well. Several behavioral disorders in man, like autism, some types of schizophrenia, and bipolar disorders, are known to have a genetic component that is dependent on the parent of origin. One well-known imprinted gene cluster is responsible for two behavioral syndromes in man: Prader–Willi Syndrome and Angelman Syndrome (PWS/AS). These affect memory, learning, mood, maternal behavior as well as embryonic growth and involve a set of genes spread over several megabases, some expressed maternally, some paternally, and controlled by common imprinting control centers and by noncoding RNAs.

Imprinted Genes and Phenotypic Inheritance

Imprinting complicates the inheritance of mutation phenotypes. This is because, depending on the parent from which a mutation is inherited, it is not necessarily expressed in the immediate progeny. As an example,

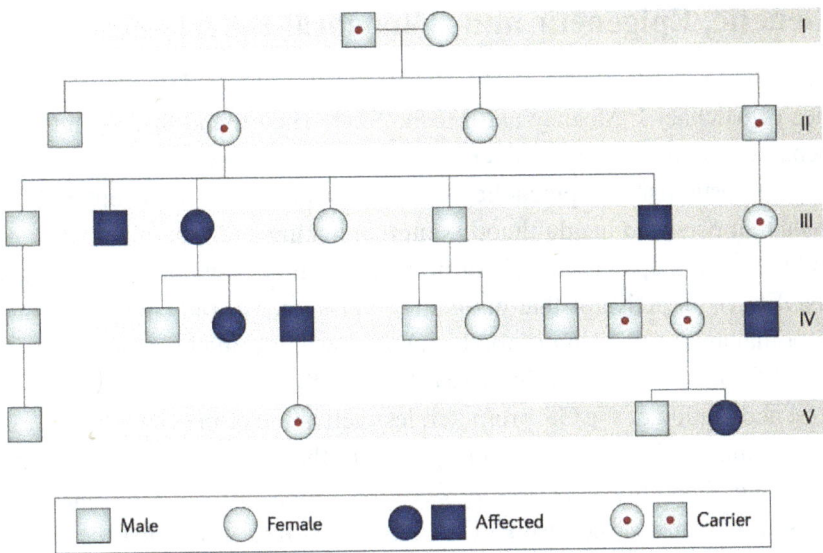

Figure 10. Inheritance of mutations in imprinted genes. Imprinting distorts the inheritance of mutant phenotypes. In this example pedigree, a loss of function mutation in an imprinted gene expressed only from the maternal allele, does not express its mutant phenotype until generation III from a paternal carrier ancestor. The gene is expressed only from the maternal allele so it is not expressed in generation II. The mutant gene is expressed only in generation III if transmitted from a carrier mother.

Source: Ferguson-Smith (2011).

we take the inheritance of a loss of function mutation in an imprinted gene, such as *Kcnq1*. This gene encodes a voltage-gated potassium channel that is not only important for placental function but is also involved in many other tissues including the heart muscle. Mutations in *Kcnq1* alter the repolarization of the action potential in the heart muscle and can cause inherited atrial fibrillation. Imprinting of Kcnq1 means that in many tissues only the maternal allele is active. If this allele is mutant, total loss of function may result. However, if the mutant allele is inherited from the father, it would be silent in any case. So, in the hypothetical pedigree shown in Figure 10, the mutation shows a phenotype only in generation III.

Genetic, Epigenetic and Behavioral Inheritance

In 2004, a remarkable set of observations were published by the laboratories of Michael J. Meaney and Moshe Szyf. They found that the nursing behavior of rat mothers was critical, over the first week of life of their pups, to establish an epigenetic state of the glucocorticoid receptor (GR) gene that persisted in adulthood. Maternal licking and grooming behavior induce in the pups high levels of nerve growth factor-inducible protein A (NGFI-A), an activator that binds to the promoter of the GR gene in the hypothalamus. Offspring of mothers with low nurturing behavior produce less NGFI-A, resulting in increased CpG methylation and decreased histone acetylation of the GR promoter, less activation of the GR gene. These effects are stably maintained and persist in the hypothalami of the adult offspring. The epigenetic marks were not genetically encoded but were caused by maternal nurturing. This was shown by the fact that they were reversed by cross-fostering the pups to a high-nurturing mother but not to a low-nurturing mother. As adults, the offspring of high-nurturing mothers continued to show high GR expression in the hippocampus, which is known to reduce hypothalamic–pituitary–adrenal (HPA) responses to stress, and remained more resistant to stress and less aggressive than the offspring of low-nurturing mothers. Adult offspring of low-nurturing mothers continue to have CpG methylation of the GR promoter, reduced histone acetylation and low GR expression. These effects and the associated behavioral responses to stress could be alleviated by infusion of an inhibitor of histone deacetylation in the brain ventricles.

We have here evidence of nurturing-induced changes in epigenetic state that are stable through development to adulthood and continue to affect behavior. It is very unlikely that this is the only consequence of maternal nurturing. Many other genes, physiological features and behavior may be similarly affected. In fact, the nurturing-induced epigenetic state of the GR gene is not very different from another kind of imprinting, so-called by Konrad Lorenz, who discovered that goose hatchlings identify as their mother the first moving thing they see in the first few hours. Lorenz demonstrated this by showing that goslings that had "imprinted" on him upon hatching would continue to follow him as they would a mother goose.

It is perhaps not surprising to find that female offspring of low-nurturing mothers in turn grow up to be low-nurturing mothers themselves. This closes a remarkable loop in which a maternal behavior induces an epigenetic response in the offspring, which is maintained through life and regenerates the maternal behavior that started the loop. It may not be far-fetched to see in this kind of loop a possible mechanism by which an epigenetic response perpetuates a behavioral perhaps even a cultural trait.

Monoallelic Expression in the Early Embryo

In the fertilized egg and for the first few cell divisions, global CpG demethylation occurs but affects the paternal genome much more rapidly than the maternal genome (see Chapters 3 and 9). Many genes are therefore expressed monoallelically from the paternal genome. Some of these are the pluripotency factors, and in fact, correct expression of OCT4 and NANOG from the paternal allele is essential for timely establishment of the pluripotent state in embryonic stem cells.

We started the discussion of imprinted genes with the idea that the imprint that determined which allele would be expressed was a differential DNA methylation mark. Increasing evidence shows that differential histone marks can also cause parent-specific monoallelic expression. It should be clear, in retrospect, that if sperm is largely depleted of histones while the oocyte retains chromatin marks reflecting maternal germ line and oocyte development, maternal and paternal alleles in the zygote will have very different histone marks at many genes. In a study of DNase I hypersensitive sites in the early mouse embryo, Inoue *et al.* (2017) identified a number of genes containing paternal allele-specific hypersensitive sites and found that the corresponding maternal allele was repressed by H3K27me3. This is then a case in which paternal-specific expression is due to the absence of repressive histone marks that are instead left over in the maternal allele from oocyte development. Most of these histone marks and the consequent imprinted expression are lost from the embryonic cell lineage but some persist in the extra-embryonic lineage and contribute to gene expression in trophoblast-derived tissues.

An extreme case of histone mark-dependent differential gene expression is not related to the parental origin of the genes but is caused by the asymmetric inheritance of histones during cell division. This was found in the germ line stem cells in *Drosophila* testes (Xie *et al.*, 2015), where the stem cells divide asymmetrically, with one daughter cell retaining stem cell identity while the other moves on to differentiate, ultimately producing spermatocytes (Figure 11). Xie *et al.* found that in this cell division, one daughter DNA copy retains all the old histones and segregates into the stem cell daughter while the other DNA copy acquires all new histones, lacking the old histone marks, and initiates differentiation. This is a remarkable departure from the usual DNA replication process, in which

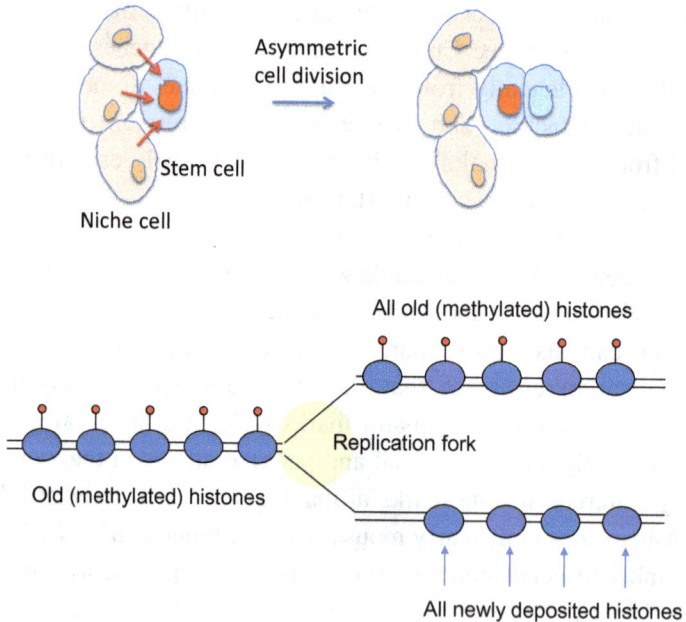

Figure 11.   Asymmetric epigenetic inheritance in *Drosophila* male germ line. The germ line stem cells in the *Drosophila* testes divide asymmetrically: one daughter cell remains in contact with niche cells and remains a stem cell; the other daughter cell moves away and starts to differentiate. Xie *et al.* (2015) found that this reflects the asymmetric replication of the stem cell DNA. One daughter DNA molecule receives all the old histones carrying the pre-existing epigenetic modifications and remains stem cell-like. The other daughter DNA receives all new, unmodified histones and drives cell differentiation.

the old histones are more or less randomly partitioned between the two daughter DNA copies (see Chapter 2, Figure 23). Though progress has been made in understanding the procedures involved in producing this asymmetric histone distribution and then segregating the daughter chromosomes so that the ones with the old histones go with one daughter and the ones with the new histones with the other daughter, the important result for our purposes is the outcome. The experiments showed that interfering with the asymmetric histone partitioning prevented correct differentiation on one hand and caused loss of stem cells on the other hand. This shows clearly that the "old" histones are instructive and determine the germ line stem cell character of one daughter cell, while the daughter cell with the "new" histones is free to respond to a new program of gene expression leading to differentiation.

Further Reading

Andergassen D, Muckenhuber M, Bammer PC, Kulinski T, Theussl H-C, Shimizu T *et al.* (2019). The Airn lncRNA does not require any DNA elements within its locus to silence distant imprinted genes. *PLoS Genet.* **15**, 1–18.

Bell AC and Felsenfeld G (2000). Methylation of a CTCF-dependent boundary controls imprinted expression of the *Igf2* gene. *Nature.* **405**, 482–485.

Eggermann T, Perez de Nanclares G, Maher E, Temple I, Turner Z, Monk D *et al.* (2015). Imprinting disorders: A group of congenital disorders with overlapping patterns of molecular changes affecting imprinted loci. *Clin Epigenet.* **7**, article 123.

Ferguson-Smith AC and Bourchi D. (2018). The discovery and importance of genomic imprinting. *eLife.* **7**, e42368.

Ferguson-Smith AC (2011). Genomic imprinting: The emergence of an epigenetic paradigm. *Nat Rev Genet.* **12**, 565–575.

Hammoud SS, Nix DA, Zhang H, Purwar J, Carrell DT and Cairns BR (2015). Transcription and imprinting dynamics in developing postnatal male germline stem cells. *Genes Dev.* **29**, 2312–2324.

Hanna CW (2020). Placental imprinting: Emerging mechanisms and functions. *PLoS Genet.* **16**, e1008709.

Hark AT, Schoenherr CJ, Katz DJ, Ingram RS, Levorse JM and Tilghman SM (2000). CTCF mediates methylation-sensitive enhancer-blocking activity at the *H19/Igf2* locus. *Nature.* **405**, 486–489.

Inoue A, Jiang L, Lu F, Suzuki T and Zhang Y (2017). Maternal H3K27me3 controls DNA methylation-independent imprinting. *Nature.* **547**, 419–424.

Ma P, de Waal E, Weaver JR, Bartolomei MS and Schultz RM (2015). A DNMT3A2-HDAC2 complex Is essential for genomic imprinting and genome integrity in mouse oocytes. *Cell Rep.* **13**, 1552–1560.

Monk D, Mackay DJG, Eggermann T, Maher ER and Riccio A (2019). Genomic imprinting disorders: Lessons on how genome, epigenome and environment interact. *Nat Rev Genet.* **20**, 235–248.

Moore T and Haig D (1991). Genomic imprinting in mammalian development: A parental tug-of-war. *Trends Genet.* **7**, 45–49.

Nativio R, Wendt KS, Ito Y, Huddleston JE, Uribe-Lewis S, Woodfine K *et al.* (2009). Cohesin is required for higher-order chromatin conformation at the imprinted *IGF2-H19* locus. *PLoS Genet.* **5**, e1000739.

Patten MM, Ross L, Curley JP, Queller DC, Bonduriansky R and Wolf JB (2014). The evolution of genomic imprinting: theories, predictions and empirical tests. *Heredity.* **113**, 119–128.

Pauler FM, Barlow DP and Hudson QJ (2012). Mechanisms of long range silencing by imprinted macro non-coding RNAs. *Curr Opin Genet Dev.* **22**, 283–289.

Peters J (2014). The role of genomic imprinting in biology and disease: An expanding view. *Nat Rev Genet.* **15**, 517–530.

Plasschaert RN and Bartolomei MS (2014). Genomic imprinting in development, growth, behavior and stem cells. *Development.* **141**, 1805–1813.

Quenneville S, Verde G, Corsinotti A, Kapopoulou A, Jakobsson J, Offner S *et al.* (2011). In embryonic stem cells, ZFP57/KAP1 recognize a methylated hexa-nucleotide to affect chromatin and DNA methylation of imprinting control regions. *Mol Cell.* **44**, 361–372.

Takahashi N, Wu J, Suzuki K, Martinez-Redondo P, Li M, Liao H-K *et al.* (2019). ZNF445 is a primary regulator of genomic imprinting. *Genes Dev.* **33**, 49–54.

Xie J, Wooten M, Tran V, Chen B-C, Pozmanter C, Simbolon C *et al.* (2015). Histone H3 threonine phosphorylation regulates asymmetric histone inheritance in the *Drosophila* male germline. *Cell.* **163**, 920–933.

Zhang H, Zeitz MJ, Wang H, Niu B, Ge S, Li W *et al.* (2014). Long noncoding RNA-mediated intrachromosomal interactions promote imprinting at the *Kcnq1* locus. *J Cell Biol.* **204**, 61–75.

Chapter 11

X Chromosome Dosage Compensation

Introduction

In all higher eukaryotes, deletions of a substantial part of the genome are lethal even if heterozygous. Although the organism can withstand a reduction in the dosage of most individual genes, it cannot tolerate a reduced dosage of a large number of genes at once, much less of one entire chromosome copy. This is thought to be due to the imbalance between the single dose of many genes and the double dose of genes in the rest of the genome. The correct relative expression of genes is important for normal development and for normal organismal function. Extra copies of chromosomes are often found in cancer cells. Trisomy of chromosome 21 is notoriously responsible for the human Down's Syndrome. Yet loss of one entire chromosome activity is what happens in species that have a male-specific chromosome such as the Y chromosome in mammals (or in insects like *Drosophila* or in nematodes). In these organisms, females have two copies of the X chromosome but males have one X and one Y. The male-specific Y chromosome is evolutionarily derived from the X chromosome and usually has lost most if not all of its protein-coding genes. Therefore, most X chromosome genes are present in two copies in XX females and only one copy in XY males. In all such species, from worm to man, a mechanism has evolved to compensate for the resulting imbalance with the rest of the genome in the autosomes. In principle, this could be done in different ways: adjusting the expression of X genes in males, or in females, or adjusting the expression of autosomes in males, or in females. Interestingly, different species have adopted sometimes very different strategies but the aim in all cases is to equalize the level of expression of X chromosome genes in XX cells and in XY cells, relative to the autosomes.

An extreme case is that of coccid insects (mealybugs) in which the entire chromosome complement derived from the father is inactivated and made heterochromatic. This could be considered a drastic case of genetic imprinting (Figure 1). In this case, the X to autosome ratio is maintained by silencing one entire set of autosomes.

More commonly, X chromosome dosage is compensated by adjusting the expression of X chromosome genes in males and females by one of three strategies: (1) decrease X expression in XX females by one half; (2) increase X expression in XY males by two-fold; (3) inactivate one X in XX females (Figure 2). Number 1 is the strategy adopted by nematodes.

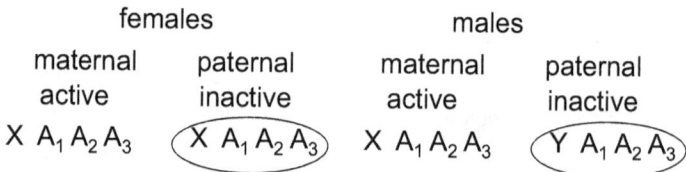

females		males	
maternal	paternal	maternal	paternal
active	inactive	active	inactive
X $A_1 A_2 A_3$	(X $A_1 A_2 A_3$)	X $A_1 A_2 A_3$	(Y $A_1 A_2 A_3$)

Figure 1.   X chromosome compensation in coccid insects. These insects compensate by the drastic method of inactivating the entire set of chromosomes derived from the father. In both males and females, only one set of chromosomes derived from the mother remains active.

1. Inactivate one set of chromosomes: coccid insects

2. Decrease X expression in females by ½ x: *C. elegans*

3. Increase X expression in males by 2x: *Drosophila*

4. Inactivate one X in females: mammals

Figure 2.   Different ways to compensate for X chromosome dosage. In most animals, X dosage compensation is done by regulating X chromosome gene expression differently in males and females. There are different ways to achieve this. Coccid insects, nematodes, flies, and mammals illustrate four different solutions to the same problem.

Number two is found in insects like *Drosophila*. The third is the strategy seen in mammals. Of necessity, the three methods have some common features. All dosage compensation requires some counting mechanism, a way to determine how many X chromosomes are present or, more importantly, the X to Autosome ratio. In many organisms, the X:A ratio is also used to determine sex so that dosage compensation is functionally linked to sex determination. The different strategies also imply different basal levels of gene expression. In nematodes and in flies, the expression of one copy of the X chromosome is adjusted so as to be compatible with one copy of an autosomal set of chromosomes. In mammals, one copy of the X is compatible with two autosomal sets. However, more recent analyses of gene expression in mammals, flies, and worms have supported the idea that a common mechanism in all three starts by upregulating X chromosome gene expression so that the expression of a single copy of an X chromosome gene is compatible with two sets of autosomes. In other words, expression is adjusted to allow for the single X in males. The problem then becomes how to reduce X activity in females to avoid a two-fold excess of activity. This is easily accounted for in nematodes and in mammals, where expression in XX animals is either down-regulated or one of the Xs is silenced. In *Drosophila*, evidence suggests that expression in XX females is initially hyperactive due to an early expression of the dosage compensation mechanism, which is then turned off when female-specific development is activated.

It is important to realize what delicate control is involved both in sensing a factor of 2 difference in the X:A ratio so that it permits a binary decision and in effecting dosage compensation of a factor of two in X chromosome gene expression. As so often when delicate control is needed, it is achieved by involving multiple antagonistic factors. Several autosomal genes activate components of the dosage compensation machinery while several X chromosome genes repress these components. These are adjusted so that a factor of 2 difference in the X:A ratio may determine both sexual development and dosage compensation.

Sex determination mechanisms vary widely in different species. In nematodes, as in flies, it is the X:A ratio. The presence or absence of a Y chromosome is not relevant. In mammals, female development is the default state that is counteracted by the expression of the SRY gene on the

Y chromosome. In some vertebrates, some fish, and some reptiles, for example, low temperature during early development results in females while higher temperature produces males. In some fish, behavioral cues may change sex: the dominant animal in a group becomes male. Sex determination in higher metazoans is extraordinarily varied and complex. We will not discuss it here except in so far as it is relevant to X chromosome dosage compensation.

X Dosage Compensation in *C. elegans*

In nematodes, XX animals are females or, more correctly, hermaphrodites and XY or XO animals are male. The mechanism that specifies sex determination in the nematode detects the ratio between X chromosomes and autosomes in the very early embryo. This is done by titrating the expression of certain key genes on the X chromosome relative to certain other genes on autosomes. The X chromosome factors act as repressors and the autosomal factors as activators of the *xol-1* gene, the regulator of sex determination (Figure 3). With two doses of repressors, *xol-1* is silenced, which allows the expression of SDC2; this is a component of a complex closely related to the cohesin and condensin chromosomal complexes. In this case, SDC2 forms a dosage compensation complex that does two things: (1) it represses the *her-1* gene, which is needed to turn on male differentiation, and (2) it is recruited to many sites along the two X chromosomes and reduces the efficiency of transcription about by a factor of 2. As a consequence, XX animals develop as hermaphrodites (rather than males) and reduce the overall expression of X chromosome genes by a half.

In XY (or XO) males, there is only one dose of the X chromosome repressors of *xol-1*, not enough to repress it, therefore enough *xol-1* is available to repress SDC2 so that *her-1* remains on and directs male development. With too little SDC2, the dosage compensation complex does not down-regulate X chromosome expression. In XX hermaphrodites, the two Xs produce enough repressors to counteract autosomal activators and repress *xol-1*. Hermaphrodite development is triggered by default, including the activation of the dosage compensation mechanism.

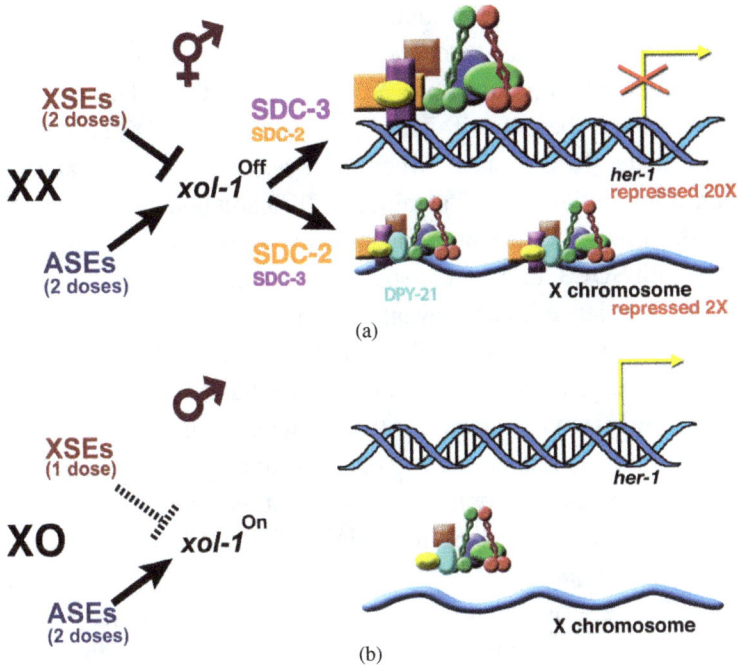

Figure 3. Regulation of sex determination and X dosage compensation in nematodes. In nematodes like *C. elegans*, the X chromosome Signal Elements and Autosomal Signal Elements regulate a key gene, *xol-1,* which controls both sex determination and dosage compensation. In XX animals, two doses of the X chromosome provide enough repressors to keep *xol-1* off. In animals with a single X, the repressive XSEs are not sufficient to silence *xol-1*.

Source: Meyer (2005).

The nematode dosage compensation complex is a specialized variant of the condensin complex, normally involved in resolving chromosomes and higher-order chromosome structures during mitotic and meiotic chromosome segregation. Both are related to the cohesin complex, responsible for sister chromatid association and for loop formation in chromatin architecture (see Chapter 8). All these complexes involve the association of two Structural Maintenance of Chromosomes (SMC) proteins, which form a ring-like structure, and a number of associated proteins that govern their association with chromatin and their loading on the chromatin fiber.

The dosage compensation complex shares some components with condensin but requires other components specific for the dosage compensation function; among these are SDC2 and SDC3. SDC2 is the key component here because it is only expressed in XX hermaphrodite embryos at the 40 cell stage, when both sex determination and dosage compensation initiate. SDC2 stabilizes SDC3 and both are needed: SDC2 targets the dosage compensation complex to the X chromosome and, together with SDC3, targets it to specific sequences in the promoter of the *her-1* gene to silence it and prevent male development.

It remains to account for the binding of the dosage compensation complex to the X chromosomes and the mechanism by which it down-regulates expression by a factor of two. Extensive analysis of the X chromosome fragments translocated to other chromosomes indicated that the dosage compensation complex detects a number of binding sites: some weaker and some stronger. Some regions of the X have no independent binding sites but nevertheless bind the complex in the context of the entire X. These experiments showed that, from a number of discrete recruitment sites, the complex spreads to occupy larger regions, involving nearly all the X chromosomes. Precisely how the complex reduces transcriptional activity by a factor of two is not yet clear. The structural relationship of the dosage compensation complex to the cohesin and condensin complexes suggests that at least part of the mechanism involves a constraint on the folding or local configuration of the chromatin fiber.

X Dosage Compensation in *Drosophila*

Flies have developed an entirely different approach to X dosage compensation, which is also tightly linked to sex determination. The key gene *Sex-lethal (Sxl)* determines both. The expression of *Sex-lethal* (reviewed by Salz and Erickson, 2010) is determined by a counting mechanism that evaluates the number of X chromosomes. It was originally thought that this occurred through the balance of activator genes on the X and inhibitors on autosomes. It appears now that it is rather the amount of activators relative to maternal inhibitors that is critical. In the presence of two X chromosomes, four principal X-linked genes accumulate enough activators to overcome maternal repressors and turn on the *Sxl* establishment

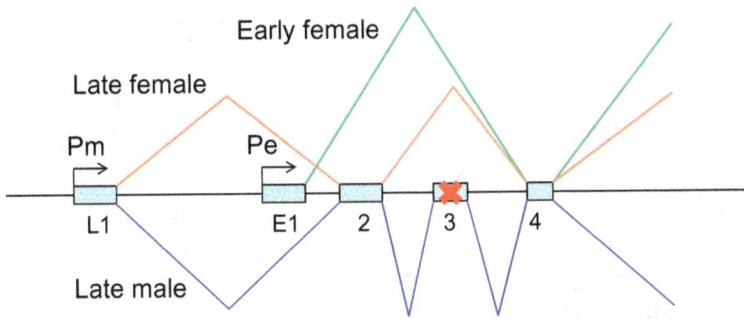

Figure 4. Expression of *Drosophila Sxl* gene. Only the first few exons of the 11 exon *Sxl* gene are shown. The early establishment promoter Pe is transiently activated in early female embryos when X-linked activators overcome maternal repressors. This produces a burst of SXL product that governs the splicing of transcripts produced by the maintenance promoter Pm. In females, splicing skips exon 3 to produce functional SXL protein. In males, the absence of SXL leads to inclusion of exon 3, which contains a termination codon and therefore produces no functional SXL protein.

promoter *Pe* (Figure 4). In males, the single X is insufficient to counteract maternal repressors and *Sxl Pe* is not turned on. The time window for *Pe* activation is very short and, by the cellular blastoderm stage (3 hours post-fertilization), enough new repressors have accumulated to block further expression.

Though brief, the early expression of SXL is sufficient to lock the *Sxl* gene into the female mode of expression. The *Sxl* product is a splicing factor that controls both sex determination and dosage compensation by regulating the splicing of the relevant genes, including its own splicing. At gastrulation, the second promoter of *Sxl* becomes active in both males and females. However, in males, the absence of the initial *Sxl* product causes the transcript to include an exon with a termination codon, while in females, the *Sxl* product splices out the offending exon. During later development then, *Sxl* product is made in females but no product is made in males. SXL controls X chromosome dosage compensation by regulating the expression of a key component of the dosage compensation complex, the *msl2* gene. In females, SXL binds to both the 5′ and the 3′ untranslated regions of the *msl2* mRNA and blocks its translation. In males, no SXL protein is available, *msl2* mRNA can be translated and

MSL2 product, key to the assembly of the dosage compensation product is made.

Most of the components of the dosage compensation complex are essentially needed only in males. In their absence, males fail to dosage compensate for their single X chromosome and die. In females, they are not needed so mutations in these components are lethal in males only. There are five known components of the dosage compensation complex: Male Specific Lethal (MSL) 1, 2, and 3, MaleLEss (MLE), and Male Absent on First (MOF), their names indicating their essential role in male viability (Figure 5). Of these components, only MSL2 is specifically regulated, the others are either constitutively present or stabilized by MSL2. In

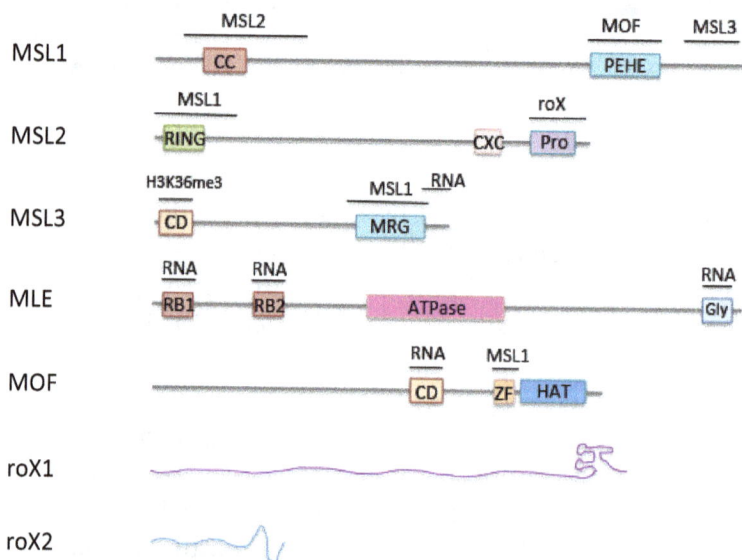

Figure 5. Components of the *Drosophila* dosage compensation complex. The Male Specific Lethal (MSL)l complex contains a set of proteins that are absolutely required in males only, hence their mutations are male lethal. The functional domains are indicated. CC: coiled coil; PEHE: rich in proline, glutamate, and histidine; RING: RING domain; CXC: cysteine-rich; Pro: proline-rich; CD: chromodomain; MRG: a protein-binding domain; ZF: zinc finger; HAT: histone acetyltransferase domain; RB1,2: RNA-binding domain; Gly: glycine-rich. The regions interacting with other components are indicated with bars above the line. The roX1 and roX2 RNAs are very different in size and sequence but they share sequence elements thought to mediate key secondary structures.

addition, the complex includes either one of two non-coding RNAs, roX1 or roX2, both transcribed from the X chromosome under control of MSL2 (Figure 6). In fact, ectopic expression of MSL2 in females is sufficient to assemble a dosage compensation complex.

The principal activity of the dosage compensation complex is to be recruited specifically to the X chromosome and to acetylate histone H4K16. The recruitment begins with the association of two MSL1 and two MSL2 to form a heterotetramer. MSL2 is a RING domain protein and, like many other RING proteins, has ubiquitin ligase activity. In fact, it ubiquitinates itself, MSL1, MSL3, and MOF components as well as histone H2BK34. Recruitment of the complex probably starts when the MSL1-MSL2 complex binds to a subset of sites on the X chromosome called High Affinity Sites (HAS), selected on the basis of sequence and local shape (Figure 7). These include the sites of the *roX1* and *roX2* genes themselves and the entire complex probably assembles as the two non-coding RNAs are transcribed. Incomplete complexes bind in a less stable way so that, when full complexes are assembled, including one or the other *roX* RNAs, they can migrate to other HAS sites to replace the incomplete complexes (Figure 8). Important for complex assembly are MSL3, a chromodomain protein that binds to RNA, and MLE, an RNA helicase that hydrolyzes ATP to power RNA folding. Interestingly, if the

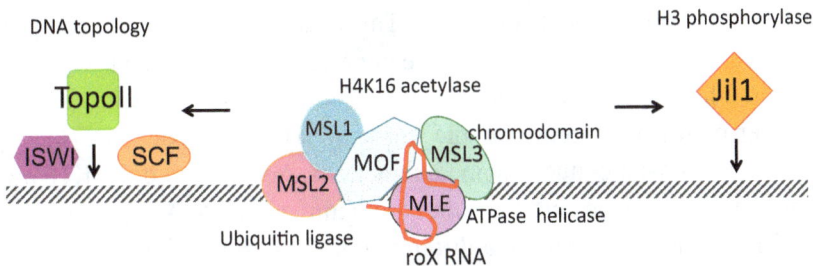

Figure 6. The *Drosophila* dosage compensation complex. The components MSL1, MSL2, MLE, MSL3, MOF, and a roX RNA are indicated together with their known biochemical functions. In addition, the complex stimulates the recruitment of the histone kinase JIL1 and a set of enzymes that modulate DNA topology. These enzymes, including topoisomerase II, SCF DNA supercoiling factor, and the ISWI nucleosome remodeler, are needed to counteract architectural changes resulting from the binding of the complex.

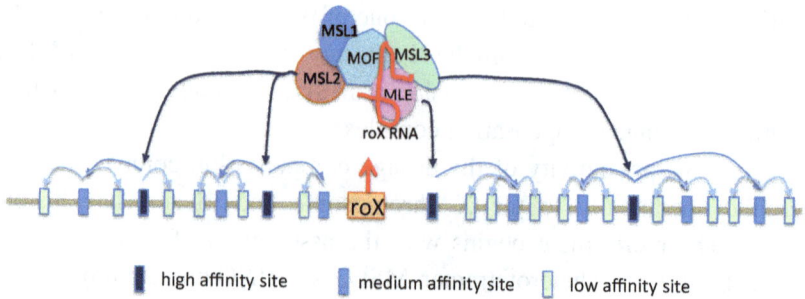

Figure 7.   Spreading of the *Drosophila* dosage compensation complex. The complex assembled at the sites of the roX genes spreads first to high-affinity sites and then to weaker binding sites aided by the affinity of the MSL3 chromodomain for H3K36me3. The spreading is therefore limited to transcriptionally active genes.

only roX RNA gene is provided as a transgene inserted in an autosomal site, this gene is the first site of recruitment, followed by limited local spreading and then by recruitment to the X chromosome HAS sites. This ability to re-localize to the X chromosome implies that the X chromosome possesses some intrinsic targeting signals. These have been identified as GA-rich sequence motifs called MSL Recognition Elements (MREs). In normal males, initial recruitment is followed by limited spreading to transcriptionally active sites on the X chromosome. This spreading is powered by the chromodomain of MSL3, which binds to histone H3K36me3, a product of transcriptional elongation. This means that the dosage compensation complex spreads only to active genes. At this point, the MOF component, a histone H4K16 acetylase, plays its role. H4K16 is a key residue in determining the ability of the chromatin fiber to condense locally through nucleosome–nucleosome interactions. Acetylation of H4K16 prevents these interactions and keeps the chromatin accessible. MOF is not male-specific; it can participate in a different complex, whose homolog is also found in mammals, that acetylates H4K16 in the promoter region of active genes and stimulates their expression. The dosage compensation complex instead binds and acetylates the gene body and 3′ end, suggesting that it may act by facilitating elongation and/or by altering higher-order chromatin conformation. Other chromatin factors such as topoisomerase II and the JIL-1 kinase play an accessory role. JIL-1, possibly recruited by the acetylation of H4K16, phosphorylates histone H3S10.

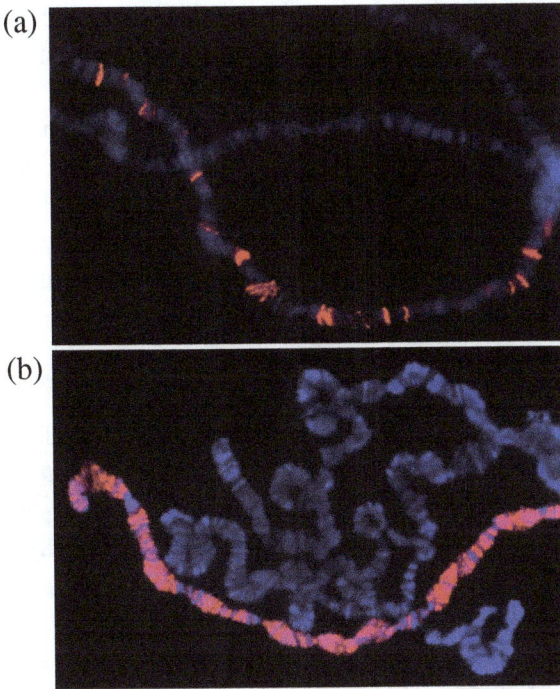

Figure 8.   Assembly of the *Drosophila* dosage compensation complex on polytene chromosomes visualized with an antibody against MSL2. (a) The assembly of the complex begins when the first component, MSL2, forms a heterotetramer with MSL1 and binds to a set of high-affinity sites on the X chromosome, two of which are the *rox1* and *rox2* genes. This initial stage is revealed here by ectopically expressing MSL2 in females mutant for *msl3* to arrest the assembly of the complete dosage compensation complex. (b) After picking up the roX1 or roX2 RNA, the complex can assemble the other components and transfer or spread to other sites. Note that the binding is not uniform on the X. Spreading requires H3K36me3 and is limited therefore to active genes. Images by Art Alekseyenko and Andrey Gortchakov, kindly provided by Mitzi Kuroda.

Antibody staining of polytene chromosomes in larval salivary glands allows the dramatic visualization of the binding of the dosage compensation complex to a single chromosome, the X chromosome, specifically in male larvae. The distribution of the complex shows that it is not uniform. Some sites clearly do not bind much, if any, complex. These sites correspond to genes transcriptionally inactive in salivary glands, hence lacking the H3K36me3 necessary for spreading, and to a subset of X chromosome genes known to lack dosage compensation.

Recent careful studies of the very early stages of embryonic development have suggested that the precise timing of events may be important. The evidence suggests that, at the earliest stage before sufficient SXL product is available, the dosage compensation complex may form in both males and females, causing overexpression of at least some X chromosome genes, such as those responsible for titrating the autosomal inhibitors. This may then be critical to allow sufficient SXL to be made to turn off the translation of MSL2 and terminate dosage compensation in females.

Mammalian X Inactivation

It was noted in the early 1940s that in the cells of mammalian females one chromosome appeared highly condensed and heterochromatic, named the Barr body from its discoverer, Murray Barr. This was shown to be an X chromosome. In 1961, Mary Lyons proposed that in cells with multiple X chromosomes, all but one are inactivated and heterochromatized during early development. Which of the two Xs becomes inactivated is chosen at random in each cell at an early embryonic stage and is then kept inactive in the cellular progeny. This insight revealed the profound consequence that female tissues are a mosaic of cells, some of which have one X chromosome active and some the other X. In females heterozygous for an X chromosome mutation, some cells have the mutant copy and some have the normal copy. This is made visible in the classical case of calico cats, females heterozygous for a mutation in an X chromosome gene that affects fur coloration (Figure 9). The *O* allele is dominant and produces red-pigmented fur. The *o* allele is recessive and results in black fur. In heterozygous *O/o* females, one of the two X chromosomes is inactivated at random, producing epidermal clones expressing the *O* allele (orange fur) and clones expressing the *o* allele (black fur).

Random X inactivation is characteristic of placental mammals. In marsupials, X inactivation occurs but it is not random but imprinted: similar to genetic imprinting, it is the parental provenance of the chromosome that specifies whether it is inactivated. In marsupials, the inactive X is always the one inherited from the father. Many mammals, for example, rodents, have a residual version of imprinted X inactivation. The paternal X is silenced in the earliest stages of embryonic development but this

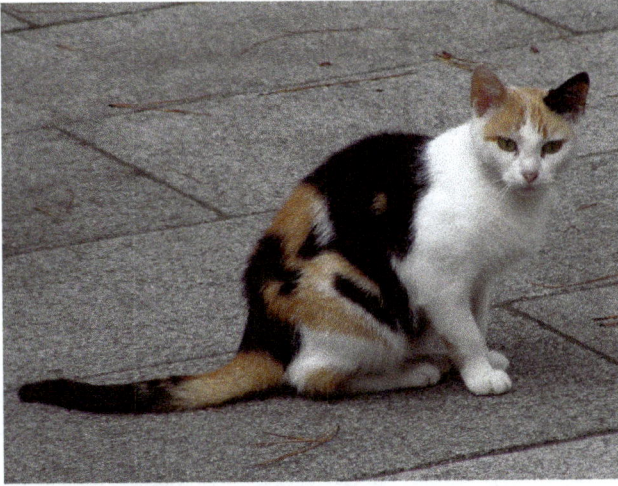

Figure 9.   Random X inactivation mosaics in calico cats. In cats, a gene important for coat color is on the X chromosome. The *O* allele is dominant and produces red-pigmented hair; the *o* allele is recessive and produces black hair. In heterozygous females *O/o*, one of the two Xs is inactivated at random when the embryonic stem cells start to differentiate, producing clones expressing the *O* allele and clones expressing the *o* allele.

inactivation is reversed in the inner cell mass by the time the embryo reaches the blastocyst stage. In embryonic stem cells, both X chromosomes are active but random X inactivation sets in as these cells leave the pluripotent stage and begin to differentiate. Crucially, X inactivation is also reversed in the germ line, as part of the process of genome demethylation that resets genomic programming. As a result, the X chromosomes in all haploid oocytes are active.

In most mammals, as in humans, there is no stage of imprinted X inactivation and random X inactivation sets in as embryonic stem cells begin to differentiate. In genetically imprinted genes, we faced the question of how to inactivate one copy of a gene while leaving the other copy on the homologous chromosome active. In genetic imprinting, the distinction is present from the beginning in the parental mark. In random X inactivation, we are dealing with one entire chromosome in which most of the genes have to be silenced but there is no prior distinguishing mark to determine which of the two Xs is to be inactivated. In addition to the problem of silencing one entire chromosome, we have the problem of counting how many X chromosomes are present: it will not do to silence an X chromosome when only one is present. Closely related is the problem of choosing which of the two Xs is to be inactivated so that when the silencing machinery is targeted upon one X, the other X is left strictly alone.

The X Inactivation Center *Xic*

A region of several hundred kb in the X chromosome, defined by genetic deletions, is the minimal region that, when present in two copies, triggers X inactivation (Figure 10). This region was called the X inactivation center (*Xic*). It contains several genes and, importantly, numerous transcription units that produce long non-coding RNAs (lncRNAs). These were once protein-coding genes that, in the course of mammalian evolution, lost coding capacity and acquired functions either as RNA molecules or through their transcriptional activity itself. In the early 1990s, a key discovery identified *Xist*, a 17 kb lncRNA transcribed from the *Xic*. This was one of the first lncRNAs characterized and its function remained enigmatic for many years. It was soon clear that *Xist* was only produced in females and was necessary for X inactivation. Furthermore, it was expressed from only one of the two Xs, the one that became inactivated, and it remained associated with that X chromosome. In fact, it spread to

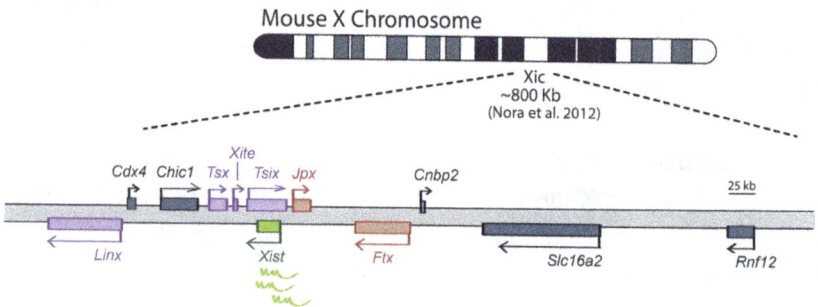

Figure 10.   The X inactivation center, *Xic*. *Jpx* and *Ftx* produce lncRNAs that have a positive effect (colored red) on the expression of *Xist*. *Tsx, Xite,* and *Linx* produce lncRNAs with a negative effect (colored purple) on *Xist*. Protein-coding genes are colored blue. *Rnf12* is a protein-coding gene that promotes Xist expression.

Source: Loda and Heard (2019).

cover much of that X chromosome and eventually condensed and hetero-chromatized it to form the Barr body. The primacy of Xist RNA in producing X inactivation is shown by the fact that transgenes expressing Xist cDNA cause inactivation of the chromosome containing the transgene, even if it is an autosome, provided the expression occurs during a time window in early development. If *Xist* expression results in inactivation of the rest of the chromosome, the problem becomes how monoallelic *Xist* expression is produced.

The *Xic* expresses several other lncRNAs, most of which are poorly understood but are thought to help regulate *Xist* expression, some in a positive and some in a negative direction. One of these lncRNAs has been better characterized and is a major negative regulator of *Xist* expression in mouse. It is called *Tsix* for two reasons: it is antagonistic to *Xist* and it is literally antisense to *Xist*, being transcribed in the opposite direction and completely overlapping the *Xist* transcript. Preventing or decreasing transcription of *Tsix* on one X chromosome in the early embryo automatically results in *Xist* expression and inactivation of that X. Similarly, mutations preventing or decreasing transcription of *Xist* on one X chromosome result in non-random inactivation of the other X chromosome. Current evidence favors the idea that it is the transcription itself of *Tsix*, rather than the *Tsix* RNA product, that interferes with *Xist* transcription. While *Tsix* plays an essential and antagonistic role to *Xist* in mouse, the human *Tsix* is not so important. A comparison of the mouse and human *Xic* regions shows that the human *Tsix* is shorter and does not fully overlap *Xist*. Human *Tsix* expression is not incompatible with *Xist* expression and lacks the key antagonistic function it has in mouse (Figure 11).

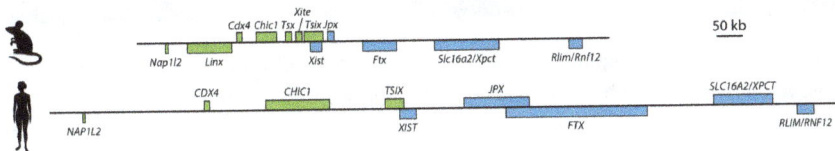

Figure 11.   Comparison of the mouse and human *Xic*s. The X inactivation centers of different species may differ in detail. In particular, the mouse *Tsix* transcript fully overlaps *Xist* and acts as a key repressor by transcribing across the *Xist* promoter. Some mammals lack *Tsix* entirely. In humans, *Tsix* does not repress *Xist*.

Source: Galupa and Heard (2018).

In mouse pluripotent embryonic stem cells, both *Xist* and *Tsix* are expressed at low levels, visible as dots of immunofluorescence localized on both X chromosomes when the cells are hybridized with fluorescently labeled *Xist* or *Tsix* probes. *Xist* is kept low by repression by pluripotency factors OCT4, SOX2, and NANOG, while OCT4, cMYC, and KLF4 stimulate expression of *Tsix*. High-level *Xist* expression cannot occur until the pluripotency factors are turned off when embryonic stem cells begin to differentiate. Inactivation of one of the two Xs also turns down the expression of pluripotency factors, which is needed for differentiation to proceed. Therefore, differentiation cannot advance until X inactivation is effective. The fact that random X inactivation is triggered when embryonic stem cells initiate differentiation has made ESCs a powerful system in which to study the regulation of X inactivation and the sequence of events that lead to the inactive X (Figure 12). In human embryonic stem cells, the choice of which X is to be inactivated occurs later than in mouse embryonic stem cell differentiation, after a stage in which both X chromosomes express *Xist* and form clouds of Xist RNA. This is probably related to the lack of antagonism between *Tsix* and *Xist*, which, in mouse, forces an early decision.

The question remains of how the counting of *Xic*s takes place and how one X chromosome is chosen to be inactivated. Evidence was

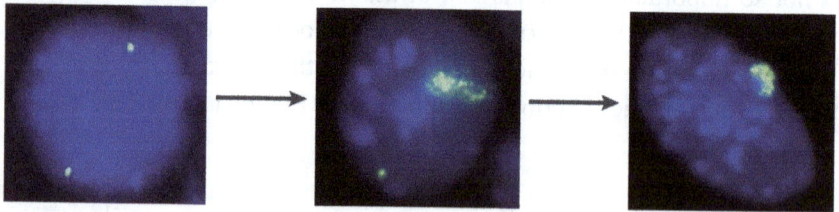

Figure 12. *Xist* transcription in mouse embryonic stem cells. In the nucleus of ES cells, Xist RNA is visualized by hybridization of a fluorescent probe. In ES cells, Xist RNA is made at low levels and remains associated with the X that produced it. When ES cells are induced to differentiate, one of the two X chromosomes is chosen to up-regulate its Xist gene. The Xist RNA remains associated in cis with the X that produced it, spreads over the chromosome, and causes its inactivation (middle picture). Eventually, the Xist gene in the active X chromosome is turned off (on the right).

Source: Avner and Heard (2001).

presented suggesting that the pairing of two *Xic* loci was involved, specifically the region upstream of *Xist* encoding the *Jpx* and *Ftx* lncRNAs. Further experiments have been inconclusive and deletions have failed to confirm a role for pairing in choice. If more than two X chromosomes are present, all but one are inactivated. Conversely, in cells with double the normal dose of autosomes, two Xs remain active. These observations suggest that inactivation is the default state and a normal dose of autosomes allows selection of just one X to remain active. The counting mechanism is still unclear but these observations suggest that, as in flies or nematodes, it involves titration of some autosomal gene products by some X chromosome products. In fact, there is evidence that the *Rnf12* gene, residing in the *Xic* near *Xist*, may play a role by inducing the degradation of REX1, another stem cell factor that helps repress differentiation genes. REX1 is a DNA-binding protein closely related to YY1, from which it derived by a transposon-mediated duplication early in mammalian evolution. REX binds to and represses the *Xist* promoter (Figure 13). A critical event in initiating X inactivation is the degradation of REX1 caused by RNF12, a ubiquitin ligase that marks REX1 for

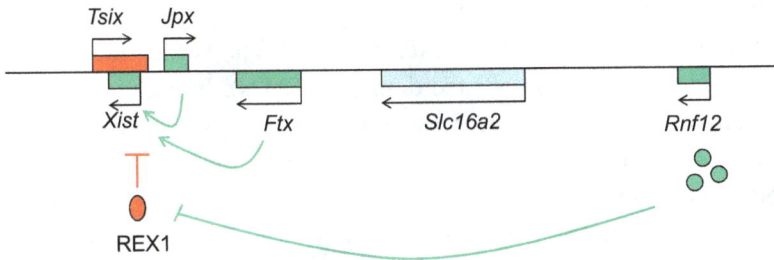

Figure 13. Model for the activation of *Xist*. REX1 is an autosomal pluripotency factor expressed in embryonic stem cells that binds to and represses the *Xist* promoter. RNF12 is a ubiquitin ligase that marks REX1 for destruction. When two X copies are present, enough RUNF12 is produced to eliminate REX1 and activate *Xist* expression. *Ftx* and *Jpx* transcription is coordinately activated with *Xist* and stimulates *Xist* expression, thus providing a positive feedback loop. Xist RNA immediately begins to silence *Rnf12*, preventing it from acting on both X chromosomes. However, if extra copies of *Rnf12* are available, both X chromosomes can be inactivated or even the single X in males.

Source: Jonkers *et al.* (2009), Barakat *et al.* (2011), and Gontan *et al.* (2012).

destruction by the proteasome. Since the *Rnf12* gene is on the X chromosome, two copies of *Rnf12* in XX females cause enough REX1 destruction to trigger *Xist* activation, while a single copy in males is not sufficient. According to this model, this is a random process that can occur on either X chromosome. The resulting inactivation of that X would silence one copy of *Rnf12*. Expression of the remaining copy is still needed to maintain the activity of *Xist*, thus excluding the possibility of inactivating both X chromosomes. In males, a single copy of the X chromosome produces insufficient RNF12 to trigger high-level *Xist* expression but adding extra copies of the *Rnf12* gene results in inactivation of the single X. Once Xist expression is activated, it is further enhanced by the lncRNAs produced by *Jpx* and *Ftx*, which are activated in parallel with *Xist*. In mouse, the effect of RNF12 is increased because REX1 stimulates expression of *Tsix*. RNF12 then both promotes *Xist* and suppresses its antagonist *Tsix*. It is not clear whether this model accounts fully for the counting and choice of X inactivation but it is very likely an important part of these two functions, aided by the multiple stimulatory and repressive effects.

Other autosomal factors are known to regulate *Xist* and *Tsix* expression. One of these is CTCF, which has multiple binding sites in the region that contains the 3′ end of *Xist*. This may help separate the region of the *Xist* promoter from that of the *Tsix* promoter. The two in fact reside in different topologically associated domains (TADs). In addition, CTCF is known to interfere with the progress of RNA Pol II transcription and could therefore inhibit *Tsix* transcription from silencing the *Xist* promoter. Another autosomal factor that contributes to *Xist* function is YY1, a DNA-binding protein known to act both as an activator and a repressor, depending on the context. YY1 may stimulate *Xist* transcription and is also involved in anchoring *Xist* RNA to chromatin. DNA methylation also plays an important role since the Xist promoter becomes DNA methylated on the active X but remains unmethylated on the inactive X chromosome. How this is achieved is not well understood. A complete account of *Xist* and *Tsix* regulation is not yet possible but what is known strongly suggests that a balance between X factors and autosomal factors is involved in mammals, as it is in flies and nematodes.

Xist-dependent Silencing of X Chromosome Genes

That *Xist* RNA is directly causative in silencing gene expression was made clear by mutational and transgene studies. An inducible *Xist* transgene inserted in an autosome can initiate and spread silencing in *cis* though less effectively than if inserted on the X. Some chromatin environments and some genes are more and some less susceptible to silencing. In all cases, *Xist* expression can only initiate silencing in a narrow window of time when embryonic stem cells begin to differentiate.

Human *Xist* RNA is 17 kb long and of similar length in other mammals but its sequence is poorly conserved. However, a conserved feature is the presence of a series of repeats, A to F, whose detailed sequence and repeat number vary but are roughly conserved among mammals. At least some of these regions fold into stem-loop structures that are conserved in many mammals and may be important for their function. Genetic deletions of some of these repeat regions have indicated their functions in X inactivation. The A element, containing 7.5 repeats of a 26 nt sequence appeared to be necessary for gene silencing. Repeats C, E, and F were involved separately and redundantly in Xist RNA spreading and localization on the X chromosome. Many studies reported the association of various proteins to these domains in attempts to account for these functions (Figure 14).

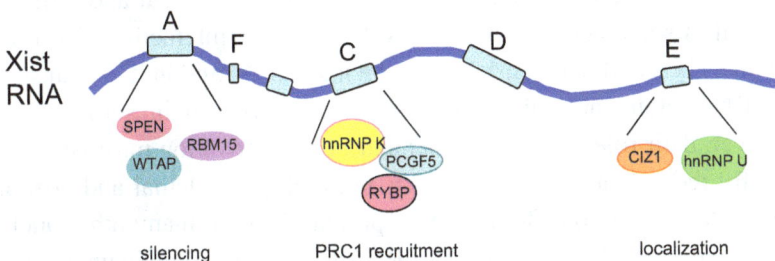

Figure 14.   Conserved repeat elements in Xist RNA and their binding proteins. Repeat A is responsible for initiating silencing. Repeat C recruits Polycomb complex PRC1. Repeat E is involved in spreading and localization of the Xist RNA on the inactive X chromosome.

Source: Loda and Heard (2019).

Repeat A was said to recruit Polycomb PRC2 complex, mediated by the chromatin remodeler ATRX. Repeat C was said to bind YY1, which would anchor it to DNA of a nucleation center. A region including repeat C and downstream of repeat E were reported to bind heterogeneous nuclear ribonucleoprotein U (hnRNP U), also known as SAF-A. More recently, several unbiased proteomic studies purified Xist RNA and characterized the associated proteins using crosslinking and immunoprecipitation approaches. It must be acknowledged that many proteins have significant non-specific affinities for RNA that confuse the picture. The more recent work has come to rather different conclusions. The Xist proteomic and mutation studies showed that the B and C repeats bind heterogenous nuclear ribonucleoprotein K (hnRNPK), an RNA-binding protein involved in RNA processing and transport. hnRNP K recruits a variant PRC1 complex by binding PCGF3 or its close relative PCGF5 (see Chapter 7). This complex, with its associated RYBP protein, ubiquitylates histone H2AK119. PRC2 is not found directly associated with Xist RNA but appears to be recruited to sites that have been marked by the variant PRC1 with H2AK119ub through the affinity of PRC2 component JARID2 for this histone mark. As described in Chapter 7, PRC2 then produces H3K27me3, which in turn recruits canonical PRC1.

Repeat E was reported to bind several RNA binding proteins whose role in Xist RNA localization is unclear or redundant. Two proteins, hnRNP U and CIZ1, have been implicated in Xist RNA spreading. The exact role of hnRNP U (also known as SAF-A) is not clear and it may be essential in some cells but not others. CIZ1 (Cip1-interacting zinc finger protein 1) is specifically enriched on the inactive X, and in its absence, the Xist RNA cloud around the inactive X is dispersed in somatic cells. However, their role in the establishment of X inactivation must be at least partially redundant since their loss is not embryonic lethal and does not prevent X inactivation. Both of these proteins bind to many other nuclear sites so their specific effects on Xist RNA localization remain unexplained at present.

Repeat E recruits a number of RNA-binding proteins (PTBP1, MATR3, TDP-43, and CELF1), which continue to aggregate through multiple heterotypic interactions to form a liquid phase condensate. This condensate persists even when new *Xist* synthesis is blocked and is clearly important for *Xist* initial spreading. Polycomb complexes, particularly PRC1, have also been reported to undergo aggregation and it is likely that these aggregates contribute to the formation of a condensate that creates a repressive nuclear compartment.

The Silencing Process

Recruitment of both PRC1 and PRC2 to the X chromosome is known to be one of the earliest steps in X inactivation and both H2AK119 ubiquitylation and H3K27 trimethylation proceed in parallel with Xist RNA spreading on the inactive X. PRC1 and PRC2 complexes maintain a repressed chromatin state but they do not generally silence active genes. How are the active X chromosome genes turned off to begin with? Consistent with the role of Polycomb complexes in maintaining but not initiating silencing, deletion of the Xist B and C repeats results in weaker gene silencing but not loss of silencing. It is the A repeat region that appears to initiate the turning off of genes. If the A repeats are deleted, PRC1 and, indirectly, PRC2 are still recruited but gene silencing is largely lost.

Recent work by Dossin *et al.* (2020) shows that the major factor that binds to the A repeat is the transcriptional repressor SPEN. SPEN is a conserved RNA-binding protein required for X inactivation. It contains a SPOC domain, which is the essential effector of silencing, as well as four RNA-binding domains that tether it to *Xist*. The SPOC domain recruits HDAC3, NCOR1, and NCOR2 (SMRT) and the NuRD chromatin remodeling complex, all known to be involved in transcriptional silencing. As *Xist* RNA begins to spread on the X chromosome, it also recruits H3K9 methyltransferases and DNA methyltransferases. As if that were not sufficient, SPOC also binds to components of the splicing machinery and to RNA Pol II itself. Furthermore, it associates with components of the m6A RNA methyltransferase. *Xist* RNA is highly m6A-methylated, mediated by the RMB15 and RMB15B factors, which recruit the m6A RNA methyltransferase complex to m6A consensus motifs. This is required for Xist-dependent gene silencing, apparently by recruiting YTHDC1, a protein containing YTH, a domain that binds to m6A nucleotides in RNA. Through this multiplicity of functions, SPEN recruits silencing complexes specifically to the active genes on the X chromosome, deacetylates them, dislodges transcription complexes, and methylates any RNA they had produced. It does not, however, silence the *Xist* gene itself. On the contrary, SPEN binding to Repeat A appears to stimulate *Xist* transcription in a way not currently understood.

X inactivation involves multiple, redundant silencing mechanisms, including Polycomb-dependent H3K27 methylation but also involving H3K9 methylation, DNA methylation, and the deposition of a histone H2A variant called macroH2A. These result in multiple and partially redundant layers of repression. Once X inactivation is established, even *Xist* RNA itself is no longer essential for its maintenance. However, in some tissues, such as in adult B-cells, the promoters of important X-linked genes may remain substantially under-DNA-methylated. In these situations, *Xist* RNA continues to be important to maintain silencing.

Spreading of *Xist* RNA

Xist RNA accumulates on the X chromosome that produced it, does not act in *trans*, and does not diffuse away. It is not hybridized to DNA but forms a cloud around the inactive X that persists even if the DNA is digested by DNase. It has been said to be associated with a poorly defined insoluble structure called the nuclear matrix or nuclear scaffold. This is not very helpful since the nuclear matrix has been a catch-all concept that includes everything in a nuclear extract that remains insoluble. The structure formed by the Xist RNA must be provisionally considered to be an assembly of proteins that together form a structure, possibly a condensed liquid phase loosely associated with the X chromosome chromatin. Many of the proteins that bind to Xist have in fact tendencies to form such condensed states. The relationship between Xist RNA and chromatin must be a close one. For example, PRC1 complexes bind to Xist RNA but evidently can act on the chromatin and ubiquitylate histone H2A. This recruits PRC2 complexes but, interestingly, the detailed localization of PRC2 and of H3K27me3 is different from and does not coincide with that of Xist RNA (Figure 15).

Spreading is not specific for X chromosome sequences since an autosomally inserted *Xist* gene can spread Xist RNA on the autosome, though

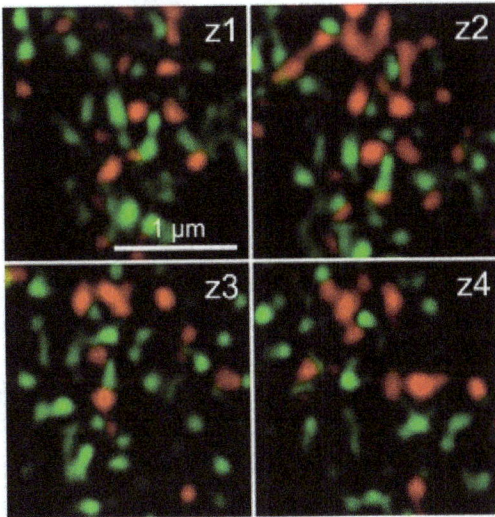

Figure 15.   Xist RNA and PRC2 complex are physically separated. The image, taken with super-resolution structured illumination microscopy, shows four serial sections of the inactive X with Xist RNA localization (red) visualized by hybridization and the EZH2 component of PRC2 (green) visualized by antibody staining. Both have discrete domains of localization but they clearly do not correspond and are physically distinct.

Source: Cerase *et al.* (2014).

less efficiently than spreading on the X chromosome. Spreading of Xist on the inactive X *de novo* occurs by a two-step process. From the initial accumulation at the *Xic*, *Xist* appears rapidly at a set of early sites called XESs. Experiments in which Xist RNA is precipitated and the associated DNA sequenced show that many of these early sites are close to the Xist locus itself but others correspond to more distant regions shown by Hi-C analysis to fold and come spatially close to the Xist locus. Recent studies have found that the XES are already marked by H2AK119ub and H3K27me3, indicating that they are sites in the X chromosome that were already repressed by PRC1 and PRC2. This suggests that the folding of the X and the pattern of Xist RNA spreading are at least in part produced by the associations of Polycomb complexes on the Xist RNA with Polycomb complexes already bound to silenced genes. These associations are produced by ther tendency of Polycomb complexes to aggregate, as discussed in Chapter7. Consistent with this, deletion of repeats B and C, which recruit PRC1, results in partial loss of Xist RNA spreading on the inactive X. In a second spreading step, Xist spreads to more distant and to gene-poor regions. Some genes are never targeted and remain active on the inactive X. In mouse, this amounts to ~5% of X genes but, in the human X, up to 15%.

Xist RNA dissociates from the inactive X at mitosis. Although the evidence was initially contradictory, live cell imaging now confirms that the Xist cloud around the inactive X chromosome disappears and the binding of CIZ1 protein is also lost. At the end of mitosis, the Xist cloud re-forms rapidly on the inactive X, consistent with the idea that it is facilitated by the Polycomb-dependent histone marks and associated Polycomb complexes previously established. Whether the reassembly of the Xist cloud involves the old Xist RNA or requires new synthesis is not known.

Xist RNA spreading is not automatically equivalent to gene silencing. In human embryos, accumulation of Xist on the X precedes signs of transcriptional silencing. While in mouse activation of *Xist* expression on the future inactive X is accompanied by repression of *Xist* on the other X chromosome, in human embryos, both Xs initially activate *Xist* and the definitive decision, as well as the onset of gene silencing occurs only after implantation or even later in some cell lineages. What controls the start of gene silencing is unclear but it is unrelated to the binding of Polycomb complexes and the deposition of the associated histone marks, which occur together with the spreading of Xist RNA.

Architecture of the Inactive X

Although the inactive X is largely heterochromatic, it does not appear to be physically very condensed and occupies a volume only slightly smaller than that of the active X. Some chromosome segments appear more condensed than others but this appears due more to changes in distribution of smaller domains than to higher condensation of local domains.

3C methodologies have shown that the inactive X forms a distinct nuclear compartment. The active X chromosome has a 3D architecture much like other chromosomes, with a TAD substructure in which local chromosome neighborhoods interact heavily within that neighborhood but to a much lesser extent with other neighborhoods. The inactive X chromosome, however, lacks a clear TAD substructure. This means that genes that, when active, contact many other sequences lose these contacts and have no preferential associations. The inactive X has instead a conserved subdivision into two mega-domains (in the mouse) separated by a region that contains the *DXZ4* satellite sequences and includes multiple CTCF binding sites that are occupied exclusively in the inactive X (Figure 16). Despite its dramatic role in the architecture of the inactive X, the *DXZ4* domain is not required for X inactivation but its deletion results in the fusion of the two mega-domains into a single chromosome-wide structure, while no effect is visible on the active X. Within the two mega-domains are regions containing genes that escape inactivation. These

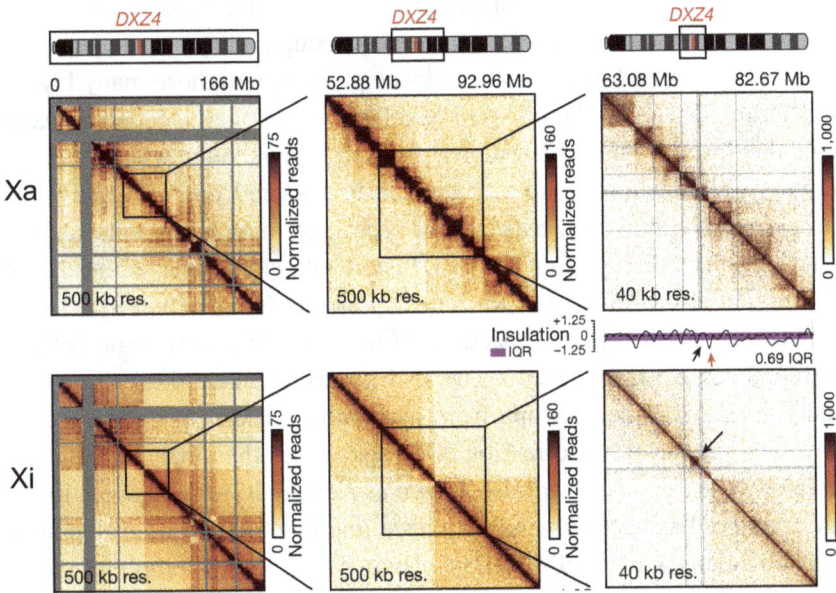

Figure 16. The inactive X chromosome is organized in two mega-domains. While the active X chromosome has a typical TAD structure, TADs are largely absent in the inactive X. In mouse, the inactive X is organized in two mega-domains separated by the *DXZ4* satellite region. Sequences within each mega-domain show here at three levels of resolution, have no preferred contacts, but associate with all other sequences of that mega-domain In the human inactive X chromosome, the presence of a centromere separates out a third mega-domain.

Source: Giorgetti *et al.* (2016).

escaper regions also tend to be delimited by CTCF binding sites and are thought to be located on the exterior of the mega-domains. Deletion of the *DXZ4* domain seems to cause increased consolidation of gene silencing such that the degree of escape is substantially reduced or lost at a number of escaper genes. In contrast, deletion of the *Xist* gene after the establishment of inactivation causes the loss of the mega-domain architecture and restoration of multiple TAD structures, all the more remarkable because X chromosome genes remain inactive due to the multiple layers of epigenetic silencing established.

Maintenance of X Inactivation

Once X inactivation is established in the very early embryo, it is very stable and the inactive state is transmitted through many cell divisions by many overlapping layers of gene silencing. Thanks to these many layers, including DNA methylation, even Xist RNA is no longer needed to maintain the inactive state. Partial reactivation occurs only when multiple repressive mechanisms are simultaneously knocked out. X reactivation occurs readily, however, by genomic reprogramming treatments such as nuclear transplantation into oocytes, fusion with embryonic stem cells, or expression of the Yamanaka pluripotency factors (see Chapter 9).

The genes that escape inactivation remain active in somatic cells to different degrees from gene to gene, in different tissues, and even from one individual to another. Escape from inactivation means that female cells have a higher level of expression of escaper genes than male cells. A few escaper genes, such as *Utx* (also known as *Kdm5c*) have been evolutionarily conserved as escapers and may have important roles in development. Certain factors, such as SMCHD1 (related to the cohesin components), are known to be important for maintenance of X inactivation but not for its establishment and may be involved in the tissue-specific degree of escape. Sporadic loss of X inactivation with age has also been observed and may be related to the general weakening of heterochromatic silencing that occurs with age (see Chapter 12). Regardless of escapers or loss of inactivation, the mere fact of X chromosome inactivation has important consequences for genetic diseases in human females. An example of this is *Mecp2*, the X-linked gene encoding a key chromatin protein that binds to

5mCpG. This protein is essential for correct gene expression, particularly in nerve cells. Loss of function mutations in *Mecp2* is lethal in males and homozygous females but causes Rett syndrome in heterozygous females manifested by devastating neurological dysfunction. This is because in roughly half the cells, the X chromosome bearing the normal allele is inactivated, leaving only the mutant allele. As a result, half of the cells lack *Mecp2* function, resulting in viable but neurologically impaired girls.

Further Reading

Avner P and Heard E (2001). X chromosome inactivation: Counting choice and initiation. *Nat Rev Genet.* **2**, 59–67.

Barakat TS, Gunhanlar N, Gontan Pardo C, Achame EM, Ghazvini M, Boers R *et al.* (2011). RNF12 activates *Xist* and is essential for X chromosome inactivation. *PLoS Genet.* **7**, e1002001.

Cerase A, Smeets D, Tang YA, Gdula M, Kraus F, Spivakov M, Moindrot B *et al.* (2014). Spatial separation of Xist RNA and polycomb proteins revealed by superresolution microscopy. *Proc Natl Acad Sci USA.* **111**, 2235–2240.

da Rocha ST and Heard E (2017). Novel players in X inactivation: Insights into Xist-mediated gene silencing and chromosome conformation. *Nat Struct Mol Biol.* **24**, 197–204.

Dossin F, Pinheiro I, Żylicz JJ, Roensch J, Collombet S, Le Saux A *et al.* (2020). SPEN integrates transcriptional and epigenetic control of X-inactivation. *Nature.* **578**, 455–460.

Galupa R and Heard E (2018). X-chromosome inactivation: A crossroads between chromosome architecture and gene regulation. *Annu Rev Genet.* **52**, 535–566.

Gelbart ME and Kuroda MI (2009). *Drosophila* dosage compensation: A complex voyage to the X chromosome. *Development.* **136**, 1399–1410.

Giorgetti L, Lajoie BR, Carter AC, Attia M, Zhan Y *et al.* (2016). Structural organization of the inactive X chromosome in the mouse. *Nature.* **535**, 575–579.

Gontan C, Achame EM, Demmers J, Barakat TS, Rentmeester E, van Ijcken W *et al.* (2012). RNF12 initiates X-chromosome inactivation by targeting REX1 for degradation. *Nature.* **485**, 386–390.

Jonkers I, Barakat, TS, Achame EM, Monkhorst K, Kenter A, Rentmeester E *et al.* (2009). RNF12 Is an X-encoded dose-dependent activator of X chromosome inactivation. *Cell.* **139**, 999–1011.

Loda A and Heard E (2019). Xist RNA in action: Past, present, and future. *PLoS Genet.* **15**, e1008333.

Lucchesi JC and Kuroda MI (2015). Dosage Compensation in *Drosophila*. *Cold Spring Harb Perspect Biol.* **7**, a019398.

Meyer BJ (2005). X-Chromosome dosage compensation. In: *WormBook*, ed. The *C. elegans* Research Community, WormBook. doi:10.1895/wormbook. 1.8.1.

Pandya-Jones A, Markaki Y, Serizay J, Chitiashvili T, Mancia Leon WR, Damianov A *et al.* (2020). A protein assembly mediates Xist localization and gene silencing. *Nature.* **587**, 145–151.

Salz HK and Erickson JW (2010). Sex determination in *Drosophila*: The view from the top. *Fly.* **4**, 60–70.

van Bemmel JG, Galupa R, Gard C, Servant N, Picard C, Davies J *et al.* (2019). The bipartite TAD organization of the X-inactivation center ensures opposing developmental regulation of Tsix and Xist. *Nat Genet.* **51**, 1024–1034.

van Bemmel JG, Mira-Bontenbal H and Gribnau J (2016). *Cis-* and *trans*-regulation in X inactivation. *Chromosoma.* **125**, 41–50.

Yu B, Qi Y, Li R, Shi Q, Satpathy AT and Chang HY (2021). B cell-specific XIST complex enforces X-inactivation and restrains atypical B cells. *Cell.* **184**, 1790–1803.e1717.

Żylicz JJ and Heard E (2020). Molecular mechanisms of facultative heterochromatin formation: an X-chromosome perspective. *Annu Rev Biochem.* **89**, 255–282.

Chapter 12

Aging

Introduction

All organisms age and at some point die. Even individual proteins can be said to age. Individual enzyme molecules accumulate changes, due to oxidation, free radicals, reactive metal ions, random unfolding, etc. that result in decrease and loss of enzymatic activity. In the cell, these processes are monitored and corrected while proteins with excessive loss of integrity are targeted for destruction. In metazoan organisms, the aging process is controlled in a variety of ways and subject to evolutionary processes but the course of aging remains to a large extent stochastic.

Human aging is characterized by a number of manifestations that have their parallels in most other metazoans from worms and flies to mice. Among these are loss of muscle mass (sarcopenia), weakening and aging of bone structure, and decreased function of the immune system. It involves a general decrease in the ability to maintain internal stability of cell and organ systems that renders the organism more prone to infections, inflammation, and cancer. Aging is the primary risk factor for many diseases including cancer, diabetes, and Alzheimer's disease. In brief, most of the organs and physiological systems suffer deterioration and dysfunction. At the cellular level, common features of aging are genomic instability, telomere attrition, epigenetic alterations, loss of proteostasis, deregulated nutrient sensing, mitochondrial dysfunction, cellular senescence, stem cell exhaustion, and altered intercellular communication

Cellular Manifestations of Aging

Genomic instability	Mitochondrial dysfunction
Telomere shortening	Cellular senescence
Epigenetic alterations	Stem cell exhaustion
Loss of proteostasis	Altered intercellular communication
Deregulated nutrient sensing	Changes in heterochromatin

Figure 1.   Some of the most prominent effects of aging at the cellular level.

(Figure 1). In this chapter, we will look at some of the elements in this dismal list in more detail.

Many theories and models have been proposed to account for organismal aging. Many of them are at least in part true but none of them offers a satisfactory account of all the available evidence in a field that is beset by vast amounts of poorly controlled experiments, contradictory data, preconceived notions, and the problems of distinguishing association from cause and cause from effect. In the aging of an organism, we can distinguish between two types of processes. One is the chronological aging of cells due to increasing damage and dysfunction of the internal homeostatic mechanisms that repair, turnover, and synthesize new proteins and intercellular matrix. This aging process affects terminally differentiated cells and tissues and is particularly important in tissues and organs that have little cell renewal capacity, for example, neural tissue. The other process is the replicative aging of dividing cells that provide maintenance and renewal of tissues. Of course, dividing cells may age chronologically as well as replicatively.

Major sources of damage to individual proteins, to organ structures, to genomic DNA, and, importantly, to mitochondrial DNA are spontaneous hydrolysis, oxidation, UV light and ionizing radiation, and environmental mutagens. Of these, an unavoidable source of damage intrinsic to metabolism is oxidation and chemical damage due to the operations of mitochondria. The mitochondrion is the cell's furnace, where carbon compounds are oxidized, storing energy in the form of ATP and releasing CO_2 and water. As energy production is a limiting factor, mitochondria regulate many other cellular functions such as cell proliferation, biosynthetic pathways, apoptosis, as well as their own replication, and the transcription and translation of their own mitochondrial genome. As the primary source of energy of the cell, mitochondria are the hub of cellular regulation and any difficulty they encounter immediately affects all other cellular processes. Energy production involves the transport of electrons through a series of steps that eventually lead to molecular oxygen and its reduction to OH- (Figure 2). In this process, there is an inevitable leakage of electrons that produces partially reduced oxygen species such as superoxide (O_2^-) and other kinds of free radicals or peroxides. These very aggressive molecules are collectively referred to as Reactive Oxygen Species (ROS) and constitute a danger for proteins, DNA, and other cellular structures. When ROS levels produce too much mitochondrial damage, apoptosis and cell death are triggered.

Cells have a variety of protection mechanisms against free radicals, peroxides, and reactive oxygen species (ROS) in general. A major

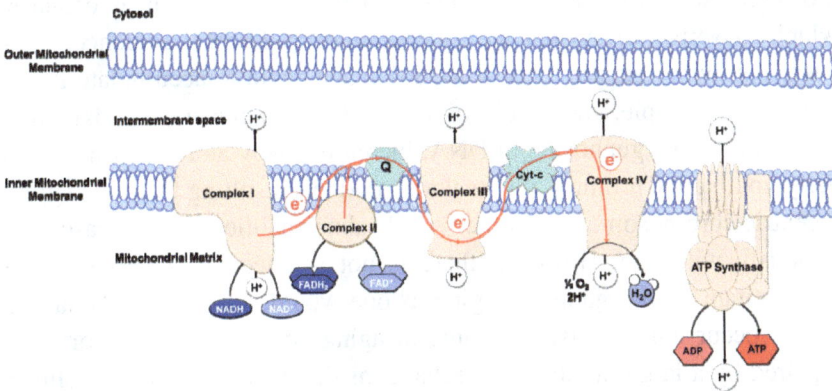

Figure 2. Electron transport chain in the mitochondrion. Electron-rich metabolic products such as NADH and succinate are used by complexes on the inner membrane of the mitochondrion to power a series of electron transfers, ultimately donating electrons to molecular oxygen, O_2, to produce water, H_2O. At each step, the energy produced is used to pump protons into the intermembrane space. The high proton concentration is relieved by using the electrochemical energy to phosphorylate ADP to ATP, thereby returning protons to the mitochondrial matrix.

Source: Dw001, Creative Commons https://commons.wikimedia.org/wiki/File:ElectronTransportChainDw001.png.

$$O_2 \xrightarrow{\text{e}^-} \cdot O_2^- \xrightarrow[\text{SOD} +O_2]{\text{H}^+} H_2O_2 \xrightarrow[\text{catalase}]{} H_2O + O_2$$

with the branch showing $H_2O_2 \xrightarrow{\text{e}^-} \cdot OH$

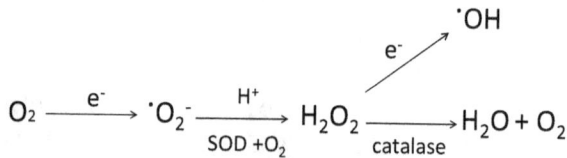

Figure 3.   Reactive Oxygen Species (ROS). Reactive oxygen species can be created by leakage of electrons from the electron transfer pathway of oxidative phosphorylation to react with molecular oxygen or other molecules, creating highly reactive free radicals. These can be neutralized by enzymes such as SOD or catalase. Two such reactions are shown here. Hydrogen peroxide, H_2O_2, can further acquire an electron and convert it to hydroxy radical, $\cdot OH$. No enzymatic detoxification exists for this very reactive free radical, which can attack all cell macromolecules. Therefore, the thorough inactivation of H_2O_2 is particularly important.

example of these protective activities is a species of enzymes called superoxide dismutases (SOD) that catalyze the conversion of superoxide to molecular oxygen and hydrogen peroxide. The latter is still a dangerous molecule but it can be further disarmed by enzymes such as catalase, which converts it to oxygen and water (Figure 3). There is evidence, however, that, with age, products of ROS damage begin to accumulate in tissues. For example, the levels of 8-oxo-deoxyguanosine, an oxidation product of deoxyguanosine in DNA, increase slowly and uniformly from early youth on. Chromosome breakage products resulting from oxidation, dicentric chromosomes, and other visible abnormalities also increase continuously with age. However, there is not a detectable sharp increase concomitant with organismal aging as one would expect. The damaging events occur continuously, not just in aging adults. They are normally repaired by a large number of mechanisms that tend to maintain cellular and organismal functions. Increased levels of ROS cause more DNA damage but do not shorten lifespan. Conversely, overexpression of superoxide dismutases lowers the ROS levels but does not by itself extend life. The homeostatic mechanisms seem to decrease in effectiveness later in life. But to say that aging occurs because homeostatic mechanisms become less effective is not a useful explanation. It just replaces the word "aging" with a phrase "decrease in effectiveness of homeostatic mechanisms". In many cases, what is called a cause of aging is just another description of part of the aging process. We know that many individual functions follow a developmental course: some genes are expressed early in development and are later turned off. Are the homeostatic mechanisms that appear to fail in aging adults developmentally turned off? It has been suggested that the energy invested in such homeostatic functions is reduced when an organism reaches post-reproductive age. The reasoning is that evolutionary drives no longer select for their continuation after reproduction has ceased. This argument is not entirely satisfactory and requires explanations for the selective trade-offs involved at the end of reproductive functions and of homeostatic functions. Why, for example, does reproduction cease at a certain age?

It is clear nevertheless that a substantial fraction of longevity is under genetic control and it is possible to select and breed longer-lived worms, flies, mice, and other organisms. However, when genetics and environment are controlled, there is still a large divergence in the aging of individuals. In the nematode *C. elegans*, for example, differences in the aging of individuals can be distinguished even within isogenic populations, sharing the same genes, reared in uniform conditions. Still, some animals grow phenotypically old sooner than others. In aging, therefore, there is much that is genetics; much that is environmental; much that depends on developmental history; but also much that is stochastic or that we cannot directly account for.

In this chapter, we will not attempt to survey all the processes that contribute to organismal aging rather we will concern ourselves with the epigenetic and chromatin mechanisms that are involved in aging and may in some cases have causative rather than just accompanying roles.

The cell cycle in brief

Dividing cells advance through a cycle of events that regulates growth, DNA replication, preparation for cell division, and mitosis (Figure 4). Cell cycle checkpoints ensure that the cell is ready to proceed to the next phase. The progress through the cell cycle is determined by cyclins and cyclin-dependent kinases (CDKs). CDKs are protein kinases that need to

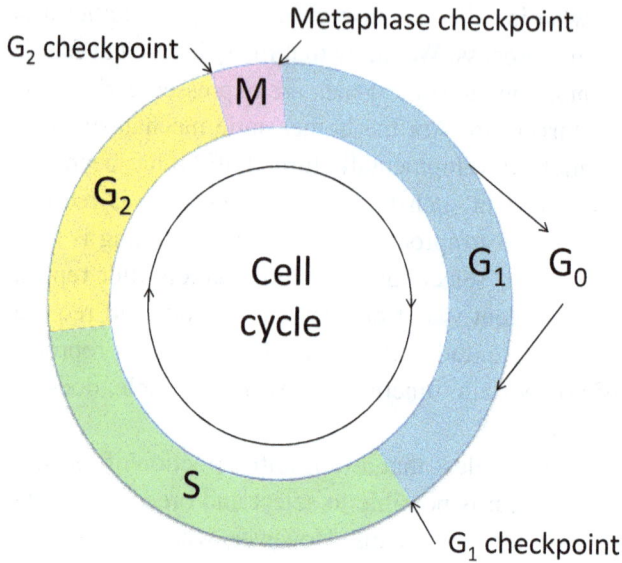

Figure 4.   The cell cycle. Cells grow during G_1 but may exit the cycle and enter a resting state G_0. The G_1 checkpoint, before entering S phase, ensures that the genome is ready for replication and contains no sites of damage. DNA replicates during S phase. After replication is completed, cells continue to grow until the G_2 checkpoint that ensures the cell is ready for mitosis. During mitosis, the chromosomes condense, attach to the spindle, at which point the Metaphase or Spindle checkpoint takes place to ensure that the chromosomes are properly attached to the spindle, aligned at metaphase, and ready to segregate to the two daughter cells. The cell cycle then proceeds to cytokinesis and mitosis.

form heterodimers with appropriate cyclins to become active (Figure 5). Cyclins are transcriptionally regulated and increase in abundance as each phase of the cycle proceeds and are then degraded. Cyclin D signals entrance into the cell cycle. Its levels are low in resting cells but increase in response to external signals by growth factors. The cyclin D-CDK4/6 complex phosphorylates retinoblastoma protein Rb. Unphosphorylated Rb causes exit of the cell cycle and maintains cells in the resting state G_0. Rb has many phosphorylation sites whose specific phosphorylation triggers different steps in the cell cycle. Phosphorylation by cyclin D-CDK4/6 permits progression to S phase. Cyclin E begins to accumulate and bind to CDK2, which hyperphosphorylates Rb and allows the expression of

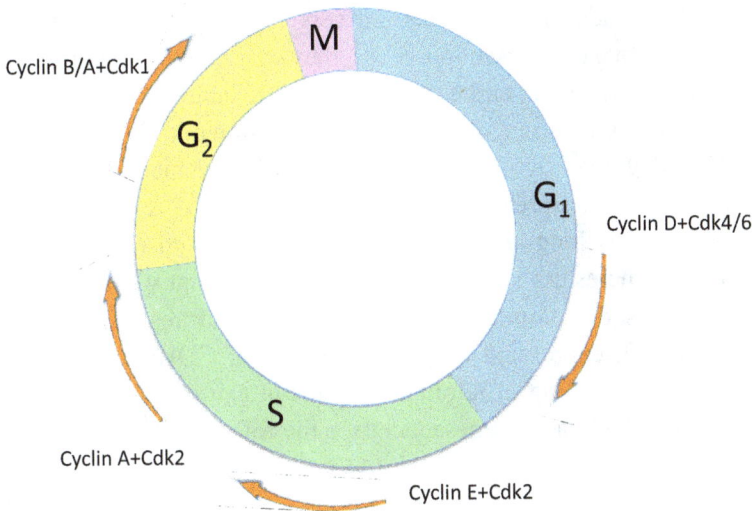

Figure 5.   Cell cycle progression requires the activation of cyclin-dependent kinases (CDKs). CDKs become active only in the form of heterodimers with the appropriate cyclin. The expression of the different cyclins is regulated during the cell cycle so that each increases gradually at the stages indicated in the figure. The activity of the CDKs promotes a complex regulative network, involving Retinoblastoma protein Rb and E2F transcription factors, which control cell cycle regulation and DNA replication.

genes necessary for DNA replication. Cyclin E is eventually replaced by cyclin A and then by cyclin B and CDK1, which initiate the process of mitosis.

The cell cycle can be arrested by a number of inhibitors of the CDKs. These provide ways to prevent replication if the cell senses a variety of stress signals. CDK inhibitors are of two kinds: one includes p21, p27, and p57, which stop the cycle at G_1. The p21 gene is activated by p53 protein, which is in turn activated by DNA damage. The other group of CDK inhibitors are produced by the INK4a/ARF locus and include p16^{INK4a} and p14^{ARF} (see Chapters 7 and 9). The latter prevents p53 degradation. These inhibitors protect cells from unregulated replication (cancer) or in the presence of cellular damage or stress conditions. If the damage cannot be repaired, in some cases, processes leading to apoptosis or cell death are activated. Not surprisingly, these inhibitors are among the first targets of pathways leading to cancer.

Double-stranded DNA breaks are very rapidly sensed and trigger a number of events. For present purposes, they cause the phosphorylation of p53, which activates the expression of the CDK inhibitor p21 (Figure 6). The result is prompt arrest of cell cycle progression until DNA is repaired and p21 is degraded by proteases. Of critical importance is the fact that telomeres can be interpreted by the cell as a break in DNA (see Chapter 1). When sufficiently long, telomeric complexes can disguise the DNA ends but when telomeres are shortened, they reach the point where these remedies fail and short telomeres trigger the DNA break response, phosphorylation of p53, expression of p21, inhibition of CDKs, and cell cycle arrest. Thus, shortening of telomeres results in exit of the cell cycle and the process of replicative senescence (see the following).

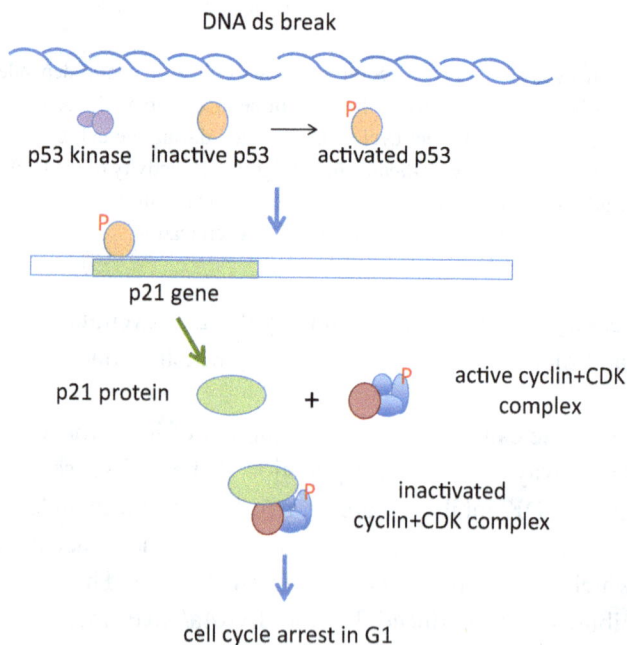

Figure 6.   DNA damage checkpoint. DNA replication will not proceed if DNA damage is detected. Double strand breaks elicit rapid signals to activate repair and to block progression into S phase. Activation of p53 protein is a rapid response to DNA damage, resulting in the phosphorylation of p53, which activates response genes, including the p21 gene. The p21 protein binds to the active cyclin + CDK complex and inactivates it, causing cell cycle arrest in G1.

Tissue renewal

Most cells in adult tissues are post-mitotic: they are terminally differentiated and have stopped dividing. In most tissues, these cells gradually age and die. Most adult tissues contain small populations of adult stem cells that are not terminally differentiated and are still able to divide: these are called somatic or tissue stem cells. These cells can replicate slowly without differentiating. They are not pluripotent because they are committed to differentiating in a manner appropriate to their tissue, but in some cases, this means that they can still produce a few varieties of cells. For example, hematopoietic stem cells in the bone marrow can differentiate into several different kinds of blood cells or cells of the immune system. In many cases, somatic stem cells are found in a **niche**: they are surrounded by cells that secrete signals which keep the stem cell from differentiating while promoting their slow replication (Figure 7). The stem cell divides to produce two daughter cells but the division can be asymmetric: one daughter cell remains in contact with the niche and continues to be an undifferentiated stem cell. The other daughter cell loses contact with the niche and starts to differentiate. In other cases, such as in the epidermis, the replicating cell has a certain probability of producing two replicating cells, or one replicating and one differentiating cell, or two differentiating cells. These probabilities may be regulated by the presence of growth factors such as

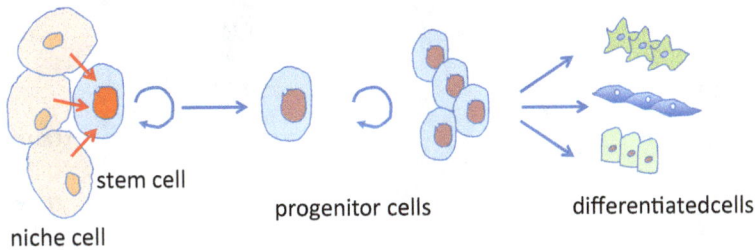

stem cell

niche cell

progenitor cells

differentiatedcells

Figure 7. Tissue stem cell differentiation. A small stem cell population resides in many adult tissues. It is maintained by interactions with niche cells that support the undifferentiated state and allow slow replication. Stem cells can reproduce themselves. Either upon reception of a signal or often by asymmetric division they can start the differentiation process. In many cases, the differentiating cell goes through a progenitor stage in which it divides to increase in cell number. Some of the cells produced then differentiate, producing one or more terminally differentiated, post-mitotic cell types.

β-catenin (also known as Wnt), which stimulates cell division, or Transforming Growth Factor beta (TGF-β), which favors differentiation.

Continuously renewing epithelia: Epidermis and intestinal lining

On one extreme of tissue stem cell types are those involved in continuously growing epithelia such as the skin or the intestinal lining. In both cases, the differentiated cells are exposed to harsh conditions and are programmed to die off and be replaced every few days in the case of the intestinal lining or a few weeks in the case of the epidermis.

Intestinal epithelium (Figure 8)

The internal lining of the gut is a single layer of cells that carry out the digestive functions: absorbing nutrients from food and keeping out undesired substances. To maximize the surface area of the gut, the cell layer forms finger-like protrusions called villi. Between villi are deep cellular wells called crypts at the bottom and sides of which are stem cells that

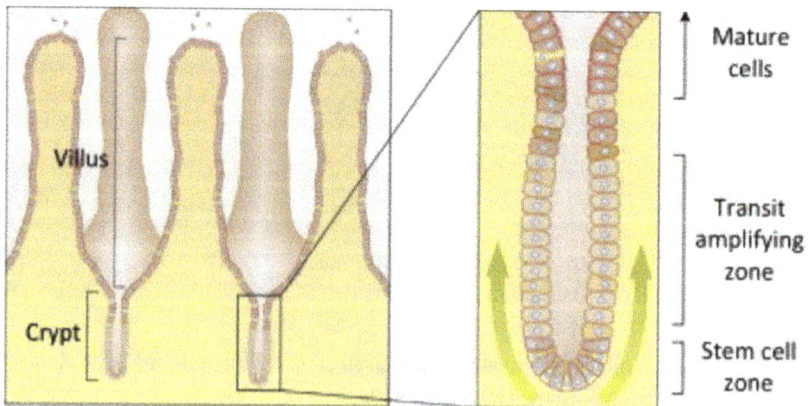

Figure 8.   Intestinal epithelium. Stem cells at the bottom of crypts divide continuously, producing new intestinal epithelial cells that migrate up to form the lining of the villus, replacing dying cells.

Source: Gerhart and Clevers (2015).

divide constantly. New cell production feeds a constant migration of cells out of the crypts and up the sides of the villi (Gerhart and Clevers, 2015). These cells are hard-working and exposed to foreign substances in the ingested food. They mature and age rapidly, undergo apoptosis, and are shed off from the villi. This constitutes a sort of treadmill constantly replacing the cells forming the lining of the intestine. The bottom of the crypt contains a dozen multipotent stem cells, which divide laterally, producing a daughter cell that stays in place and remains a stem cell, and one that moves up the side of the crypt. As cells move up the sides, they may divide a few more times (transit-amplifying cells), and differentiate, producing some of the different types of cells forming the intestinal lining. Intestinal epithelium cells work very hard and are exposed to harsh conditions. They need to be renewed frequently. The rate of cell division of the stem cells is one of the highest in the human body and the epithelium is renewed every 4–5 days. Nevertheless, the division of the stem cells is tightly controlled and escape from this regulation is responsible for most bowel cancers. Intestinal stem cells, isolated and cultured, can be used to produce intestinal organoids (Meneses *et al.* 2016). That is, in the appropriate media, they can regenerate the crypt-villus structure and the different types of cells normally found in the lining of the gut.

Epidermis (Figure 9)

The epidermis is the outer layer of the skin, lying above the dermis and separated from it by a basement membrane. The dermis contains sense organs, sweat glands, hair follicles, and blood vessels. The epidermis lacks blood vessels and is nourished from the dermis. It consists of a series of layers, the innermost of which is the basal or germinative layer, consisting of proliferating keratinocytes. These cells, so named because of the keratin granules they contain, are attached to the basement membrane and constitute the stem cells of the epidermis. As they divide, they produce the spinous layer of proliferating keratinocytes, the thickest layer of the epidermis. These cells continue to divide, in turn producing the next layer, the granular layer. Here, the keratinocytes stop dividing, lose their nuclei, and start differentiating. The next layer, the clear or translucent layer, found only in the palm of the hand and soles of feet, consists of dead,

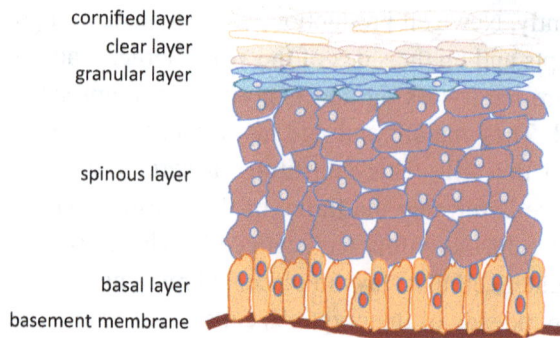

cornified layer
clear layer
granular layer

spinous layer

basal layer
basement membrane

Figure 9.   Epidermal cell layers. The basal layer consists of germinating keratinocytes that divide continuously, producing the spinous layer. These new cells differentiate progressively and die, forming a cornified, waterproof outer layer that protects the skin and the internal organs.

flattened keratinocyte cell bodies. The outer layer of the epidermis, the cornified layer, forms a tight barrier of dead cells whose envelope proteins and keratins surrounded by lipids protect the underlying tissues from loss of water, chemical and physical damage, and pathogens. The dead cells of the cornified layer are continuously shed and replaced from the lower layers. The role of Polycomb repression is essential for the progressive differentiation of the proliferating keratinocytes to form the different layers of the epidermis (see Ezhkova *et al.*, 2009 and Chapter 7). Polycomb repression is gradually turned down, derepressing the differentiation genes, including the INK4A and B inhibitors of cell cycle progression, resulting in proliferation arrest. *De novo* DNA methylase DNMT3A is also important and its loss results in excessive proliferation of keratinocytes and a pre-cancerous state. Aging and sun exposure are factors that promote loss of DNMT3A expression in the epidermis.

Neural Stem Cells and Cognitive Functions

Mutations in certain functions tend to be found with particular frequency in different kinds of aging tissues. In particular, mutations in genes involved in DNA methylation such as DNMT3A, a *de novo* DNA CpG methyltransferase, and TET2, a CpG DNA demethylase (see Chapter 3), are frequently found at higher rates in aging tissues, though it is not clear in what way they might have to do with clonal expansion or replicative advantage. What is clear is that these genes are particularly important for the function of neural tissues.

Neural stem cells are known to exist in the human central nervous system and are responsible for neurogenesis: the formation of new nerve cells. However, human neural stem cells decrease precipitously after childhood. One place where they are thought to remain is the hippocampus, a brain structure believed to be involved in learning and the formation of new memories. TET2 and 5hmC, the product of its action on 5mC, are both highly abundant in the hippocampus and decrease with age in parallel with the decrease in adult neurogenesis. In mice, low levels of TET2 in the hippocampus are associated with aging and cognitive impairment. Recent work shows that knocking down TET2 expression in the hippocampus of young mice results in loss of neurogenesis and impaired learning and memory. Conversely, expressing exogenous TET2 in the hippocampus of aging mice restores neurogenesis and rejuvenates cognitive processes. Along similar lines, studies of the hippocampus of elderly patients with Alzheimer's disease found an increase in DNA methylation in the promoter of many genes that are normally in a bivalent state in the hippocampus of control individuals. The genes affected by this differential methylation are preferentially involved in neurogenesis and neural differentiation and become repressed as a result. This holds out the possibility, exciting for some of us, to rejuvenate aging intellects. The role of DNA demethylation in the hippocampus may be unusual and due to the loss of neural stem cells very early in development. Reactivation of some of the neurogenesis-associated genes might relieve aging effects in the hippocampus but have little bearing on general organismal aging.

Somatic Mutations and Clonal Expansion

DNA replication is a marvelously complex and remarkably exact mechanism that includes error correction features. Furthermore, cells are provided with many DNA damage repair mechanisms. Nevertheless, sequence errors can occur, escape correction, and be transmitted to daughter cells at a rate estimated around 6×10^{-10} per base per cell division. Since the haploid human genome consists of 3×10^9 base pairs, this means about two mutations every cell division, though the frequencies vary in different cell types. An intrinsic risk associated with tissue stem cells is the generation of mutations in every round of DNA replication. The more cell divisions, the more mutations accumulate in the genome, estimated from studies with adult stem cells to add up to ~40 mutations/genome/year. Somatic tissues are therefore mosaics of cells with different mutations at different genomic sites. It has even been argued that the frequency of cancer of all types in any given tissue is directly related to the number of divisions cells undergo in that tissue (Tomasetti and Vogelstein, 2015).

Traditionally, the frequency of mutations in tissues is said to increase with age. However, this is based on the number of mutations found by genomic sequencing of a tissue sample, not by measuring the frequency at which new mutations arise. What has become clear from recent advances in DNA sequencing technology, including single-cell genome sequencing, is that certain mutations or constellation of mutations can confer proliferative advantage to the cell carrying them. As a result, the cell carrying such mutations undergoes what is called Aberrant Clonal Expansion (ACE). This means that such mutant clones get larger and represent a larger fraction of the cells in a tissue (Figure 10). In some cases, more than 10% of the cells in a tissue come in fact from an expanded clone. For this reason, just counting the frequency of a particular mutation in a tissue does not tell you about the frequency with which the mutation arises but rather about how much the clone carrying that mutation has expanded. Such clones expand with time, giving the impression that the frequency of mutation increases with age. As a result, it is not clear at this time whether the frequency of mutagenesis really increases with age.

Mutations that confer proliferative advantage are one of the features of tumors. Such mutations and the resulting clonal expansions are therefore pre-cancerous. Clonal expansion affects also whatever other mutations the expanding clone contains. Any other mutation present in the original cell that acquires the expansion-driving mutation will also expand. These other mutations are passengers that have "hitched a ride" with the driver mutation. In addition, the expanding clone will acquire

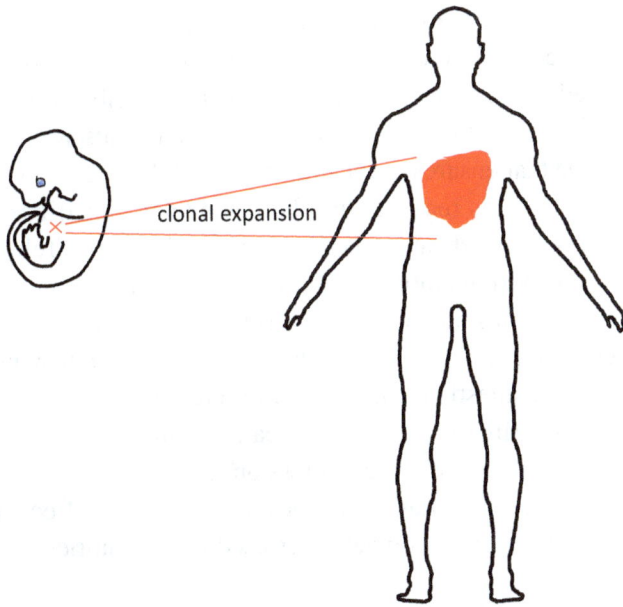

Figure 10. Aberrant clonal expansion. A mutation in a single embryonic cell, if it confers a growth advantage on other cells, can expand to constitute a large percentage of the adult tissue.

additional mutations every round of cell division. Adult stem cells and the tissues they feed will tend to increase their mutational burden and make it more likely that some of the mutations (or combinations of mutations) acquired will be harmful in various ways ranging from loss of function, lower ability to respond to signals, or loss of commitment to a differentiated state and uncontrolled neomorphic growth.

Loss of Tissue Renewal

The risk of uncontrolled growth is a major biological hazard. For this reason, cell proliferation in adult tissues is hedged-in with multiple controls to avoid it or to minimize its consequences. Primary cultures of growing embryonic cells can be maintained as replicating cultures *in vitro* but, as discovered by Leonard Hayflick in the 1960s, they can only undergo a limited number of cell divisions (Figure 11). After 50–60 doublings, human cells slow down, change appearance, and stop dividing. Hayflick called this cellular senescence. It is now attributed to a gradual shortening of telomeres every replicative cycle in the absence of telomerase, the enzyme that ensures replication of the DNA ends (see Chapter 1). When a critical limit is reached, the shortened telomeres trigger the process of cell cycle arrest and senescence (see Figure 6). Telomerase is abundantly expressed in embryonic stem cells but is absent or at very low levels in most human somatic tissues. It is still expressed, however, in tissue stem cells such as those that produce continuously renewing tissues: the epidermis, the intestinal lining, or proliferating T and B cells of the immune system. Primary cell cultures can be "immortalized" by treatments that reactivate telomerase expression, including viral infection or expression of certain cellular oncogenes and this is, in effect, what has occurred in most tissue culture cell lines used in laboratories.

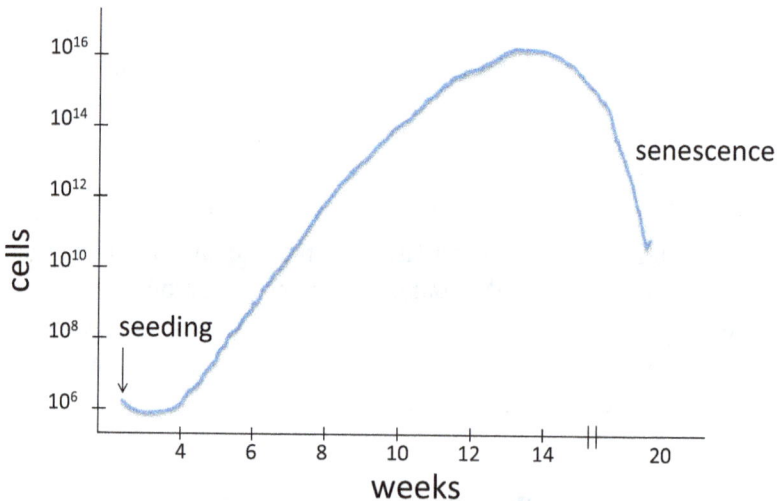

Figure 11.   Primary cell cultures — Hayflick limit. Primary cell cultures, seeded from cells taken from growing tissue *in vivo*, start slowly as the cells adjust to the culture medium and then start doubling. In a cell culture, the cells are passaged when they reach a certain density to avoid overcrowding and exhausting the medium. Under these conditions, they keep proliferating until they reach 40–60 doublings, the Hayflick limit. Then, they slow down and start to become senescent.

Cellular Senescence

Telomere shortening is not the only possible cause of cellular senescence. Stem cells can become senescent if exposed to a variety of stresses such as persistent DNA damage, intercellular stress signaling, unfolded protein toxicity, and oxidative stress. The effects are similar. Interestingly, inhibition of histone deacetylases and therefore inhibition of heterochromatin formation also induces senescence. RNAi knockdown of lamin B1 can induce senescence independently of telomere dysfunction, while overexpression of lamin B1 delays the onset of normal senescence.

Typical features of the senescent state (Figure 12) include a change in cell morphology and a decrease in Polycomb proteins and H3K27me3 with consequent derepression of many genes. Important among these is the *INK4/Arf* locus (see Chapters 7 and 9), where loss of Polycomb repression results in the expression of inhibitors of cyclin-dependent

Features of senescent cells

Cell cycle arrest in G_1

Decrease in RNA and protein synthesis

Accumulation of unfolded, nonfunctional proteins

Increased secretion of pro-inflammatory cytokines (SASP)

Enlarged cell size

Markers of DNA damage

Shortening of telomeres

Loss of lamin B

Expression of β-galactosidase

Decrease in transcriptional repression

Loss of heterochromatin

Figure 12.   Features of senescent cells. The features listed are indicative and the list could be made much longer and more detailed. Not all these features are present in all types of senescent cells.

kinases, principally p16 (CDKN2A), and therefore cell cycle arrest. Other specific features of senescent cells are short telomeres, reduced histone biosynthesis, loss of Lamin B1, and consequent partial detachment of heterochromatin from the nuclear lamina, expression of β-galactosidase, senescence-associated secretory phenotype (SASP). SASP is manifested by the secretion of inflammatory cytokines, proteases, and growth factors, sometimes in the form of exosomes, vesicles that behave like a cellular garbage heap, containing enzymes, RNAs, and DNA fragments. Exosomes can be taken up by surrounding cells and therefore can transmit signals to other cells. The detailed composition of the secreted material varies with the cell type and the cause of the senescence. Some of the secreted material taken up by surrounding cells can cause them to become senescent in turn. Probably for this reason, removal of senescent cells from mouse tissues was found to delay the onset of organismal aging.

A prominent feature of a common type of senescence induced by expression of oncoproteins such as Ras is the formation of prominent senescence-associated heterochromatin foci (SAHF) (Figure 13), strong concentrations of heterochromatin not attached to the nuclear lamina but rather associated with each chromosome. These are not seen in typical replicative senescence, where most heterochromatin remains at least

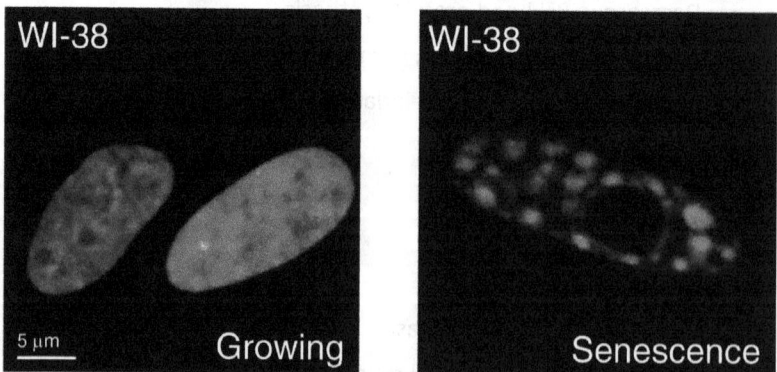

Figure 13.   Senescence-Associated Heterochromatin Foci (SAHF). The cells whose nuclei are visible on the left are growing cultured cells. Upon activation of the cRAF oncogene, the cells become senescent and display typical senescence-associated heterochromatin foci.

Source: Chandra *et al.* (2015).

partially attached to the lamina but this could be just a matter of degree. SAHFs have caused much confusion because they have often been taken as newly formed heterochromatin while all measures of total heterochromatin indicated that heterochromatin actually decreases. Studies of the chromatin architecture of oncogene-induced senescence as well as of replicative senescence show that the difference is due to a much stronger loss of lamin B and lamin B receptor in oncogene-induced senescence. While heterochromatin remains partially associated with the nuclear lamina in replicative senescence, it becomes totally detached in oncogene-induced senescence and loses internal cohesion forming SAHFs in the interior of the nucleus. This changes the pattern of chromatin contacts in parts of the nucleus: some heterochromatic regions come in contact with some euchromatic regions containing active genes, causing their reduced expression. Other changes bring together euchromatic regions, resulting in increased expression of other genes.

Senescent cells tend to be larger and have a characteristic flattened appearance. Both cellular and organismal senescence display changes in **nuclear morphology** and chromatin modifications. Typically, nuclei become larger and less condensed due to loss of heterochromatin, with larger and more prominent nucleoli. Loss of lamins makes the nuclei more easily deformed. These effects have stimulated much interest in the possible role of heterochromatin and of the **nuclear lamina**, its components, and their interactions with chromatin in aging. We will see some of the results further down.

Chromatin and Aging

The idea that loss of heterochromatin might underlie many of the manifestations of aging was behind one of the earliest models for the aging process. There are now many other models for aging, not necessarily incompatible with the chromatin model. In recent years, much new evidence has accumulated on the effects of aging on chromatin. In human cells induced to enter replicative senescence, a decrease in the expression of the replicative histone genes has been reported, accompanied by an increase in levels of histone variants such as H3.3, which are non-replicative and expressed throughout the cell cycle (see Chapter 2). This was taken to suggest that the decrease of histone levels slows down and then arrests DNA replication. Much more likely, however, is the reverse: slowdown of replication causes a corresponding decrease in expression of replicative histone genes. More significant is an apparent change in micrococcal nuclease sensitivity, with aged fibroblasts showing a more irregular nucleosome positioning, lower levels of HP1, and instability in X chromosome inactivation. However, reports of changes in heterochromatin marks such as H3K9me2,3 or in active histone marks such as H3K4 methylation or H3 and H4 acetylation are confused, inconsistent, and contradictory. If heterochromatic silencing systematically decreases in senescence, we would expect a general loss of heterochromatic silencing. Reports of changes in the transcriptome with replicative senescence suggest that some genes increase while some decrease. Gene expression is said to become more "noisy", which would be consistent with decreased suppression of random gene activity by heterochromatic silencing. Similarly, DNA methylation was found to be reduced in certain regions, often corresponding to heterochromatin, while other regions, often corresponding to CpG islands, showed inappropriate increases in DNA methylation. Part of this confused situation may be due to the different models used and to the reliance on oncogene-induced senescence, which often causes a detachment of heterochromatin from the lamina and the formation of heterochromatin aggregates juxtaposed to euchromatic regions. This would cause a collection of variable effects: some heterochromatic regions become less, while some euchromatic regions become more repressed by the proximity of heterochromatin.

In addition, the question remains to what extent effects seen *in vitro* senescence are relevant to the behavior of post-mitotic cells and to organismal aging. What happens to the chromatin and gene expression in senescent tissue stem cells may not necessarily hold for post-mitotic differentiated cells. However, some arguments can be made for the relevance. One is that if tissue stem cells start to become senescent, the differentiated cells that they produce may show the consequences of any dysfunctional gene expression in the senescent stem cells. Second, of course, the reduction or loss of stem cells that have become senescent and unable to replicate means that the corresponding tissues lose the ability to replenish and renew their cells. A third consequence of senescence in tissue stem cells is the abovementioned senescence-associated secretory phenotype (SASP) which can be shown to affect surrounding cells. In fact, removal of senescent cells from tissues demonstrably delays organismal aging. Despite the inconclusiveness of much of the research on replicative senescence and its relevance to organismal aging, we will return further down to what is probably the most solid and reliable result of that body of work, which is that senescent cells lose expression of lamin B. This could be the primary cause of alterations in the physical status of heterochromatin and transcriptionally silent genes.

Transposon Derepression

Loss of histones, loss of heterochromatin, loss of or inappropriate DNA methylation, and loss of or inappropriate PcG silencing, all of these can lead to increased sensitivity to DNA damage, loss of chromosome integrity, replicative senescence, transposon mobilization, inappropriate gene expression, accumulation of junk proteins, etc.

If some aspects of heterochromatic silencing decrease, many genomic regions may become more transcriptionally active, including repetitive elements and transposable elements, which make up more than 50% of the human genome. This would lead to increased transpositional activity, and, in fact, transposon mobilization has been proposed to be responsible for age-induced cellular degeneration. This appears to happen normally in the nervous system, where LINE element L1 has been reported to become mobilized in neural progenitor cells and has even been claimed to be an important factor in neuronal plasticity. This last seems exceedingly unlikely: such a mechanism would be beneficial only in situations where a large fraction of cells is expendable and justifiable by the production of very rare beneficial events. The mobilization of L1 elements has been reported in senescent fibroblasts. A generalized derepression of transposable elements could well have cumulative deleterious effects due not just to new insertions but even more to the increased rate of DNA breaks associated with high transposase activity. In fact, a relative opening of hitherto silenced chromatin has been reported in senescent cells. Transcription of transposable elements and even of satellite sequences increases. Transposition activity increases distinctly but only at late stages of cellular senescence. It seems unlikely therefore that transposon mobilization contributes significantly to neural degeneration, as has been proposed. It does, however, confirm further the idea that cellular aging is associated with derepression of heterochromatin and an increase in indiscriminate transcriptional activity.

The Role of Lamins

We have seen that loss of lamins and of lamin attachment is one of the effects of cellular senescence. We saw also in earlier chapters that lamins and proteins associated with the nuclear lamina form a major attachment site for heterochromatin (see Chapters 4 and 8). Loss of lamins or changes in lamin expression would therefore be expected to reduce the association of heterochromatin with the nuclear periphery where it is concentrated with the associated proteins and enzymes. Heterochromatin would become less associated with the structures and proteins that maintain its stability and more likely to come in contact with transcriptionally active chromatin. Work on genome architecture in the past few years has made it clear that the higher-order folding of the genome in the nucleus has important consequences for the local expression of individual genes and larger genomic domains (see Chapter 8). The fact that cellular senescence is accompanied by reorganization of genomic architecture in large part attributed to the loss of lamins raises numerous concerns. What are the direct and indirect consequences of loss of lamins and of attachment of silent chromatin to the nuclear envelope? What is the significance of the normal segregation of heterochromatin to the nuclear periphery?

Lamins are intermediate filament proteins that polymerize to form a meshwork of fibers that is the main constituent of the nuclear lamina (see Chapter 4). There are two kinds of lamins: lamin A/C and lamin B. Lamin A and lamin C are the product of the same gene. Structurally, B-type lamins are the most important. In fact, embryonic stem cells lack lamin A/C and their lamina is composed of B lamins only. Lamin A is expressed and required only when embryonic stem cells start to differentiate. Lamins bind to many kinds of proteins that interact with heterochromatin, in particular LAP and LBR proteins that bind to HP1 and other heterochromatin proteins. They also bind other repressive proteins, including histone deacetylases and form a repressive environment that promotes heterochromatin and tends to silence genes that are artificially targeted to the lamina. To assess the consequences of loss of lamin B1, several laboratories looked at the distribution of histone marks associated with transcriptional activity (H3K4me3) or Polycomb repression (H3K27me3) in proliferating and senescent human cells. They found major changes occurring in large-scale domains (Figure 14). Chromatin immunoprecipitation (ChIP) showed strongly elevated H3K4me3 in domains normally associated with the nuclear lamina (LADs). Loss of H3K27me3 occurred in regions between LADs, particularly associated with genes and enhancers. Both kinds of changes are indicative of increased transcriptional activity. This is often correlated with activation of senescence genes. Knockdown of lamin B1 expression in proliferating cells produces the same kinds of changes, implying that loss of lamin B1 does not simply accompany senescence but actually triggers the changes in chromatin organization and in gene expression that are characteristic of senescence.

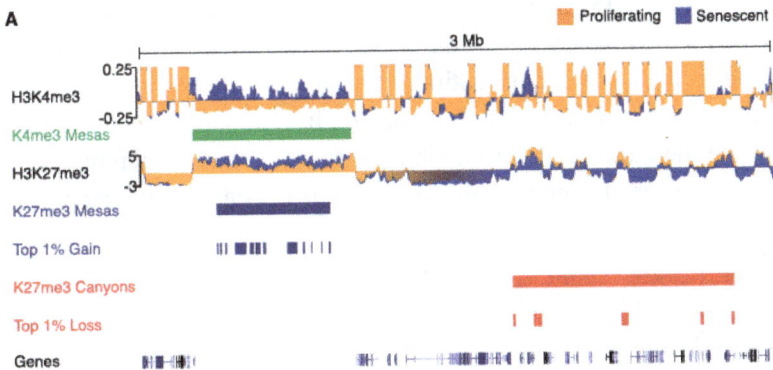

Figure 14. Changes in histone marks occur in senescent cells. Chromatin immunoprecipitation results show changes in H3K27me3 and H3K4me3 in senescent compared to proliferating cells. "Mesas" are regions of increase and "canyons" are regions of decrease. Many of these regions correspond to lamin-associated domains (LADs). Mesas of both marks are well correlated with lamin attached domains (LADs).

Source: Shah *et al.* (2013).

LADs and Changes in Senescence

Regions of chromatin that are associated with the nuclear lamina can be identified by immunoprecipitating chromatin with antibodies against lamins or individual lamin-associated proteins. Another technique called DamID (see Chapter 13) labels DNA associated with the nuclear lamina by fusing lamin with a bacterial Adenine DNA methylase called Dam methylase. This allows any genomic region that comes in the near vicinity of the lamin-Dam methylase to acquire adenine methylation, which can then be identified through enzyme action and DNA sequencing. These techniques have shown that precisely defined genomic regions are associated with the nuclear lamina. These regions are called Lamin Associated Domains (LADs). They generally have lower levels of transcription, lower levels of active chromatin marks (H3K4me3, H3K36me3, and histone acetylation), lower density of genes or longer intergenic regions, and more heterochromatin proteins. Studies have shown that LADs contain different kinds of genes with different degrees of silencing. Some are more loosely associated with the lamina and retain some transcriptional activity. Some become transcriptionally active when removed from contact with the lamina and placed in a euchromatic context. Others are more intrinsically repressed and remain silent when moved to euchromatin. Still others correspond to deep heterochromatin and are most strongly associated with the lamina and also most heterochromatic in character. Experiments also show that these different chromatin regions would have different effects if they were released from the lamina and came in contact with euchromatic regions.

LADs show changes in senescent cells: they generally acquire more active histone marks and redistribute H3K27me3. Some LAD regions acquire H3K27me3 while others lose it. These changes are consistent with the interpretation that gene-poor regions are heterochromatic in proliferating cells but tend to lose heterochromatin marks in senescent cells, acquiring more histone acetylation and H3K4me3 instead (H3K4me3 "mesas" in Figure 14). In proliferating cells, LADs that contain genes have both some active marks and some H3K27me3 (consistent with some gene expression). These regions become more transcriptionally active and lose H3K27me3 (H3K27me3 "canyons") (Figure 15). Overall, therefore

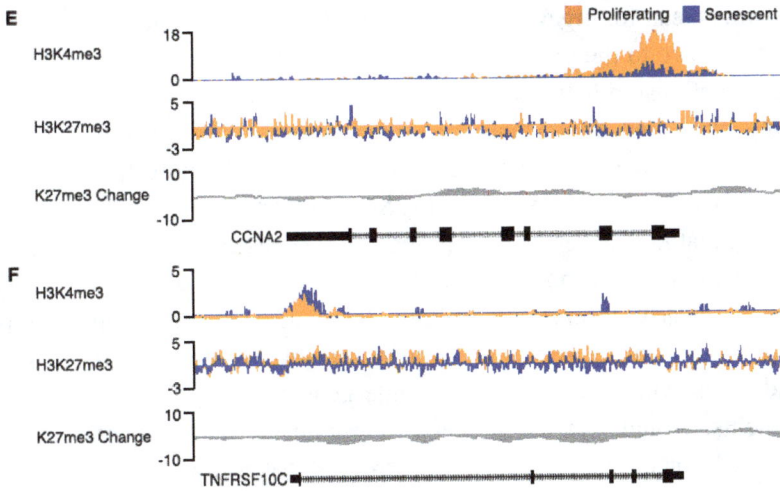

Figure 15.   Chromatin changes found in senescent cells are correlated to changes in gene expression. Genes in Lamin-Associated Domains of proliferating cells frequently acquire mesas of H3K4me3 in senescent cells and increased expression. Among these genes are those typically expressing proteins involved in the senescence pathway, including senescence genes, anti-proliferation genes, and cell death/stress genes. (E) shows the profiles of CCNA2, a gene downregulated in senescent cells. (F) shows profiles of TNFRSF10C, a gene upregulated in senescent cells.

Source: Shah *et al.* (2013).

there is a trend for these heterochromatic regions to lose heterochromatin and become more active. In fact, some LADs lose lamin association and dissociate from the nuclear envelope. Furthermore, in senescent cells, lamin B1 is strongly depleted. But is this a cause or a consequence of senescence and loss of heterochromatin?

If expression of Lamin B1 is knocked down by means of RNAi in proliferating cells, the same changes in histone marks and heterochromatin proteins are produced, indicating loss of heterochromatin, and the classical phenotypes of cellular senescence are induced. This implies that loss of lamina or lamina attachment **causes** the heterochromatin and gene expression changes and senescence rather than being caused by senescence. But what causes the loss of lamins? And, granted that cellular senescence involves the loss of lamins and then of heterochromatin, what does this mean for organismal senescence? How do we know that this has any relevance to the visible effects of aging that we see around us? What is the relationship between cellular senescence, which affects only replicating cells, and organismal senescence? Arguments can be made that many organismal phenotypes can be attributed to failure to adequately renew tissues from tissue stem cells. Some evidence suggests that cellular stresses that induce senescence in replicative cells can also induce similar chromatin effects in post-mitotic, terminally differentiated cells. Indeed, aging is clearly observed in nematodes, whose entire adult life is post-mitotic. The most convincing argument, however, is provided by progeria syndromes, where failures due to single-gene mutations recapitulate large segments, though not the entirety, of organismal aging manifestations. The study of progerias, genetic syndromes that result in premature and accelerated aging, is a powerful source of evidence. Perhaps the most dramatic of these is Hutchinson–Gilford Progeria Syndrome (HGPS), caused by a mutation in the LaminA/C gene. Children with HGPS begin to show symptoms of aging in their first few years and generally die of cardiovascular failure in their teens. Dramatic as the symptoms of HGPS are, before we look into this progeria in mechanistic detail, it is useful to consider another progeria syndrome called Werner Syndrome (WS).

Werner Syndrome

WS is often called "adult progeria" because its symptoms set in in early adults. WS is caused by loss of function of the WRN gene. WRN protein is a RecQ DNA helicase important for many processes that involve DNA: DNA replication, DNA damage repair, transcription (which also causes DNA damage), and genetic recombination. Loss of WRN function causes difficulties in DNA replication, in the repair of double-strand DNA breaks, in the maintenance of telomere length, and, because WRN binds to p53, in reduced p53-dependent apoptosis. WS patients show premature cellular senescence setting in around age 20. This is accompanied by genome instability, DNA breaks, deletions, rearrangements, high frequency of tumors, and degeneration of mesodermal tissues. The common interpretation of these effects has been that the increased DNA damage is responsible for increased tumors, telomere shortening, and senescence, and WS has been widely used as evidence for models of aging based on DNA damage. But why do these effects occur principally in mesodermally derived tissues? If they are caused by DNA damage and replication difficulties, they should affect all tissues. And why are the symptoms not manifested until early adulthood?

Recent work has opened a different way to interpret the effects of WS. Research by Zhang *et al.* (2015) shows that WRN binds to a complex that contains SUV39H1 (a major H3K9 methylase in heterochromatin), HP1α, and LAP2β (a lamin-binding protein that binds HP1α and recruits heterochromatin to the lamina) (Figure 16). Embryonic stem cells express principally SUV39H2, rather than SUV39H1; they have less heterochromatin and what they have does not bind WRN and their heterochromatin formation does not require WRN. The mesenchyme is a mesodermal connective tissue from which the circulatory system, the muscle, and bone tissues are developed. In mesenchyme cells, normal aging results in typical loss of heterochromatin structures and histone marks: lamin and lamin-associated proteins, HP1α, SUV39H1, and H3K9me3, all are drastically reduced and so is WRN itself (Figure 17). Mesenchymal stem cells are particularly dependent on SUV39H1 and, when they lack WRN, they develop all the expected syndromic symptoms of normal aging: premature senescence,

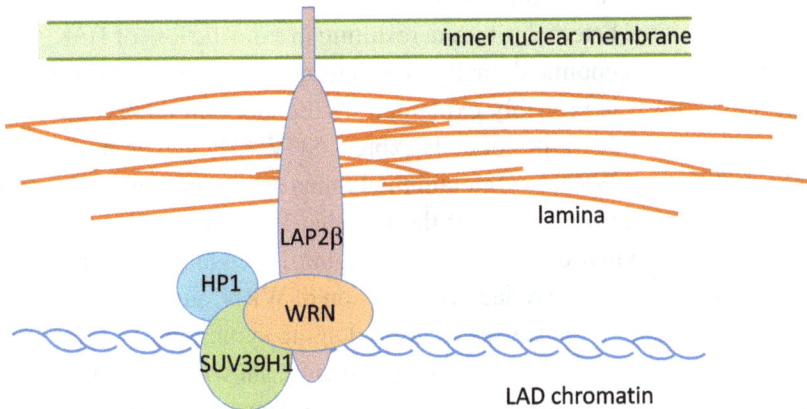

Figure 16.   WRN is an integral component of a complex connecting chromatin to the nuclear lamina. WRN forms a complex with HP1, SUV39H2, and lamin-associated protein LAP2β, which recruits and maintains heterochromatin to the nuclear lamina.

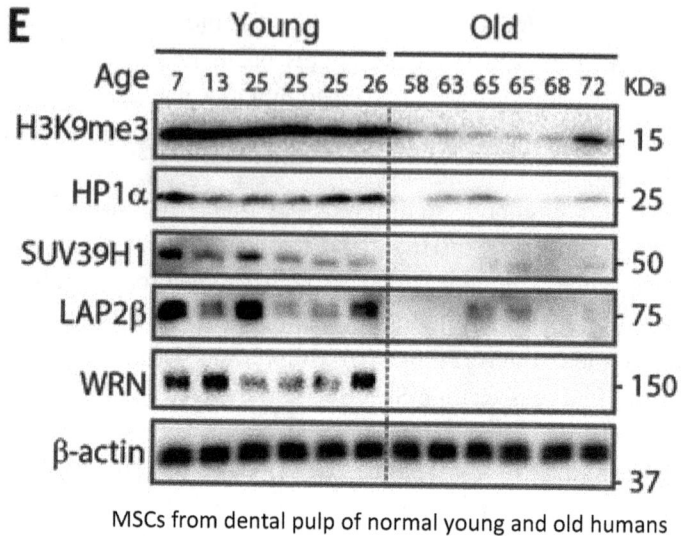

Figure 17.   Normal aging produces loss of heterochromatin marks in humans. Western blots for H3K9me3 and several heterochromatin-associated proteins show major decreases in older individuals compared to younger ones. Actin is included for comparison.
Source: Zhang *et al.* (2015).

shortening of telomeres, and increased DNA damage. In addition, they lose the lamina-associated proteins LAP2β and Lamin B receptor (LBR) and the associated heterochromatin, resulting in a drastic loss of H3K9me3 and HP1 in large genomic domains. The late appearance of WS symptoms after adolescence is probably explained by the fact that embryonic stem cells and certain other types of cells express SUV39H2 and do not depend on SUV39H1 and WRN to maintain the lamina association of heterochromatin. This may also account for the fact that WS affects principally tissues of mesenchymal origin. In normal aging individuals, mesenchymal stem cells appear to have reduced expression of WRN, suggesting that this might also be one of the causes of normal aging symptoms.

Not all heterochromatin is equally affected, showing once again that there are functionally different kinds of heterochromatin. What is most altered is the heterochromatin in many pericentromeric regions and in many subtelomeric regions. These are not just disease-dependent effects; they are closely paralleled by effects seen in normal aging. When mesenchymal tissues of old humans are compared with those of young people, the same loss of H3K9me3, HP1α, SUV39H1, LAP2β, and WRN itself is observed. Crucially, if the SUV39H1 gene or the HP1α gene are knocked down or mutated in mesenchymal cells, the same loss of hetero-chromatin and premature senescence and derepression of heterochromatic satellite sequences occur as in WS. What does not occur is the increased DNA damage. In contrast, overexpression of HP1α in WRN mutant mes-enchymal stem cells suppresses cellular senescence. These results strongly suggest that WS reflects at least a part of the symptoms of organismal aging. They also imply that loss of heterochromatin and/or inner mem-brane/lamina association, not direct effects on telomeres, is responsible for premature senescence. What remains possible, however, is that tel-omere shortening might in some way independently induce loss of hetero-chromatin or its lamina association.

Hutchinson–Gilford Progeria

In contrast to WS, HGPS sets in early childhood. Death ensues before the age of 20, usually from heart disease. HGPS is therefore often called "childhood progeria". For a dramatic illustration of this condition, which can nevertheless co-exist with full intellectual capacity, the reader is invited to visit https://www.hbo.com/movies/life-according-to-sam. This is a reportage on the life of Sam Berns, a child affected by HGPS, viewed at the age of 13. HGPS shows some of the same cellular symptoms as WS: reduced expression of lamin B2, loss of H3K9me3, HP1, and heterochro-matin, cellular senescence, and affecting primarily mesodermal tissues such as bone, muscle, skin, and the circulatory system. HGPS does not involve increased DNA damage and tumor incidence. Neither HGPS nor WS involves cataract formation or neural degeneration and cognitive defi-ciencies and therefore these two progerias do not represent the full range of symptoms of true organismal aging.

HGPS affects the nuclear lamina itself. Lamina composition and structure change from embryonic stem cells, which have only the B lamins, to differentiating cells, which start to express also lamin A/C (Figure 18). When cells differentiate, lamin A and C as well as lamin B are essential to assemble the normal lamin network. Different parts of the

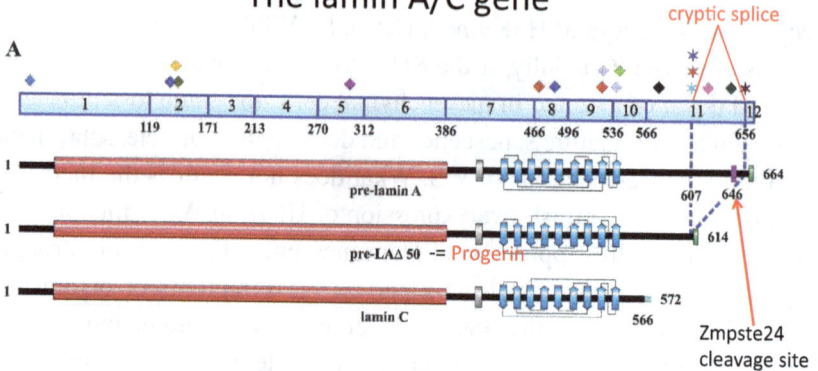

In HGPS, a mutation activates what is normally a cryptic splice site and produces **Progerin**: a Lamin A protein with 50 amino acids deleted removing an important cleavage site. This cryptic splice site is occasionally used in normal cells, producing a small amount of Progerin. This small amount has been shown to increase with age.

Figure 18.   The lamin A/C gene. Lamin A and Lamin C are produced by the same gene by alternative splicing. They interact with Lamin B proteins to make up the nuclear lamina. In the normal pre-lamin A protein, a cleavage site for the Zmpste24 protease normally cleaves off the C-terminal tip. In HGPS, a point mutation in intron 11 activates a cryptic splice 5′ donor site, resulting in pre-LADelta50, a slightly shorter protein with an internal deletion of 50 amino acids but with the normal C-terminal exon. This protein lacks the Zmpste24 cleavage site and therefore retains the C-terminal. This protein will give rise to Progerin.

Source: Dechat *et al.* (2008).

lamin proteins bind different sets of proteins that act on chromatin, for example, LAP and LBR that bind to HP1, or histone deacetylases. In fact, mutations in different parts of the lamin genes cause different genetic syndromes. The mutation in HGPS affects the lamin A/C gene (Figure 19). Lamin A and lamin C are produced from differential splicing of the 3′ terminal region of the same transcript. The mutation does not affect the shorter lamin C but it activates a cryptic splice site near the 3′ end, causing a small deletion. This small deletion removes a proteolytic cleavage site that normally would allow the C-terminal region of lamin A to be clipped off. This is important because the C-terminal is the site of **farnesylation**, the attachment of a 15-carbon isoprenoid chain that targets the lamin to

The Lamins and the nuclear Lamina

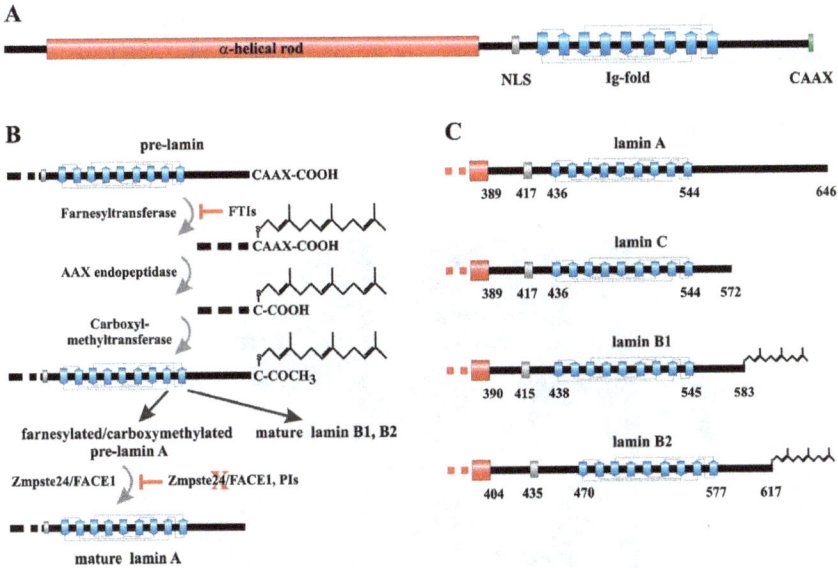

Figure 19. C-terminal farnesylation of lamin proteins. Lamins A and B are modified at the C-terminal by addition of a farnesyl hydrocarbon. This is associated with the proper positioning and interactions of the lamin Bs. In the case of lamin A, it must be cleaved off by the Zmpste24 protease to prevent inappropriate positioning with respect to the nuclear membrane. Lamin C lacks the farnesylation site. In HGPS, the novel splicing removes the Zmpste24 cleavage site resulting in Progerin: a slightly shorter protein that retains the farnesylated end. Therefore, Progerin is targeted to the nuclear membrane, where it accumulates and interferes with proper assembly of the nuclear lamina.

Source: Dechat *et al*. (2008).

the nuclear membrane. Both lamin A and lamin B are farnesylated, but the farnesylated tip of lamin A is then cleaved off to allow lamin A to come off the membrane and form complexes networking with lamin B. The mutation in HGPS results in a slightly smaller protein called **Progerin** that retains the farnesylated C-terminal. As a result, the lamina does not assemble properly, and lamin B is also depleted because it fails to assemble with lamin A. The nuclear envelope is weakened and the nucleus shows characteristic deformations of the nuclear envelope, which collapses or causes "blebbing" out of the nucleoplasm (Figure 20). Importantly, there are significant losses of heterochromatin marks, hetero-chromatin proteins, and heterochromatin itself.

It has been possible to produce induced pluripotent stem (iPS) cells, the equivalent of embryonic stem cells, from HGPS patients. These grow and proliferate normally (embryonic stem cells do not express lamin A/C) but, when induced to differentiate, they start producing lamin A/C and

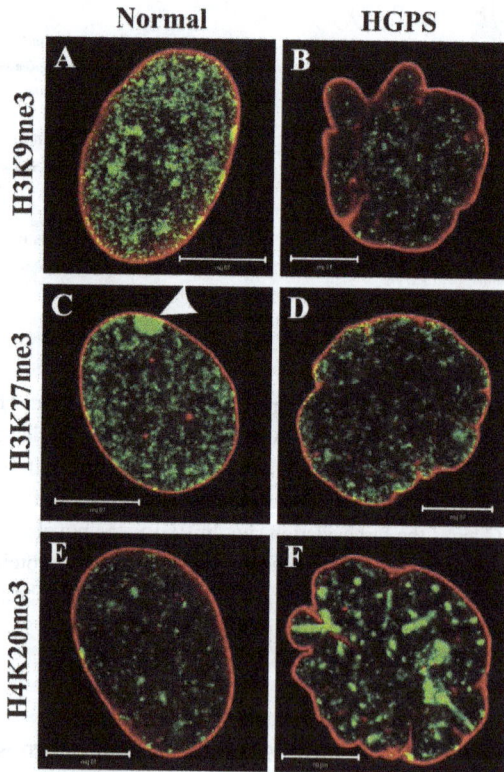

Figure 20.   Changes in morphology and histone modifications in HGPS nuclei. HGPS nuclei lose the rigid envelope of normal nuclei and show local weaknesses or "blebbing". Changes in histone marks are also prominent, in particular loss of H3K9me3 and H3K27me3 repressive marks. In C, D notes the loss of the H3K27me3-binding inactive X (arrowhead). H4K20me3, normally found in pericentric heterochromatin, increases with normal aging and in HGPS.

Source: Dechat *et al.* (2008).

HGPS iPS cell

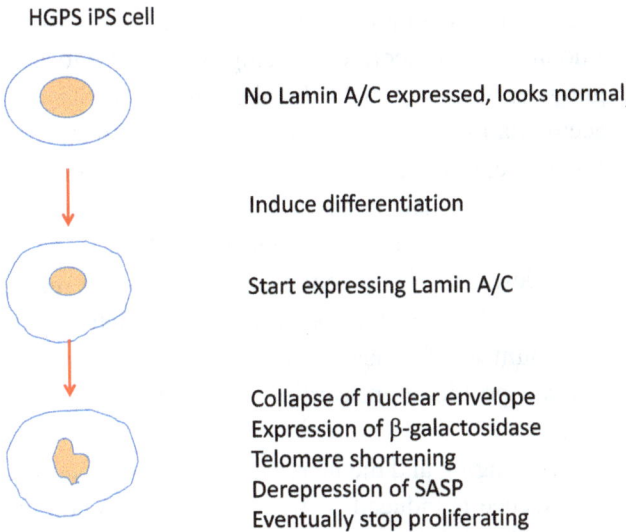

No Lamin A/C expressed, looks normal

Induce differentiation

Start expressing Lamin A/C

Collapse of nuclear envelope
Expression of β-galactosidase
Telomere shortening
Derepression of SASP
Eventually stop proliferating

Figure 21.   Induced pluripotent cells derived from HGPS patients. iPS cells can be produced from HGPS and look and function normally. No lamin A/C is expressed in normal
embryonic stem cells. When they are induced to differentiate, they start expressing lamin
A/C and acquire all the HGPS features.

Progerin. The results become rapidly apparent: the cells develop premature senescence marks, including reduced telomere length, changes in
nuclear shape, loss of heterochromatin, and changes in gene expression
associated with senescence (Figure 21). Knockdown of Progerin expression by targeted RNAi alleviates these effects. The converse is true when
a transgene expressing Progerin is introduced into normal differentiated
cells: typical senescence sets in, including reduced proliferation, decrease
of heterochromatin, nuclear morphological defects, and expression of
senescence markers.

Splicing Selectivity and Aging

What is the cause and what is the effect of these events? The fact that the
expression of a Progerin transgene produces the progeria phenotypes
strongly implies that it is causative. The interesting discovery that
some Progerin is made in normal cells showed that the cryptic splice site

that is activated by the mutation in HGPS is occasionally used in normal cells. The amount of this incorrect splicing was shown to increase with age. An oligonucleotide that blocks the aberrant splice site was shown to reduce the accumulation of Progerin and significantly restore normal cellular phenotypes in cultured cells from HGPS patients. This approach has not been tried in live animals to see if it might reduce organismal aging symptoms. However, increased heterogeneity in RNA splicing has been found to be a widespread phenomenon that affects many genes, not just the Lamin A/C gene. Increased intron retention associated with aging has been found in a number of genes and is associated with vascular pathology, blocks in cell proliferation, cardiac stress, and other similar aging-related defects.

These effects of aging and the increase in Progerin in normal cells are not seen if senescence is induced by treatments that do not affect telomeres, for example, by expression of oncogenes such as *ras.* These treatments arrest the cell cycle without involving telomere length or heterochromatin. Conversely, telomere shortening induced by interfering with telomerase function increased Progerin production, as well as changes in alternative splicing of numerous other genes. Independently of the frequency at which it occurs genome-wide, alternative splicing of specific genes may specifically promote aging. For example, alternative splicing of p53 increases with age, producing the truncated p44 variant that lacks the transactivation domain and is known to lead to increased senescence and aging phenotypes. Other factors tell similar stories.

The interesting question is therefore as follows: What links telomere length, the nuclear lamina, heterochromatin, and reduced stringency in RNA splicing? By its nature and evolution in vertebrates, alternative splicing is heterogeneous, its mechanisms are gene-specific and chromatin features may affect different genes differently, which has made it more difficult to discern systematic relationships. Increases in intron retention have been found associated with age in nematodes, flies, and humans. This, in principle, implies less splicing activity, which could result from faster transcription, less pausing, and less expression of splicing factors. Splicing is targeted by consensus sequences at 5′ and 3′ splice sites and depends also on the branch-point sequence in the intron (see Chapter 4). These are not fixed recognition sequences: they vary considerably from one splice site to another. There are better splice sites and less optimal splice sites. The order in which introns are spliced depends therefore on many factors and may vary in different tissues and under different conditions, leading to alternative splicing patterns (Figure 22). Splicing is produced by the spliceosome, a multisubunit complex containing proteins and small nuclear RNAs. Additional sequences in the primary RNA transcript may promote or suppress the use of specific splice sites. *Trans*-acting factors binding to chromatin may enhance or inhibit splicing. Importantly, transcription speed, chromatin structure, and histone marks can also affect splice site selection. Changes in spliceosomal components and in other splice factors occur with aging. The expression of some splicing regulators is correlated with longevity in mouse and humans. However, there is no consensus about which splicing factors correlate with age in different settings and no evidence about their causal link with aging. So, although there is general agreement that there are age-associated changes, there is no clarity about what changes are significant, which go up or down, whether they have general effects or are specific for certain genes or tissues. Therefore, functional studies are still needed to determine if they are causally linked to aging phenomena.

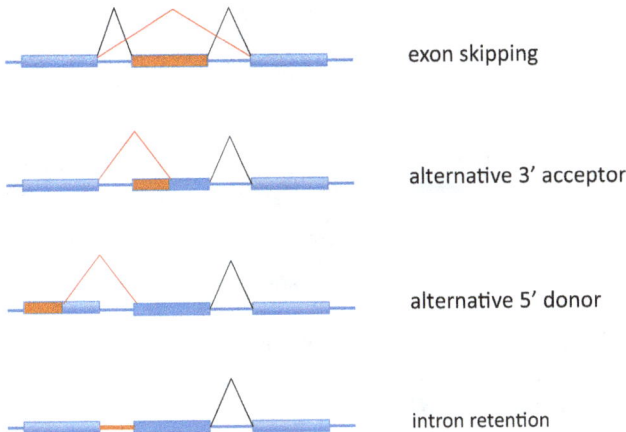

Figure 22. Alternative splicing. Splicing involves the recognition of splice donor and splice acceptor sites and their accessibility if the RNA transcript has time to assume a folded structure. Alternative splice donor or acceptor sequences, rate of transcription elongation, and availability of splice factors are among the factors that determine splicing choices.

Aging-associated changes in alternative splicing have generally focused on the spliceosome and splicing factors but it is becoming increasingly recognized that a key role is played by the speed of transcriptional elongation. This is not just due to allowing splice factors more time to carry out their work. Critical for the controls of splicing is the time allowed for the growing RNA to fold. The nascent RNA secondary and tertiary structures may mask splice sites through base pairing, expose them in unpaired loops, or bring in proximity to alternative 5′ and 3′ sites. This implies that the effects of the rate of transcription on splicing would vary from one gene to another, depending on the sequence and the possibilities of secondary structure formation (Figure 23). Higher transcription rates usually increase the skipping of splice sites and therefore the inclusion of alternative exons or even the retention of introns within the mRNA.

DNA damage caused by UV is known to substantially slow down transcription elongation. Increased frequency of DNA damage might

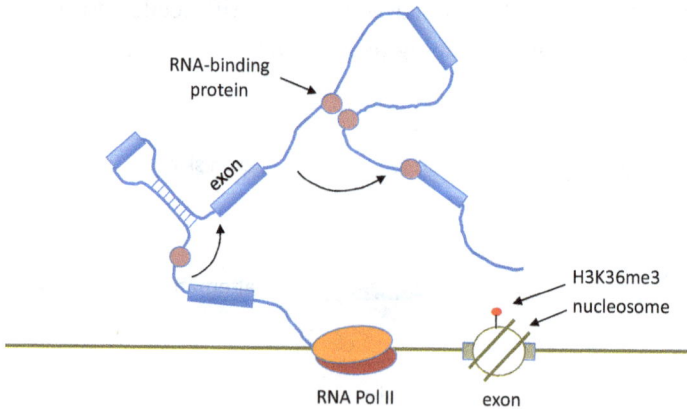

Figure 23.   Some factors affecting RNA splicing. Splicing occurs co-transcriptionally and the state of the chromatin has important effects on splicing patterns. The transcript elongation rate is affected by DNA methylation, sequence biases, and histone modifications. The elongating RNA polymerase recruits transcription factors. A slower rate of transcription gives the nascent RNA more time to fold and bind RNA-binding proteins and splicing factors. RNA-binding proteins may occlude sequences important for splicing in the exons or in the introns. Or they may form loops causing exon skipping. RNA secondary structure may prevent access to some splice sites and result in intron retention, may bring two exons close, and facilitate exon skipping.

therefore be responsible for some of the changes in splicing patterns observed with aging. In addition, a lower elongation rate could have catastrophic consequences for very long genes such as the longest known human gene, the dystrophin gene, which encodes a component of a complex that connects muscle fibers to the extracellular matrix. With a primary transcript length of 2.3 megabases, this gene would normally require more than 24 hours to transcribe. DNA damage could increase this to several days. This opens vast opportunities for RNA folding and splicing anomalies to take place but it would also greatly reduce the rate at which dystrophin could be made available to anchor muscle fibers.

DNA Methylation and HP1 in Splicing

DNA methylation can either promote or inhibit exon recognition and splicing of many genes, affecting alternative splicing sites, which have less optimal consensus sequences, but not constitutively spliced exons. Exons normally have higher levels of DNA methylation than introns. Constitutive exons have a higher level of DNA methylation than alternative exons. Exons also have higher nucleosome density, which means a higher density of H3K36me3, which promotes DNA methylation. The distribution and density of CpGs in a gene would also affect the DNA methylation levels. Here again, exons display a sharp increase in CpG density and in DNA methylation (Figure 24).

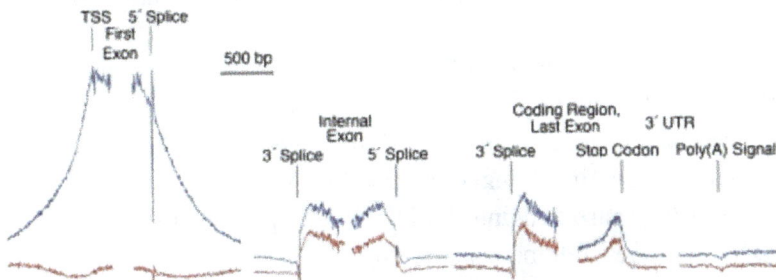

Figure 24.   CpG density and 5mCpG density across human genes. The density of CpGs (blue) and of 5mCpG (red) is plotted across the average gene, showing the sharp rise in CpGs in entrons and rapid drop at the 5′ intron boundary.

Source: Edwards *et al.* (2010).

DNA methylation slows down transcription elongation in a way dependent on CTCF binding, Me2CP recruitment, and HP1 recruitment. Sequence-specific binding of the CTCF insulator protein (see Chapter 8) slows down RNA polymerase hence promoting splicing. The CTCF binding consensus contains CpGs whose methylation prevents CTCF binding. So, by preventing CTCF binding, DNA methylation speeds up polymerase and decreases splicing. DNA methylation recruits the 5mC-binding protein MeCP2 (see Chapter 3). MeCP2 is a highly abundant chromatin protein and an important mediator of the repressive effects of DNA methylation. One of the activities of MeCP2 is the recruitment of histone deacetylases. Loss of histone acetylation makes transcription elongation more difficult and therefore slower. Finally, DNA methylation recruits dimers of heterochromatin protein HP1. Though prototypically found in heterochromatin, HP1 or its paralogs are also found in euchromatin and specifically in transcribed genes (see Chapter 5 and 6). That HP1 is important in splicing is clear but its role is somewhat ambiguous. Depletion of HP1γ in cultured cells causes genome-wide aberrant splicing. HP1β has been shown to recruit splicing factors, which suggests that it promotes splicing. HP1 paralogs apparently enhance exon recognition when bound immediately upstream of the exon but lower exon recognition when bound to the exon itself. These different effects apply specifically to alternatively used splice sites rather than normally used splice sites. This is because normal splice sites have strong sequence determinants while alternative splicing sites have more ambiguous sequences and are therefore more affected by other factors such as rate of elongation or HP1 presence.

Overall, then, the effect of DNA methylation on individual splice sites could be positive or negative but changes in DNA methylation can certainly produce changes in individual sites and therefore in exon usage, particularly exons involving weaker splice sites. Can we then say that progerin is the cause of aging? Or alternative splicing? Or loss of lamins? Or DNA damage? Telomere shortening? The preceding discussion shows that aging can have multiple primary causes and many contributing factors, often linked in complex ways. In addition, there are the many and complex arguments based on metabolism, on protein homeostasis, on mitochondrial dysfunction, and on nutrition, each argued vociferously by a committed core of proponents. At present, I do not see that any single answer provides a unitary account of organismal aging. On the contrary, it might be argued that there are many possible pathways and that each of the many mechanisms that have been proposed might play a role, sometimes greater, sometimes smaller. The multiple links among the different pathways also argue that you cannot proceed far along one pathway without involving one or more of the others.

Further Reading

Bhadra M, Howell P, Dutta S, Heintz C and Mair WB (2020). Alternative splicing in aging and longevity. *Hum Genet.* **139**, 357–369.

Booth LN and Brunet A (2016). The aging epigenome. *Mol Cell.* **62**, 728–744.

Chandra T, Ewels PA, Schoenfelder S, Furlan-Magaril M, Wingett SW, Kirschner K *et al.* (2015). Global reorganization of the nuclear landscape in senescent cells. *Cell Rep.* **10**, 471–483.

Dechat, T, Pfleghaar K, Sengupti K, Shimi T, Shumaker DK, Solimando LR *et al.* (2008). Mutant nuclear lamin A leads to progressive alterations of epigenetic control in premature aging. *Genes Dev.* **22**, 832–853.

Deschênes M and Chabot B (2017). The emerging role of alternative splicing in senescence and aging. *Aging Cell.* **16**, 918–933.

Edwards JR, O'Donnell AH, Rollins RA, Pecham HE, Lee C, Milekic MH *et al.* (2010). Chromatin and sequence features that define the fine and gross structure of genomic methylation patterns. *Genome Res.* **20**, 972–980.

Ezhkova E, Pasolli HA, Parker JS, Stokes N, Su IH, Hannon G *et al.* (2009). Ezh2 orchestrates gene expression for the stepwise differentiation of tissue-specific stem cells. *Cell.* **136**, 1122–1135.

Feser J and Tyler J (2011). Chromatin structure as a mediator of aging. *FEBS Lett.* **585**, 2041–2048.

Gerhart H and Clevers H (2015). Repairing organs: Lessons from intestine and liver. *Trends Genet.* **31**, 344–351.

Gorbunova V, Seluanov A, Mita P, McKerrow W, Fenyö D, Boeke J *et al.* (2021). The role of retrotransposable elements in ageing and age-associated diseases. *Nature.* **596**, 43–53.

Hayflick L (1965). The limited in vitro lifetime of human diploid cell strains. *Exp Cell Res.* **37**, 614–636.

Hug N and Lingner J (2007). Telomere length homeostasis. *Chromosoma.* **115**, 413–425.

Ito T, Teo YV, Evans SA, Neretti N and Sedivy JM (2018). Regulation of cellular senescence by polycomb chromatin modifiers through distinct DNA damage- and histone methylation-dependent pathways. *Cell Rep.* **22**, 3480–3492.

Lev Maor G, Yearim A and Ast G (2015). The alternative role of DNA methylation in splicing regulation. *Trends Genet.* **31**, 274–280.

López-Otin C, Galluzzi L, Freije JM, Madeo F and Kroemer G (2013). The hallmarks of aging. *Cell.* **153**, 1194–1217.

Melzer D, Piling LC and Ferrucci L (2020). The genetics of human ageing. *Nat Rev Genet.* **21**, 88–101.

Meneses AMC, Schneeberger K, Kruitwagen HS, Penning, LC, van Steenbeek FG, Burgener IA *et al.* (2016). Intestinal organoids — current and future applications. *Vet Sci.* **3**, 31.

Rando TA and Chang HY (2012). Aging, rejuvenation, and epigenetic reprogramming: Resetting the aging clock. *Cell.* **148**, 46–57.

Schultz MB and Sinclair DA (2016). When stem cells grow old: Phenotypes and mechanisms of stem cell aging. *Development.* **143**, 3–14.

Shah PP, Donahue G, Otte GL, Capell BC, Nelson DM, Cao K *et al.* (2013). Lamin B1 depletion in senescent cells triggers large-scale changes in gene expression and the chromatin landscape. *Genes Dev.* **27**, 1787–1799.

Shumaker DK, Dechat T, Kohlmaier A, Adam SA, Bozovsky MR, Erdos MR *et al.* (2006). Mutant nuclear lamin A leads to progressive alterations of epigenetic control in premature aging. *Proc Natl Acad Sci USA.* **103**, 8703–8708.

Tomasetti C and Vogelstein B (2015). Variation in cancer risk among tissues can be explained by the number of stem cell divisions. *Science.* **347**, 78–81.

Tomasetti C, Li L and Vogelstein B (2017). Stem cell divisions, somatic mutations, cancer etiology, and cancer prevention. *Science.* **355**, 1330.

Vlaming H and van Leeuwen F (2012). Crosstalk between aging and the epigenome. *Epigenomics.* **4**, 5–7.

Zhang W, Li J, Suzuki K, Ou J, Wang P, Zhou J *et al.* (2015). A Werner syndrome stem cell model unveils heterochromatin alterations as a driver of human aging. *Science.* **348**, 1160–1163.

Chapter 13

Methods

ATAC: Assay for Transposase-Accessible Chromatin

This method uses a hyperactive variant of the transposase enzyme from the bacterial Tn5 transposon. Tn5 is a compound transposon, consisting of a core containing antibiotic resistance genes flanked by two Insertion Sequence 50 (IS50) elements in inverted orientation (Figure 1). IS sequences are themselves elements that can transpose independently and consist of a coding sequence for a transposase and a regulatory protein framed within 19 bp related but non-identical sequences (Outer End and Inner End) that are recognized by the transposase. When Tn5 is mobilized from an insertion site, one transposase binds to each of the Outer End sequences and the two transposases then bind to each other with the body of the Tn5 transposon looping out (Figure 2). Each transposase cuts the flanking DNA of the opposite end, liberating the Tn5 with its two ends still bound to the transposase dimer. This complex then attacks a DNA target site, inserting the Tn5 between the transposase dimer into the target DNA. In fact, only the transposase and the Outer End 19 bp are necessary for the enzymatic activity of the transposase. So, if instead of the transposon flanked by the 19 bp OE sequence, just the OE sequence is used, bound to transposase, the result is fragmentation of target DNA with the OE sequence to the 5′ end of the DNA fragments. In addition, a hyperactive variant of the transposase has been produced by introducing some amino acid changes. This makes a powerful, highly efficient, and flexible

447

Tn5

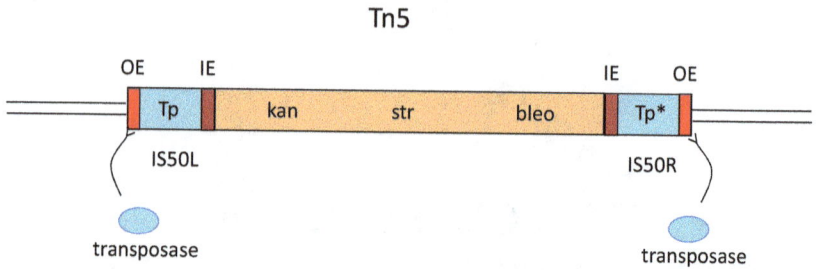

Figure 1.   The Tn5 Transposon. Tn5 is a compound transposon in which an insertion sequence IS50 in inverted orientation at each end flanks three antibiotic resistance genes. The IS50 sequence encodes the transposase Tp but a mutation in IS50R makes inactive transposase Tp*. The IS50 element is flanked by 19 bp Outside and Inside Ends (OE and IE) that bind to the transposase.

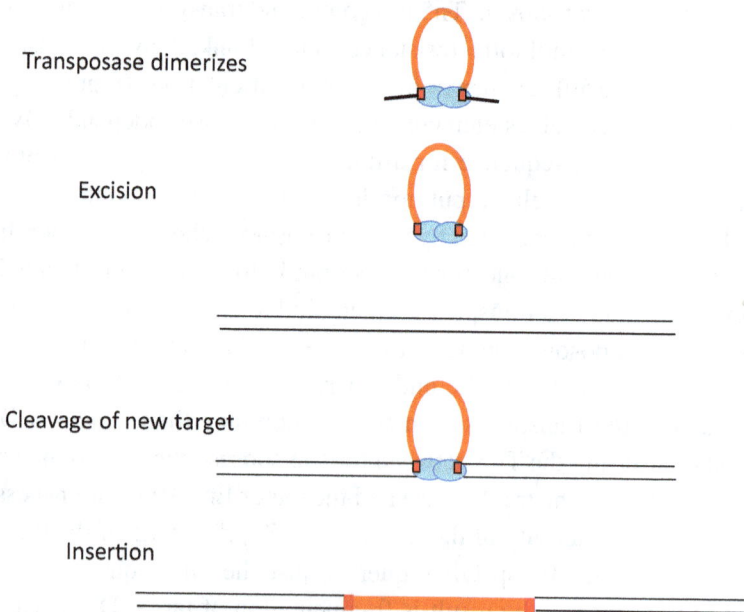

Figure 2.   Tn5 transposon insertion. A transposase binds to each OE and the two transposases dimerize. This activates their nucleolytic activity, which excises the transposon from its insertion site. The complex now looks for a new target site into which to insert. It does so by activating cleavage and rejoining of the appropriate strands, resulting in insertion of the transposon sequence.

tool for genomic manipulations and, through different strategies, it has been utilized for a variety of operations.

In the basic application, called Tagmentation, the purified transposase is bound to a 19 bp double-stranded fragment representing the Outer End. Just as tinkering with the transposase has produced the hyperactive variant, modification of the OE sequence has produced a more efficient version, called Mosaic End or ME. The transposase with bound fragment dimerizes and is ready to attack DNA. The transposase dimer cleaves the DNA at each site to which it binds, attaching the 3′ end of each ME to a 5′ end of the target site at sites staggered by 9 bp. This produces a DNA fragment with an ME attached at each 5′ end and a 9 nucleotide gap on the opposite strand (Figure 3). By suitably designing the sequences that can be attached to the obligatory ME, the transposase method can be

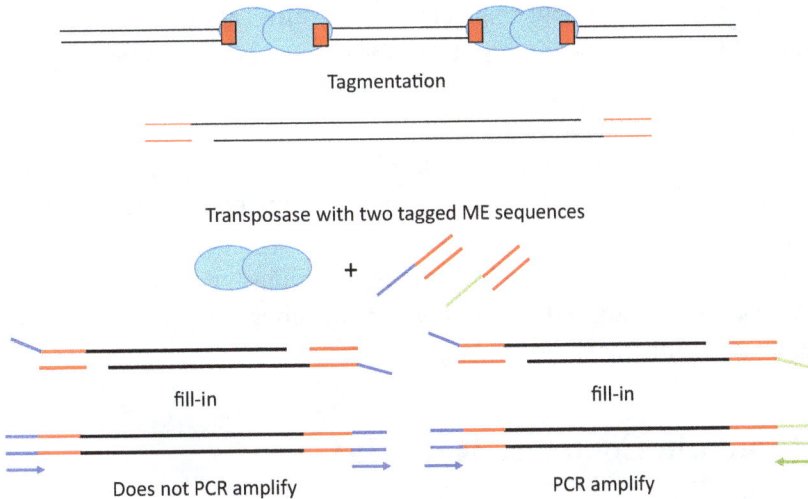

Figure 3. Application of ATAC. Transposase only requires the 19 bp OE sequence for function. A modified OE sequence called Mosaic End, ME, is much more effective than the wild-type OE. Transposase bound to double-stranded ME produces a staggered cut in target DNA and attaches the 3′ ME to the 5′ of the DNA fragment (tagmentation). The ME sequences can be tagged with any desired additional sequence, commonly including adapters used for Next Generation Sequencing (blue and green tags). Transposase incubated with a mixture of the two tagged MEs can bind two of the same or one of each. Only fragments with two different tags will PCR amplify.

exploited for a variety of purposes. Perhaps the most widely used is simply to cleave chromatin at sites accessible to the transposase, producing a collection of fragments whose ends represent accessible sites such as nucleosome-free regions, displaced nucleosome sites, and DNA hypersensitive sites. The extreme efficiency of the transposase method permits the analysis of even very small quantities of chromatin, even single cells.

In the example procedure shown in Figure 3, the transposase is incubated with a mixture of double-stranded ME sequence tagged at the 5' end with either of the two primer sequences. The transposase dimer will bind either one of each or two of the same to make an active transposome. The transposomes will attack accessible sites on chromatin and produce fragments with the tagged ME sequence at each end. These fragments will then be filled in by a brief elongation to produce fully double-stranded fragments. Now the fragments can be PCR-amplified with forward and reverse primers. Fragments that had the same sequence tag at the two ends will not PCR-amplify but fragments with a different tag at each end will amplify the product and are suitable for sequencing. Additional tags can be introduced, including T7 promoters for PCR-free amplification, "barcoding" tags, and fluorescent tags.

ATAC fragmentation is often used as a sequencing approach and is then called ATAC-seq. The Tn5 transposase preferentially targets accessible chromatin sites and therefore is the method of choice to identify and sequence genome-wide nucleosome-free regions, nucleosome-depleted regions, regions targeted by chromatin remodeling activities, or sites rendered accessible by DNA-binding factors.

Chromatin Contacts: 3C to Hi-C

In a 2002 paper that was to open a vast field of studies on genome architecture, Job Dekker *et al.* introduced the technique of Chromatin Conformation Capture (3C) to determine whether and how frequently one part of the genome contacts any other part. They expected that the local folding as well as the higher-order organizational features of genomic chromatin was likely to have important roles in gene expression, DNA replication, DNA repair, and other activities of the genome in the nucleus. To determine the local folding as well as the higher-order architecture, Dekker *et al.* wanted a high throughput approach that could be applied to the entire genome. The concept was that chemical crosslinking with formaldehyde, such as was used for Chromatin Immunoprecipitation (ChIP), would very rapidly freeze the configuration by crosslinking chromatin at the sites of contact at the moment of treatment. To identify the sites of contact, the genomic DNA was cut with a restriction enzyme, producing a collection of fragments some of which were crosslinked with other fragments (see Chapter 8, Figure 19). The DNA was then diluted and ligated to favor ligation of ends within a crosslinked fragment and prevent ligation between unlinked ends. Crosslinks were then reversed, yielding linear fragments in which the end of one fragment was fused to the end of another fragment with which it had been in contact. At this point, with the DNA sequencing techniques available, the only option to identify the contacts was to ask for each fragment pair whether a PCR product could be obtained by suitable primers directed outwards from each fragment end. Different fragments might have different ligation frequencies and different PCR amplification efficiencies. To estimate the frequency of contacts, a control ligation was done *in vitro* with all the restriction fragments of interest and PCR reaction was carried out to evaluate the amount of each resulting product. The contact frequency for each pair of genomic fragments was then evaluated as the ratio of the product obtained from the crosslinked genomic fragments to the product obtained from the control template.

As predicted from a chromatin model that combines the freely jointed chain and the elastic rod description, Dekker *et al.* showed that contacts are high within a local region largely dependent on the persistence length of the chromatin fiber. This will vary depending on the G+C content of the sequence, with GC-rich regions more flexible than AT-rich regions. The highest crosslinking frequency for the yeast chromosome 3 occurred at a genomic separation of about 9 kb. In addition, the results showed that the chromosome tended to fold so that the two telomeres were held close to one another. The polymer approximation and the parameters evaluated by curve-fitting allowed the estimation of the physical distance between two genomic sequences.

The 3C approach was particularly fruitful when applied to local interactions, such as those between enhancers and promoters, and the effects of features such as chromatin insulators, or the binding of chromatin proteins. In such cases, the relative rather than the absolute crosslinking frequency was the relevant result.

A problem arose, however, if more general more extensive regions were to be analyzed. By the PCR method, if all the relevant genome sequences were known, each possible contact had to be interrogated individually. The technique was therefore in principle high-throughput but in practice limited to one contact at a time. More general approaches were quickly devised and the application of massively parallel sequencing (or Next Generation Sequencing) made it possible to generalize the technique.

The 5C Technique

One of the first variations was the Chromatin Conformation Capture Carbon Copy or 5C method. This method starts with the 3C procedure to obtain a collection of the ligated, de-crosslinked fragments. This collection is then hybridized to primers designed for each restriction enzyme fragment end in the region of interest, directed outwards. Forward primers hybridize to the 5′ end of a restriction fragment, including half of the restriction site; the primer 5′ end includes the sequence of a T7 promoter. Reverse primers hybridize to the opposite strand of a restriction fragment, thus their 5′ end includes half of the restriction site and is provided with a 5′ phosphate. Their 3′ end includes the sequence of a T3 promoter. When annealed to two ligated restriction fragments, the two primers will be adjacent and can be ligated together. The products are then amplified using T7 and T3 polymerases to produce an amplified library representing all the ligation products of fragments for which primers are provided. These can be sequenced by Next-Generation sequencing to yield the sequences of the ligation products in proportion to the original crosslinking frequency. The 5C approach is a significant improvement that does not require a separate reaction for each possible contact. However, it is still limited by the number of primers that can be used in a single reaction and requires the synthesis of a primer for each possible contact.

The 4C Techniques

Some of these limitations are addressed by a type of variation collectively referred to as 4C techniques. These approaches still start from the viewpoint of a single site but now can ask about this site's interactions with the entire rest of the genome. The idea is based on the circularization of the ligation fragments produced as in the standard 3C method and then the use of outgoing primers from the two ends of the fragment of interest to amplify the entire ligated sequence. To do this, the de-crosslinked ligated products have to be trimmed with a frequent cutting restriction enzyme or similar method to make the ligated sequence short enough to be efficiently PCR amplified. The resulting amplified products, representing all ligated sequences from all genomic contacts with the site of interest, are then sequenced by Next-Generation Sequencing methods.

The Hi-C Technique

This approach is the most general. The concept is the same as in 3C: The chromatin is crosslinked to freeze all contacts, then cut with a restriction enzyme, and the DNA ends associated with each fragment are ligated under dilute conditions. The Hi-C approach wants to select and sequence all the possible contacts that any genomic sequence enters into. To do this, all DNA fragments that have become ligated need to be tagged and recovered for sequencing. This is done by using a restriction enzyme that leaves a 5′ overhang and filling in the fragment ends before ligation with a suitable biotin-tagged nucleotide (depending on the restriction enzyme used to cut the genomic DNA). After biotin tagging, the blunt ends are ligated as in 3C. The total DNA is then broken into small fragments, usually by shearing, and the biotin-labeled fragments are recovered with streptavidin linked to beads. Now, all the recovered fragments can be sequenced by Next-Generation Sequencing. Computer power identifies and keeps track of all genomic sequences linked to other genomic sequences. These are usually displayed in a heat map matrix of any desired genomic region against its own sequence, where the number of times a given local sequence is found ligated to any other sequence in that genomic region is proportional to the intensity of the spot in the matrix (see, for example, Figures 20, 21, 27 *et cet.* in Chapter 8).

Subsequent improvements were aimed at increasing the efficiency of the process and the resolution of the mapping. These included a higher ligation efficiency and recovery of the fragments as well as reducing the intervening steps by performing the restriction enzyme cleavage, labeling, and ligation *in situ* on permeabilized nuclei. This also reduces the frequency of random contacts due to ligation in solution. Increasing the efficiency and the number of contacts sequenced to 4.9 billion permitted mapping the human genome in tissue culture cells with a resolution of 950 bp.

Chromatin Immunoprecipitation, ChIP

This technique and its various modifications have become a fundamental tool to map binding sites for chromatin proteins or protein modifications throughout the genome. The concept is straightforward: chopping up genomic DNA and using antibodies to select those fragments bearing the desired protein. To stabilize the binding of the protein so that it will resist the immunoprecipitation process, the proteins are crosslinked to DNA.

When first developed by John Lis and David Gilmour in 1984, UV radiation was used as a crosslinking reagent. In 1988, Alexander Varshavsky introduced formaldehyde as a quicker, more convenient, reversible crosslinking agent. The technique was made popular in 1993 by Valerio Orlando and Renato Paro to analyze the distribution of Polycomb proteins in the *Drosophila* bithorax complex. It was followed by many years of improvement and refinement but it came into its own with the availability of whole genome sequences that accompanied the achievement of the human genome sequencing project in the early 2000s. The key to the exceptional value of chromatin immunoprecipitation or ChIP lies in the analysis of the immunoprecipitated chromatin fragments. The earliest applications of the genome sequences was the construction of microarrays containing millions of oligonucleotides representing the entire genome. Carefully designed oligonucleotides that avoided repetitive motifs could be chosen to form an overlapping tiled array of microdots at high density. These arrays could then be hybridized with the immunoprecipitated chromatin fragments, usually after amplification and labeling with a fluorescent probe. The result was read by a scanner and interpreted by a computer program. The resulting technique was known as "ChIP-on-chip". Immensely useful as the ChIP-on-chip results were, they were still limited by hybridization efficiencies of different sequences, the choice of oligo-nucleotides, and most of all by the limited signal range of the fluorescence detected.

The ChIP technique came into its own with the advent of efficient and affordable Next-Generation Sequencing machines. Direct sequencing of the immunoprecipitated fragments gave much sharper resolution, limited only by the size of the genomic fragments. It also gave a direct readout of the enrichment of a particular sequence in the total immunoprecipitated genome fragments and could be directly analyzed by statistical methods. Next-Generation Sequencing was particularly suited for ChIP-seq because only relatively short reads of the order of 100 nucleotides are required to identify unique fragments. Paired-end sequencing can also be used to reduce costs by sequencing short segments from each end of a fragment.

The basic ChIP procedure starts with crosslinking chromatin. This can be done by adding formaldehyde directly to the tissue culture medium, usually to 1% for a few minutes at room temperature. Crosslinked chromatin is next fragmented, usually by sonication to an average fragment size of 200–400 bp. Problems with fragment size arise due to the different susceptibility of different genomic regions to sonic disruption. Heterochromatin and highly condensed chromatin are more resistant. Certain regions are particularly sensitive. In particular, though not commonly appreciated, binding sites of Polycomb complexes are unusually sensitive to sonication, achieving a fragment size of 200–300 bp when most of the genome is still in fragments longer than 1kb.

Chromatin fragments that include the desired protein are then immuno-precipitated with a suitable antibody. The quality and specificity of the antibody are key to the success of ChIP. Many commercially available antibodies are not sufficiently specific or free of contaminating cross-reacting activities. Sufficient affinity is also important for adequate immunoprecipitation, particularly when small numbers of cells are used. The antibodies are often pre-attached to beads coated with protein A. It should be noted that the immunoprecipitation buffer usually contains 0.1% SDS and 0.1% deoxycholate and is thus mildly denaturing or unfolding for many proteins. This is an advantage since many antibodies are raised against protein fragments or denatured proteins. It is a disadvantage in that it requires antibodies that are resistant to these conditions. After collecting the immunoprecipitated fragments, the crosslinking is reversed and proteins are removed by phenol extraction. For analysis or sequencing, the DNA fragments are usually amplified by a whole-genome PCR amplifying method.

An alternative procedure is native ChIP, in which crosslinking is avoided and the chromatin is fragmented using micrococcal nuclease. This tends to cleave between nucleosomes and in nucleosome-free regions. It is therefore particularly suited for mapping histone modifications. Many DNA-binding proteins bind in nucleosome-free regions, so care must be applied to avoid losing these. Often, however, DNA-binding proteins or protein complexes protect a subnucleosomal DNA fragment, in which case the binding sites can be recovered and mapped with high precision. A particular variety of native ChIP is that developed by Skene and Henikoff (2017), which they called Cleavage Under Targets and Release Using Nuclease (CUT&RUN). This procedure can be carried out *in situ*, using micrococcal nuclease to release DNA fragments bound to proteins. Using carefully controlled conditions, the nuclease digestion cleaves on either side of a bound complex, releasing subnucleosomal fragments. Fragments of 120 bp or smaller are taken to represent the binding sites. The actual binding site can be localized more precisely by mapping the fragments on the genomic sequence. At any given genomic site, the sequence common to all the fragments from that site can narrow down the binding to less than 20 nucleotides.

Cryo-Electron Microscopy of Single Particles

Structure determination of biological macromolecules has been acknowledged to be of enormous value, not just for the intrinsic understanding of structural principles but for the insight and practical applications that result from the knowledge of the physical structures of proteins and nucleic acids. The techniques utilized to solve the structures to high resolution have been traditionally two: crystallography, usually using X-ray diffraction, and nuclear magnetic resonance (NMR). Both approaches have enjoyed considerable success and have produced a large number of protein structures and have revealed structural principles that in the past year have allowed accurate prediction of protein structure from amino acid sequence using artificial intelligence computations. Both approaches have serious limitations. Crystallography requires the production of crystals and has therefore been limited to molecules that are readily purified and crystallized. NMR works with proteins in solution and requires soluble proteins. Both are limited to small proteins beyond which the computations become too difficult to handle. Both cannot readily handle the large multiprotein complexes that are almost the general rule in chromatin research. In principle, electron microscopy offers an alternative approach that bypasses these difficulties.

A beam of electrons is diffracted by a specimen and can be focused by electromagnetic lenses to form an image much as light is focused by glass lenses. The effective wavelength of the electron beam used in microscopy is orders of magnitude smaller than that of visible light and permits therefore a vastly higher resolution. However, electron bombardment is highly destructive for organic materials. Electron microscopy has dealt with this problem in the past by staining the organic specimen with heavy metal salts, which coat the material, producing an outline of the specimen. This gives high contrast but limits the resolution and dehydrates and distorts the structures. Reducing the temperature of the specimen to that of liquid nitrogen or liquid helium and using very low beam intensities are alternatives to reduce the beam damage. In the high vacuum required for electron microscopy, hydrated samples can only be studied at very low temperatures. Cryo-electron microscopy combines these features. In cryo-EM, samples are flash-frozen to vitrify the material and prevent distorting formation of ice crystals. These techniques were worked out in the 1980s but extensive applications of cryo-EM hit their stride only in the 2010s, as new electron detectors, powerful image processing algorithms, and 3D reconstructions have become available. Useful introductory overviews of the cryo-EM revolution can be found in Nogales and Scherer (2015) and in Milne *et al.* (2013).

Cryo-EM can be used in many varieties of biological research to study cells, bacteria, viruses, and other biological materials but its blooming influence in recent years has been its application to the structures of large macromolecules and molecular complexes. Its major relevance to chromatin study and epigenetics is through the imaging of the large protein and nucleic acid complexes that are active in the nucleus. Only small quantities of the target macromolecule are needed, sometimes even in mixtures or unpurified extracts. Proteins difficult to crystallize or membrane proteins are equally well handled. In contrast to crystallography or NMR, cryo-EM relies on single-particle imaging. Transmission electron microscopy gives an image of the projection of the particle observed on the plane perpendicular to the electron beam. Electron-dense parts of the target scatter the electron beam producing changes that are imaged by the electron detector placed on the other side of the target. To reduce the electron beam damage, very low beam intensities are generally used, which results in low image to noise ratios. This is compensated by averaging the images of many particles in the same orientation. The 3D structure is then reconstructed from the averaged projections in different orientations.

This requires the search for the images of thousands or even millions of individual particles and extensive computations to determine the orientation of each. Both are now carried out by sophisticated algorithms. The classification of single-particle images is facilitated by a variety of approaches to tilt the target relative to the electron beam and recover several images from the same particle at different angles. This is complicated by the fact that large proteins and particularly macromolecular complexes have inherent flexibilities and alternative conformations that exist in equilibrium. The use of partial structures or proteins genetically tagged with well-characterized substructures has provided alternative information to resolve configurations. For example, tagging a protein by fusion with a fluorescent protein helps not only to orient single images but also to relate them to images from optical microscopy. Despite the difficulties, resolutions reached have continuously improved, sometimes reaching atomic visualization. The structures of large complexes can also profit from the crystallographical structures of component proteins that can be docked onto the larger structure obtained from cryo-EM.

Some of the striking successes of the cryo-EM approach in recent years are the structures of the PRC2 complex in different states and with alternative components. The large assemblies of the human transcription pre-initiation complex (PIC) containing RNA Pol II, general transcription factors, and Mediator as well as promoter DNA have been recently published at 2.9 Å resolution (see, for example, Schilbach *et al.*, 2021).

The fact that cryo-EM does not require crystallization but permits the assembly of structures in near-physiological conditions allows the study of functional states and mechanistic intermediates. The high-resolution structures produced allow the study of molecular interactions, conformational changes, and reaction intermediates and lend themselves to studies of drug discovery. Cryo-EM has its shortcomings and difficulties, not least among which are the high costs of acquisition and maintenance of the EM equipment and of the sophisticated high-power computer infrastructure involved. Continuing improvements in the hardware and software have made it easier to expand the applicability of cryo-EM to increasingly higher resolution and smaller particles or molecules.

DamID

Like chromatin immunoprecipitation (ChIP), DamID is a method devised to identify the genomic sequences associated with a particular protein of interest. Unlike ChIP, DamID requires no antibody to the protein of interest and does not involve precipitation. Also unlike ChIP, DamID measures cumulative contacts of the protein with DNA over time rather than the association of the protein at the time of immunoprecipitation. Originally devised by Bas van Steensel and Steve Henikoff (2000), it requires instead the genetic fusion of the protein of interest with a bacterial adenine methyltransferase, which will then tag with methylation the DNA that finds itself in the vicinity of the protein binding site. The transgenic fusion protein is generally a chromatin component whose genomic localization is to be investigated. The adenine methyltransferase was chosen because the N6-methylation it produces is infrequently found in metazoan DNA. Its target is the A in the GATC sequence. The fusion protein will therefore methylate a GATC in the vicinity of the protein's binding site. Such a sequence occurs on the average every 256 bp but, occasionally, the nearest GATC may be more distant. In addition, the range of Dam methylation from any binding site extends up to 5 kb. This, together with the variability in the distance of GATCs, limits the precision with which the protein binding site is localized.

To identify the sites methylated by the fusion protein, two cognate restriction enzymes are used: DpnI and DpnII. DpnI cuts DNA at GATC sites only if the A is methylated, while DpnII cuts GATC only if it is not methylated. Genomic DNA is cut first with the DpnI, producing 5′ ATC ends. These are ligated to adapters that will be used for PCR. The product is then digested with DpnII to cut all fragments that were not flanked by methylated GATCs. PCR amplification is then carried out with primers complementary to the adapters. The amplified product, which contains only fragments that had both ends methylated, is then sequenced. To minimize background methylation and to avoid physiological artifacts due to higher than normal levels of the protein of interest and the toxic effects of high Dam methylation, the Dam fusion protein is usually expressed at low levels. In addition, the background level of methylation is determined by expressing the Dam methylase alone. The DamID results are then expressed as the ratio of methylation by the Dam fusion protein to the Dam methylase alone.

The method requires the introduction of a transgene expressing the protein of interest fused to the Dam methylase. This is a disadvantage in many cases but it can also be turned into a powerful advantage if the transgene is placed under control of a regulated promoter. For example, a heat shock promoter permits the turning on and off of the transgene. Even more valuable is a promoter that is regulated by tissue- or cell-specific factors to produce Targeted DamID, sometimes known as TaDa. This allows the use of the whole animal or unpurified tissues to carry out DamID because the transgene is only expressed in a specific tissue or cell.

Improvements and variations in the approach include the use of mutant Dam methylases with higher activity and specificity; the use of other methylases, including enzymes that are not sequence-specific, combined with immunoprecipitation with antibodies against N6A methylation; targeting of the methylase by CRISPR-Cas9 methodologies.

The Polymerase Chain Reaction (PCR)

The polymerase chain reaction (PCR) is probably the single most valuable and powerful tool in molecular genetics. The technique was foreshadowed by techniques developed in the laboratory of H. Gobind Khorana in the 1970s and then independently developed by Kary Mullis in 1983. PCR exploits the ability of DNA polymerases to elongate a complementary oligonucleotide primer annealed or hybridized to a longer single-stranded DNA molecule to synthesize a complementary copy of that DNA molecule. This first reaction cycle is followed by heating to "melt" the double-stranded DNA product and then by a second cycle in which a second primer complementary to the end of the just-completed DNA strand primes a second round of synthesis in the opposite direction, producing the complementary sequence, which is in effect a copy of the first single-stranded DNA molecule. As a result, these two cycles have doubled the original DNA molecule. The process can be repeated *ad libitum*, given a supply of the two oligonucleotide primers and of the polymerase enzyme, doubling the number of DNA molecules each time and thus exponentially increasing the number of DNA copies. The procedure relies on the processivity of the DNA polymerase, which enables it to elongate the primer to the end of the template DNA strand and on a method to separate the double strands at the end of each cycle to enable a new round of priming and elongation. This is achieved by raising the temperature above the melting temperature of the double-stranded DNA molecule, then cooling to allow annealing of the primers and a new round of synthesis. The process is made possible by the use of DNA polymerases derived from bacteria able to grow at high temperatures and therefore resistant to temperatures above the melting temperatures of double-stranded DNA. Typically, such a DNA polymerase can be isolated from thermophilic bacteria such as *Thermus aquaticus*, derived from hot springs and able to grow in water near the boiling point. Such polymerases survive multiple cycles of heating above the melting temperature and followed by cooling to allow primer annealing and DNA synthesis. The whole process is carried out in a thermocycler programmed to cycle between a synthetic stage of a few minutes, heating to a melting stage, cooling to an annealing stage, followed by a new synthetic stage. The cycles are repeated a pre-set number of times, using temperature settings optimized for each given DNA sequence.

The practical use of the PCR technique was made possible not only by the development of temperature-resistant DNA polymerases and programmable thermocyclers but also by the increasingly rapid and inexpensive synthesis of oligonucleotides. Programmable, automated oligonucleotide synthesizers dependent on chemistries originally established in Khorana's laboratory have been essential for the adoption of PCR as the pre-eminent tool in genome studies of all types. The efficient amplification made possible by PCR means that it is in principle possible to detect a single DNA molecule in a highly complex mixture of genomic DNAs. The detection can be applied to RNA if preceded by reverse transcription with a reverse transcriptase. This class of enzymes use self-priming of RNA molecules or oligonucleotide-dependent priming to produce a complementary DNA strand on an RNA template. As a result, a desired DNA or RNA sequence can be singled out and selectively amplified from a complex mixture of DNA or RNA molecules.

Quantitative Real-Time PCR

Quantitative real-time PCR or qPCR is a technique to determine the amount of a particular sequence present in a mixture of DNA or RNA molecules using the Polymerase Chain Reaction (PCR) in a thermocycler machine equipped to monitor continuously the amount of product present in the reaction.

The basic PCR reaction requires suitable oligonucleotide primers directed in converging directions, a thermostable DNA polymerase and a thermocycler machine that can be programmed to cycle through a high-temperature stage to melt the double-stranded DNA, an annealing cycle to allow hybridization of the single strands with excess primers, and a synthesis stage in which the thermostable DNA polymerase extends the primers sufficiently to replicate the region of the convergent primer, usually selected to be no more than two or three hundred nucleotides apart (Figure 4). The cycle is repeated 20–40 times. For qPCR, the reaction takes place in the presence of a suitable fluorophore dye specific for double-stranded DNA, and the fluorescence is monitored after each synthesis step to allow quantitative measurement of the product accumulated.

After a few cycles, the product begins to be detected and the product accumulation enters the exponential phase, doubling every cycle. The number of cycles required to first detect the product above the background is called the quantification cycle C_q (Figure 5). This can be used to calculate the concentration of template sequence present in the initial sample, knowing the exponential rate of increase. Different sequences have

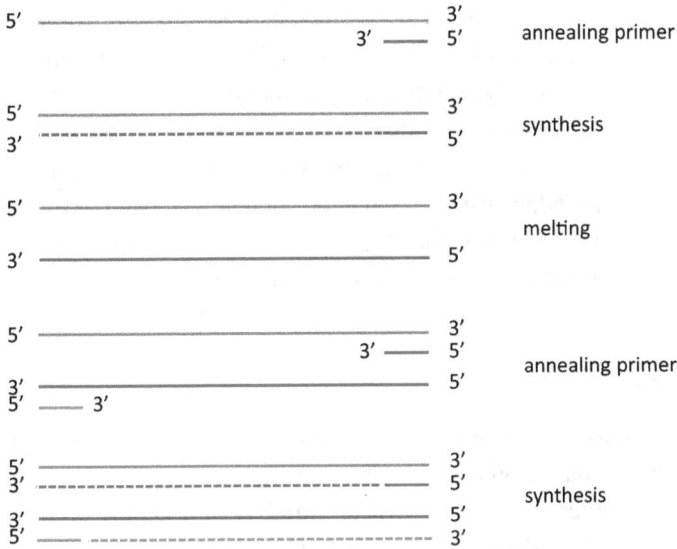

Figure 4.   Two cycles of the polymerase chain reaction (PCR). After two cycles of annealing and synthesis, an initial single strand has become two double-stranded molecules.

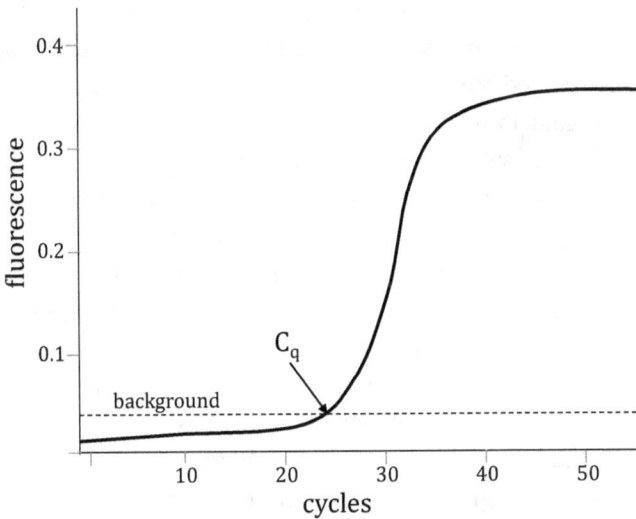

Figure 5.   Real-time PCR. Double-stranded product DNA is monitored by the binding of a suitable fluorescent dye. The fluorescence shows an exponential increase, which then slows down and plateaus as the primers or nucleotide triphosphates are exhausted. Cq, the number of cycles needed for the fluorescence to rise above the background, can be used to calculate the initial number of template molecules.

different efficiencies of amplification so absolute quantification requires a calibration curve with a known DNA sample with the same amplification efficiency. Alternatively, relative quantification can be determined with respect to another sequence known to be abundantly present in the sample. qPCR is frequently used to determine the level of expression of a gene relative to an abundantly expressed gene such as a ribosomal protein gene. For quantification of RNA, the PCR is preceded by a reverse transcription step to produce cDNA with a reverse transcriptase.

RNAi Knockdown

An early approach to transient interference with the expression of a specific gene was based on the idea that an oligonucleotide with the complementary sequence to all or part of the mRNA of a gene would hybridize with the mRNA and prevent its translation. Introducing such a complementary oligonucleotide into a cell would then produce the equivalent of a mutation in the corresponding gene. This would obviously be a very powerful tool, particularly for cultured cells or for organisms in which genetics is impractical or not possible. Early attempts to apply this approach yielded very mixed results for various reasons, including the fact that double-stranded RNA elicits a powerful immune response in vertebrates. The organism treats this as a viral attack and produces interferon and other defensive substances. Studies in invertebrates and particularly in *C. elegans* revealed a whole new world of protective mechanisms that are now collectively referred to as RNA interference or RNAi (see Chapter 5).

Discoveries for which Andrew Fire and Craig Mello received the Nobel Prize in 2006 showed that the effective agent in the antisense RNA approach to gene silencing was not the antisense RNA itself but the small amount of double-stranded RNA that usually accompanied the antisense RNA. As we now know, double-stranded RNA is chopped into 21–23 bp fragments by the Dicer RNase, often referred to as small interfering RNAs or siRNAs. These fragments are then bound by a complex called RNA-induced Silencing Complex or RISC, which includes an Argonaute protein. The Argonaute, one of a family of Argonaute proteins, is responsible for selecting the appropriate strand, degrading the complementary or passenger strand, and using the guide strand to bind and then cleave an mRNA molecule containing the complementary sequence. This cleavage or "slicing" destroys the mRNA and therefore prevents functional expression of the corresponding gene. The efficiency with which a double-stranded siRNA prevents the expression of a gene is highly variable and the gene-silencing process is called knockdown rather than knockout, a term reserved for the total gene inactivation resulting, for example, from a gene deletion.

For knock-down purposes, siRNAs can be synthesized chemically to order by commercial services and introduced into cells. This can be done by transfection or electroporation protocols in the case of cultured cells. In some organisms like *C. elegans*, the RNA can be fed directly to the animals and is taken up readily from the gut. Alternatively, particularly if whole organisms are targeted, the siRNA can be produced *in vivo* by viral, transposon, or plasmid vectors in the form of short hairpin transcripts that are then processed to siRNAs in the cells.

Different siRNAs have very different knockdown efficacies and the choice of sequence for a given mRNA target is critical. Three kinds of criteria are involved. One is the selection of the region in the mRNA to which to target the siRNA. Another is the avoidance of sequence motifs frequently found in other cellular RNAs. A third concern is the half-life of the siRNA in the cell. Algorithms are available to aid selection of the sequence. It is commonly found that no more than one-fourth of the siRNAs results in knockdown efficiencies better than 80%. In general, it is desirable to use multiple siRNA sequences, directed against different parts of the target mRNA. The knockdown efficiency can be tested by reverse-transcription PCR using primers from a different part of the target mRNA. Although it is still the simplest and least expensive way to produce loss of gene function, it is now under strong competition by CRISPR-Cas methods (see Chapter 13, CRISPR-Cas Genome Editing section).

Sequencing

If any single technological advance can be said to have dominated biomedical research in the past 20 years, it is undoubtedly DNA sequencing.

Advanced sequencing technologies have revolutionized many fields by providing DNA (or RNA) sequencing power on a scale previously inconceivable and at steadily reducing costs per base pair.

Also known as Next-Generation Sequencing (NGS) and other laudatory designations and third or fourth-generation methods, these technologies are revolutionary approaches to polynucleotide sequencing that replaced the single-molecule Sanger chain termination sequencing that dominated the original human genome sequencing technology. These methods have made possible a variety of other technologies, such as whole genome sequencing of any species or mixture of species, chromatin immunoprecipitation, transcriptome sequencing, single-cell sequencing, 3C genome architecture, and a range of other methods, that produce large numbers of DNA fragments that need to be identified. Several excellent review articles explain and compare the different approaches and commercial services currently available (Shendure *et al.*, 2017; Slatko *et al.*, 2018). The sequencing field has been driven by biotechnology companies and the technologies and instrumentation are now entirely proprietary. Here, I will survey the main features of the most important of these sequencing techniques.

Massively Parallel Next-Generation Sequencing

Distinct from another post-Sanger sequencing approach such as single-molecule or nanopore sequencing, massively parallel sequencing is based on the concept of microscale sequencing reactions carried out simultaneously in one million to one billion separate molecules. Although a variety of platforms are available today, employing procedures differing in design and detail, they are all based on DNA polymerase synthesis carried out in parallel in one million to several billion spatially separated sequencing foci. By far the most widely used technology is the Illumina, which employs fluorescently tagged nucleotides, monitored microscopically and individually tabulated by computer.

Each single-stranded DNA molecule, generally 150–250 nt long, is attached to a support slide. DNA synthesis proceeds in a series of steps in which the slide is flooded with different solutions, providing DNA polymerase and four chain-terminating nucleotides, each with a different color fluorescent label. After the incorporation step, an image of the slide is taken, resulting in a myriad of colored points corresponding to the DNA molecules with the first nucleotide added. A computer keeps track of the nucleotide incorporated at each spot in each cycle of the sequencing procedure. To prepare for the next cycle, the chain terminating group and the fluorescent labels are removed and the next cycle takes place.

Two alternative technologies are the Roche 454 and the Ion Torrent. Roche 454 uses pyrosequencing, a sequential synthesis in which incorporation of a nucleotide is monitored by detecting pyrophosphate release in picoliter chambers. The pyrophosphate release is monitored by a light-producing reaction of a different frequency for each of the four nucleotides. Commercial sequencers based on this technology reached sequence runs of 600–800 nt. In the early days, these were longer runs than obtainable with other methods, which made Roche 454 the preferred instrument for whole genome sequencing. They were discontinued in 2013 when long sequence reads became possible with other technologies.

Ion Torrent relies on the release of H^+ when a nucleotide is incorporated, when the reaction microchamber is supplied with one nucleotide at a time. The release of H^+ is detected by monitoring the pH with an ion-sensing semiconductor, one in each microchamber. This distinguishes the Ion Torrent technology from all the previously mentioned ones in that it relies entirely on electronics and requires no modified nucleotides or bulky and expensive optics. Millions of microchambers, each with its detector, are integrated into chips, the largest of which permits 100–130 million reads with read lengths of 200nt.

Single-Molecule Technologies

Although the read length of massively parallel biosynthetic sequencing technologies has greatly increased, it is still limited to under 1kb. This is more than adequate to identify sequences of known genomes for techniques such as ChIP, DamID, or 3C; it is not optimal for whole genome sequencing or for applications that need to investigate the state of a single DNA molecule over long distances. For this kind of application, technologies are needed that can sequence single molecules many tens of kb long.

Pacific Biosciences

Generally known as PacBio, this is the pre-eminent technology for large fragment sequencing, permitting single molecule read lengths of 50 kb. Key to the method is the design of reaction wells called zero-mode wave-guides (ZMWs), small relative to the wavelength of the light used. The design of ZMWs is such that detection occurs only at the bottom of the well, where a modified DNA polymerase is attached. Synthesis occurs with four nucleotides whose terminal phosphates are tagged with different fluorophores. When a nucleotide is incorporated, the fluorescent pyroph-osphate is released and is no longer detected at the bottom of the ZMW. The real-time readout allows, in principle, to follow the rate of each nucleotide incorporation so that the slower rates for modified nucleotides can be monitored. In principle, this can allow the detection of methylated nucleotides. In practice, however, 5mC cannot be readily identified yet because the difference in rate for this modification is too small. The latest PacBio chip now contains up to 8 million ZMWs that can be read simultaneously.

Another innovation of the PacBio method is in sample preparation. DNA molecules are circularized, including an adaptor sequence. Primers complementary to the adaptor initiate DNA synthesis, which proceeds around the circularized template, allowing each molecule to be sequenced repeatedly. Primers for either strand can be used and therefore both strands are sequenced. The final sequence is produced by a consensus of the numerous reads from each ZMW.

The disadvantages of the PacBio system at present are its high error rate and relatively high cost. The intrinsic error rate of the method can be compensated by the multiple reads for each molecule.

Nanopore systems

A completely different approach to single-molecule sequencing is to thread long single-stranded DNA molecules through a narrow passage and sense the different bases by the different current changes induced in a detector as they pass by. The approach can be used for DNA or RNA sequencing and, in principle, even for protein sequencing. The two key aspects of this approach are the nature of the nanopore and the mechanism by which the nucleic acid is passed through it.

Biological solutions for the nanopore have turned to transmembrane proteins embedded in a lipid membrane, mostly α hemolysin or porin A from *Mycobacterium smegmatis* (MspA). Solid-state sensor versions produce nanopores from metal alloys with nanometer pores. Simple diffusion tends to make the polynucleotide move too rapidly through the pores for good resolution. An important question is therefore how to achieve a constant, slow passage of the nucleic acid. Motor proteins such as DNA polymerases, helicases, and exonucleases have been utilized.

The most successful, commercially advanced nanopore sequencing system is that of Oxford Nanopore Technologies. This system uses a polymer membrane in which are embedded α hemolysin nanopores. New versions of the nanopore protein are under development for specific purposes. Double-stranded DNA molecules are bound to a motor protein, generally φ29 DNA polymerase, which is targeted to the nanopore protein. When the polymerase-bound DNA is loaded onto the nanopore, a single strand is progressively unwound and passed through the pore. A different motor protein is used for RNA sequencing. The pore generally senses a current change as nucleotides move through. This is dominated by a nucleotide but affected by flanking nucleotides. Base calling algorithms have been developed to interpret the current change signatures. Different pore protein variants allow a narrow or broader region to be sensed, which can be beneficial in reading homopolymer tracts. Certain algorithms allow nucleotide modifications to be decoded. Sequence readout occurs in real time, as a molecule passes through a nanopore. Each pore in an array reads independently. A DNA molecule typically takes seconds to pass through the pore. As one molecule leaves a pore, a new molecule is loaded. Each read is potentially hundreds of kb long but typically only reads of several tens of kb can be expected.

One of the remarkable advantages of the nanopore technology is the small size, low cost, and portability of the instruments. Oxford Nanopore's typical instrument is the MinION, a portable, cell phone-sized instrument that can be connected to a portable computer for direct sequence analysis in the field. The MinION contains a flowcell, which is an array of up to 512 nanopore channels. Each channel contains a membrane and nanopore.

Each has its electrode connected to a channel in a sensor array chip. In principle, this allows an output of up to 50 Gb of sequence (72 hours at 420 bases per second for each of 512 channels). A larger instrument contains up to 48 flow cells for a nominal 14 terabases of sequence output in 72 hours.

The Oxford Nanopore technology and the long-read sequencer approaches, in general, have two major weak points. One is the relatively high error rate, compared to short-read sequencing. Current error rates are 5–20%, depending on the type of molecule, reading speed, and library preparation. This can be compensated by base-calling and sequence assembly algorithms and by the large number of molecules that can be rapidly sequenced. The second drawback is sample preparation. Single reads as long as 3 Mb have been claimed but to obtain average read lengths of a few tens of kb requires high quality and high molecular weight input DNA. A variety of sample preparation kits are available but all are limited by the quality of the input.

Nanopore approaches have also been applied to protein sequencing. With 21 amino acids instead of four nucleotides, and many more post-translational modifications, this is a much more complicated business than nucleic acid sequencing. For progress in single-molecule protein sequencing, see Bošković and Keyser (2021).

CRISPR-Cas Genome Editing

Ever since the dawn of what was then called genetic engineering, in the 1970s, it has been the dream of every genetic engineer to be able to target protein factors, activators, sequence modifications, DNA cleavage, or any other conceivable event to any specific sequence in the vast sequence forest that constitutes the mammalian genome. Many technologies have been developed to target, for example a DNA-binding protein to any desired nucleotide sequence. The most recent and by far the most general, flexible, precise and amenable to a large variety of applications is the CRISPR-Cas family of methods. To understand the details of the methodology and to appreciate the amazing biology that underlies it, it is well worth the effort to consider how it came about.

In the space of less than 10 years, tools based on CRISPR-Cas mechanisms have appeared and imposed themselves on molecular genomics as the most powerful and versatile approaches to manipulate the genome, the functioning of cells and the achievement of a degree of control that is truly extraordinary. In acknowledgment of the importance of CRISPR-Cas techniques in modern biology, the Nobel Prize in Chemistry was awarded in 2020 to Jennifer Doudna and Emmanuelle Charpentier.

Discovery of CRISPR mechanisms

In the late 1980s, while cloning an enzyme gene from the ordinary and well known lab bacterium *E. coli*, Ishino *et al.* noted a repetitive, palindromic 29 nucleotide sequence alternating with non-repetitive short segments of unknown origin. As genome sequences of many bacteria began to accumulate, similar repetitive structures were noted in many other species. About half of the bacteria examined and 90% of archaea have at least one such locus now called CRISPR (Clustered, Regularly Interspersed Palindromic Repeats). In brief, the non-repetitive sequences, originally called "spacers", derive from invasive genetic elements such as plasmids or bacteriophage. CRISPR clusters contain a few to several hundred such spacers and their presence is associated with a degree of resistance to the corresponding genetic elements. This suggested that such snippets of sequence were used as part of an acquired immunity mechanism. CRISPR loci are flanked by a set of genes called *cas* (CRISPR-associated) genes that turn out to be responsible for the acquisition and utilization of the CRISPR repeats to attack invading DNA. CRISPR mechanisms vary considerably in different organisms, some are simpler, some complex. In essence, however, the RNAs derived from the spacer sequences bind to a Cas effector complex and serve as guides that recognize homologous invading DNA and target an endonuclease activity to it.

In the most common, so-called type II systems, the CRISPR locus is constitutively transcribed starting from a promoter in the Leader sequence and producing a long transcript that is then processed to form small crRNAs, each including one of the spacer sequences (Figure 6). The processing occurs with the help of a trans-activating crRNA or tracrRNA,

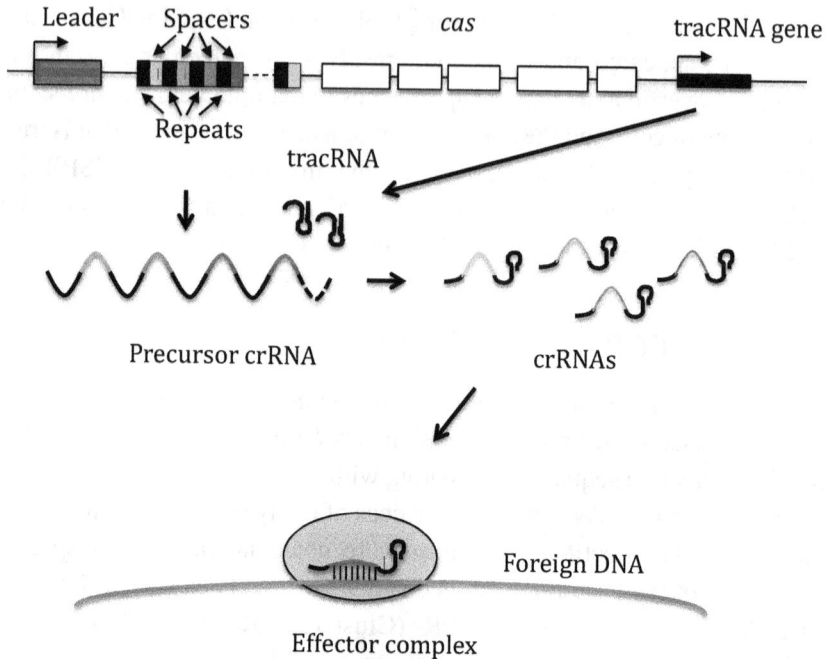

Figure 6.   The CRISPR locus contains a number of repeated sequence elements separated by spacers with a variety of sequences. Genes encoding Cas proteins involved in the creation and utilization of the CRISPR mechanisms are adjacent as is a gene (tracRNA gene) encoding sequences complementary to the repeat elements. The repeats and spacers are transcribed as a long RNA, which is processed with the help of tracRNA to generate individual crRNAs, each containing one spacer sequence. These crRNAs are incorporated in a complex with appropriate Cas proteins and serve as guides to target foreign DNA molecules.

transcribed from a flanking region of the CRISPR locus, which contains a sequence complementary to that of the CRISPR repeats. The 5' end is produced by cleavage near one end of the repeat sequence preceding the spacer while the 3' end is more variable but may contain much of the palindromic part of the repeat sequence and therefore able to form a stem-loop structure. The crRNA is incorporated in a complex with Cas proteins, in the simplest case with the Cas9 protein, which includes a nucleolytic activity. The crRNA serves as a guide for the complex to search double-stranded DNA for target sequences to cleave. Target recognition requires,

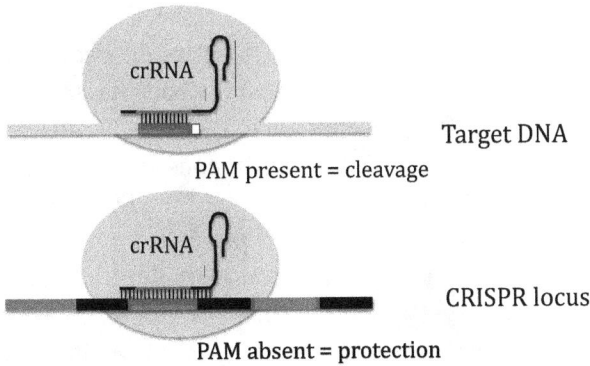

Figure 7. Self *vs* non-self discrimination. Recognition of target DNA requires correct pairing of the spacer sequence in the crRNA with a sequence in the target DNA. It also requires the presence of a PAM motif on the target DNA (small white square). This results in cleavage of the target DNA. The absence of the PAM motif and a more extensive sequence homology with the crRNA results in protection of the endogenous CRISPR locus.

in addition to the spacer homology, the presence of a short Proto-spacer Adjacent Motif (PAM) at the 3' end of the homology. This is a critical requirement not only for recognition but also to distinguish a legitimate target sequence from the sequence present in the CRISPR locus itself (Figure 7). PAM sequences vary in different bacteria but, in a commonly used system from *Streptococcus pyogenes*, the motif is NGG. When a suitable target sequence is identified, the crRNA-Cas complex cleaves the target DNA with the nuclease activity that resides in the Cas9 protein.

In essence, the CRISPR-Cas mechanism provides an RNA guide to target virtually any desired sequence in a genome and a protein handle that can be functionalized to direct to that target sequence any of a variety of functions. For ease of use, in genomic applications, the tracrRNA sequence is often incorporated in the desired crRNA guide sequence. Therefore cells must be supplied with the tracrRNA-crRNA fusion, often called short guide or sgRNA, and a Cas9 protein. These can be provided by transfection or by introducing transgenes expressing the sgRNA from an RNA pol III promoter and the Cas9 gene from a pol II promoter.

Less well studied but potentially equally interesting is the process by which the CRISPR immunity is acquired. This involves a spacer acquisition complex that contains the Cas1, Cas2, Csn2 and Cas9 proteins and takes place immediately as the DNA enters the bacterium, as shown by studies using the *Staphylococcus aureus* bacteria and bacteriophage *φ12* by Modell *et al.* (2017). In addition to PAM motifs, spacer acquisition seems to initiate near a free DNA end. In consequence, spacers are predominantly acquired from the leading edge of the DNA entering the bacterium. Acquisition during replication is possible but much less frequent.

Different CRISPR systems vary considerably in the details of their mechanisms. Some target single-stranded DNA or RNA. Some have different PAM requirements. Some require no PAM. While the type II system described above has been used most widely, interest is now expanding to the new features available in alternative CRISPR systems.

CRISPR-Cas applications

The original application of CRISPR-Cas technology was simply to exploit the endonucleolytic activity of Cas9 to direct DNA cleavage at specific sequences to generate targeted mutations. Double stranded DNA breaks are frequently repaired by the error-prone Non-Homologous End-Joining (NHEJ) pathway, which generally results in small deletions or insertions and therefore loss of function, if introduced in a coding region. This approach and the plasmid tools needed was rapidly applied by many laboratories to knock out genes in many organisms and proved to be highly efficient, generally requiring little selection to obtain knockout mutations. Soon, however, concerns arose about the frequency of undesired untargeted mutations. Although these are reduced by the PAM requirement, some PAMs are more stringent than others and PAM occurrence is dependent on the target genome. Mutations introduced in the Cas9 protein have significantly reduced the frequency of off-target mutations. A related approach employs Homology Directed Repair (HDR) in which the double strand break is repaired by incorporating sequences from a homologous DNA fragment. In this approach, an exogenous DNA fragment is provided that can include desired insertions or mutations flanked by homologous sequences. This approach greatly reduces the likelihood of off-target effects and allows the introduction of desired modifications or additions into the sequence of interest.

CRISPR versatility for genome manipulations

Given the basic CRISPR-Cas tools, i t was not long before a large variety of novel applications were devised (for a review, see Mali et al., 2013) and many more imaginative uses have been found more recently . First, it should be noted that the system permits parallel targeting of a Cas complex to a variety of genomic sites, limited only by the number of guide sgRNAs that can be expressed in a cell. The original Cas9 protein includes a nucleolytic activity but this can be deleted for other applications that do not require DNA cleavage. Instead, the Cas9 protein can be fused to any desired protein or enzyme moiety to target a desired function to the desired genomic site. Among the variety of functionalities that can be thus targeted to specific genomic sites are transcriptional activators or repressors, histone modifying activities, green fluorescent protein or other chromophore, protein-protein interacting domains. The guide RNAs themselves can serve as functional elements by attaching to them additional RNA sequences to drive RNA-RNA interactions, RNA-protein interactions and other functions.

Prime sequence editing

An application of particular interest is genomic editing. This has become a fine art that has gone far beyond the creation of simple knockouts. A particularly ingenious and powerful method to edit the genome sequence to introduced desired changes was developed by Anzalone *et al.* (2019). They used a Cas9 modified to produce a nick rather than a double strand cut in the target DNA. In addition, the Cas9 was fused to a modified reverse transcriptase. The guide RNA, called prime editing guide RNA or pegRNA incorporates a short edit sequence that is to be inserted in the genome at the nick site. The pegRNA annealed to the DNA is then extended by the reverse transcriptase activity. The displaced DNA strand is trimmed of and the remaining nick is ligated by normal DNA repair activities. After a round of DNA replication, the editing is completed. With this approach, editing efficiency varies with the target sequence, the length and sequence of the primer binding site and the length and sequence of the reverse transcriptase template. Efficiencies of 10-40% were obtained with reached sequence errors (indels) of a few %. Clearly the design of the pegRNA is critical and the higher efficiencies were obtained if a second nick was introduced in the non-edited strand to bias the repair of the sequence mismatch towards the edited sequence. Further improvements continue to be added but this technique is currently the most efficient and versatile genome editing tool available.

Further Reading

Anzalone AV, Randolph PB, Davis JR, Sousa AA, Koblan LW, Levy JM et al. (2019). Search-and-replace genome editing without double-strand breaks or donor DNA. *Nature*. **576**, 149–157.

Aughey GN and Southall TD (2016). Dam it's good! DamID profiling of protein-DNA interactions. *WIREs Dev Biol*. **5**, 25–37. doi: 10.1002/wdev.205

Aughey GN, Cheetham SW and Southall TD (2019). DamID as a versatile tool for understanding gene regulation. *Development*. **146**, dev173666.

Bošković F and Keyser UF (2021). Toward single-molecule proteomics. *Science*. **374**, 1443–1444.

de Wit E and de Laat W (2012). A decade of 3C technologies: insights into nuclear organization. *Genes Dev*. **26**, 11–24.

Deamer D, Akeson M and Branton D (2016). Three decades of nanopore sequencing. *Nat Biotech*. **34**, 518–524.

Dekker J, Marti-Renom MA and Mirny LA (2013). Exploring the three-dimensional organization of genomes: interpreting chromatin interaction data. *Nat Rev Genet*. **14**, 390–403.

Drexler HL, Choquet K and Churchman LS (2020). Splicing kinetics and coordination revealed by direct nascent RNA sequencing through nanopores. *Mol Cell*. **77**, 985–998.e988.

Ishino Y, Shinagawa H, Makino K, Amemura M and Nakata A (1987). Nucleotide sequence of the iap gene, responsible for alkaline phosphatase isozyme conversion in Escherichia coli, and identification of the gene product. *J Bacteriol*. **169**, 5429–5433.

Kono N and Arakawa K (2019) Nanopore sequencing: review of potential applications in functional genomics. *Develop. Growth Differ*. **61**, 316–326.

Mali P, Esvelt KM and Church GM. (2013). Cas9 as a versatile tool for engineering biology. *Nat Meth* **10**, 957–963.

Marshall OJ, Southall TD, Cheetham SW and Brand AH (2016). Cell type-specific profiling of protein-DNA interactions without cell isolation using targeted DamID with next-generation sequencing. *Nat. Protocols.* **11**, 1586–1598.

McCord RP, Kaplan N and Giorgetti L (2020). Chromosome conformation capture and beyond: toward an integrative view of chromosome structure and function. *Mol Cell.* **77**, 688–708.

Milne JLS, Borgnia MJ, Bartesaghi A, Tran EEH, Earl LA, Schauder DM *et al.* (2013). Cryo-electron microscopy — a primer for the non-microscopist. *FEBS J.* **280**, 28–45.

Modell JW, Jiang W and Marraffini LA (2017). CRISPR-Cas systems exploit viral DNA injection to establish and maintain adaptive immunity. *Nature.* **544**, 101–104.

Nagano T, Lubling Y, Stevens TJ, Schoenfelder S, Yaffe E, Dean W *et al.* (2013). Single-cell Hi-C reveals cell-to-cell variability in chromosome structure. *Nature.* **502**, 59–64.

Nogales E and Scheres SHW (2015). Cryo-EM: a unique tool for the visualization of macromolecular complexity. *Mol Cell.* **58**, 677–689.

Restrepo-Pérez L, Joo C and Dekker C (2018). Paving the way to single-molecule protein sequencing. *Nat Nanotech.* **13**, 786–796.

Saibil HR (2022). Cryo-EM in molecular and cellular biology. *Mol Cell.* **82**, 274–284.

Schilbach S, Albara S, Dienemann C, Grabbe F and Cramer P (2021). Structure of RNA polymerase II pre-initiation complex at 2.9 Å defines initial DNA opening. *Cell.* **184**, 4064–4072.e4028.

Shendure J, Balasubramaniam S, Church GM, Gilbert W, Rogers J, Schloss JA *et al.* (2017). DNA sequencing at 40: past, present and future. *Nature.* **550**, 345–353.

Skene PJ and Henikoff S. (2017). An efficient targeted nuclease strategy for high resolution mapping of DNA binding sites. *eLife.* **6**, e21856.

Slatko BE, Gardner AF and Ausubel FM (2018). Overview of next-generation sequencing technologies. *Curr Prot Mol Biol.* **122**, e59–e59.

van Steensel B and Henikoff S (2000). Identification of in vivo DNA targets of chromatin proteins using tethered Dam methyltransferase. *Nat Biotech.* **18**, 424–428.

Yin Y, Jiang Y, Lam K-WG, Berletch JB, Disteche CM, Noble WS *et al.* (2019). High-throughput single-cell sequencing with linear amplification. *Mol Cell.* **76**, 676–690.

Yip KM, Fischer N, Pakhia E, Chari A and Stark H (2020). Atomic-resolution protein structure determination by cryo-EM. *Nature.* **587**, 157–161.

Glossary of Terms

Actin-related protein ARP: One of a number of proteins with strong similarity to cytoskeletal actin, including the ATPase domain. Several ARPs are found in the nucleus, for example components of nucleosome remodeling complexes.

allele-specific expression: Condition in which only one of the two alleles of a gene in a diploid organism is active. Associated with genetic imprinting in mammals.

allosteric shift: Conformational shift in a protein or enzyme induced by the binding of a small molecule or another protein, often resulting in a functional change.

Alu element: A small Interspersed Nuclear Element (SINE) evolved from the 7SL RNA. It utilizes a reverse transcriptase and transposase produced by a different element to insert in new genomic sites.

Argonaute (Ago) protein: One of a family of proteins that modify and mediate the action of small RNAs in RNA interference (RNAi) mechanisms.

ATAC sequencing: Assay for Transposase-Accessible Chromatin using Sequencing. This method uses a hyperactive mutant of the Tn5 transposase to cleave accessible DNA in chromatin.

bivalent chromatin state: The state of certain genes in stem cells, whose promoters have both active histone marks (H3K4me3) and repressive histone marks (H3K27me3).

blastomere: A cell of the early embryo, constituting the hollow sphere called blastocyst.

blastocyst: The hollow cell sphere stage of the early mammalian embryo. An internal clump of cells, the inner cell mass, gives rise to the embryo itself while the outer cell layer, the trophoblast produces the placenta and embryonic membranes.

bromodomain: A conserved protein domain that binds to specific histone lysines when they are acetylated.

budding yeast: A yeast microorganism that replicates by budding rather than symmetric fission. Baker's yeast (Saccharomyces cerevisiae) is the prototype.

CTD (C-Terminal Domain) of RNA polymerase II: The C-terminal domain of the largest subunit of RNA polymerase II, consisting of numerous repeats or near-repeats of a consensus sequence YSPTSPS. This sequence can be phosphorylated at specific sites and binds a variety of proteins that regulate transcription.

CAGE, Cap Analysis of Gene Expression: A technique that assesses gene expression by identifying sequences associated with the 5′ cap of RNAs.

cell-autonomous: A function that acts autonomously on the cell that expresses it rather than on neighboring cells.

cellular senescence: An age-associated process in stem cells or growing cell tissues, caused by telomere shortening, DNA damage, stress signals, unfolded proteins, overexpresson of oncoproteins. Results in arrest of proliferation, loss of lamin, secretion of cytokines, and other factors (Senescence-Associated Secretory Phenotype, SASP).

centromere: A chromosomal region to which bind proteins forming the kinetochore, a complex structure to which spindle fibers attach at mitosis to segregate homologous chromosomes to the daughter cells.

CHD nucleosome remodeling complex: A family of nucleosome remodelers characterized by two chromodomains, a SNF2-like ATPase domain, and a DNA binding motif.

ChIP: Chromatin Immuno-Precipitation. A technique to identify chromatin sequences associated with specific proteins using a specific antibody.

chromatin: A general term for the form of DNA found in the nucleus, characterized by packaging with histones into nucleosomes.

chromodomain: a conserved protein domain that binds to specific trimethylated lysines residues in histones.

chromoshadow domain: A structural domain found in the C-terminal region of HP1 proteins. So-called for a distant similarity to the chromodomain and involved in dimerization.

Chromosome Conformation Capture (3C): A type of technique that relies on crosslinking chromatin and recovering the crosslinking sites to map contacts between distant DNA sequences and eventually determine chromatin architecture in the nucleus. Variants include 4C, 5C, Hi-C.

clonal expansion: Mutations occurring in growing tissues that give cells a growth advantage, forming an expanding clone in the tissue.

cohesin: A protein complex that can bind two DNA molecules and translocate along them. Involved in sister chromatid cohesion and DNA loop extrusion.

condensin: A protein complex that can bind two DNA molecules and translocate along them. Involved in folding and condensing chromatin in mitotic chromosomes.

CpG island: Genomic regions enriched in CpG dinucleotides in vertebrate genomes. Typically associated with transcriptional promoter activity.

CRISPR (Clustered Regularly Interspaced Short Palindromic Repeats): Sequence features found in many bacterial species. Produce RNA guide molecules involved in targeting invasive genomes. Now a mechanism used for genome editing and targeting technologies.

CTCF: A DNA-binding factor/insulator protein that interacts with cohesin and plays an important role in genome architecture.

CXXC domain: A modified zinc finger protein domain that binds to CpG-rich DNA regions such as CpG islands.

DamID: A technique in which a DNA methylase domain is fused to a protein of interest to tag genomic regions in physical proximity to that protein.

DNA methyltransferase or methylase (DNMT): A class of DNA methyltransferases that methylate genomic DNA. They include maintenance methylase (DNMT1) and *de novo* methylases (DNMT3).

dosage compensation: A mechanism that seeks to equalize the expression level of a gene present in one copy in males and two copies in females. Generally applies to X chromosome genes.

DSIF, DRB Sensitivity-Inducing Factor: A factor that, together with NELF, is responsible for promoter-proximal pausing of RNA polymerase II.

Embryonic Stem Cells (ESCs): Undifferentiated cells of the inner cell mass in the early embryo, which are pluripotent: they have the potential to differentiate into all the different types of adult tissues.

endonuclease: A type of enzymatic activity that cleaves DNA internally.

eRNA: enhancer RNA. Non-coding RNAs transcribed from enhancer regions. In some cases eRNAs have been found to play regulatory roles in transcription.

euchromatin: A part of genomic chromatin originally defined by the fact that it decondenses after mitosis. Generally, decondensed, non heterochromatic part of the genome containing active genes.

exon: A part of a gene sequence representing mRNA protein-coding regions after splicing out intronic sequences.

exonuclease: A type of enzymatic activity that removes terminal nucleotides sequentially from DNA or RNA.

FACT (Facilitates Chromatin Transcription): A heterodimeric protein complex that binds to nucleosomes and facilitates the passage of transcribing RNA polymerase II.

FAIRE (Formaldehyde-Assisted Isolation of Regulatory Elements): A technique that partitions chromatin fragments depleted of nucleosomes and hence likely to be regulatory sites or active promoters.

fission yeast: A yeast microorganism that replicates by symmetric cell division rather than asymmetric budding. *Saccharomyces pombe* is the prototype.

FRT (Flippase Recognition Target): A short recognition sequence that is the target of site-directed recombination by the Flippase recombinase. Can be used to excise a DNA sequence framed by two FRTs.

G-quadruplex: A non-helical DNA structure that forms in sequences rich in Gs. Often found at telomeres.

General Transcription Factor GTF: One of a number of transcription factors that are recruited to a promoter region to help recruit RNA polymerase II and initiate transcription.

genome browser: A computer application that utilizes a genome sequence and gene annotations to display genes, transcription units, splicing patterns or other specific inputs over the whole genome.

genomic programming and reprogramming: A pattern of genomic epigenetic marks and regulatory factors that determines the state of differentiation, lack of it or pluripotency of a cell. Reprogramming alters the programming state, for example by returning a differentiated cell to a pluripotent cell (induced pluripotency).

Hayflick limit: The number of cell divisions before a human differentiated cell population stops dividing. Usually 40–60 divisions.

helicase: A class of enzymes that moves along and unwinds double-stranded DNA through ATP hydrolysys. RNA helicases carry out a similar activity in base-paired RNA regions.

Helix-Turn-Helix (HTH): A protein domain consisting of two α-helical segments linked by a short polypeptide that is often a DNA-binding domain in many transcription regulatory proteins.

hemimethylated: Refers to a symmetric DNA sequence targeted by a methyl transferase but is methylated on one strand only.

heterochromatin: A chromatin region that remains condensed during interphase. Generally associated with histone H3K9 methylation and binding of repressive heterochromatin proteins.

Hi-C: The most general type of 3C (Chromosome Conformation Capture) technique in which all sites of contact between two DNA sequences in the genome are identified.

HMG (High Mobility Group) proteins: A class if small, highly charged chromosomal proteins that affect the structural features of chromatin and participate in the regulation of chromatin events.

histone: One of four small, positively charged proteins, aH2A, H2B, H3 and H4, that form the core of the canonical nucleosome.

histone acetyl transferase HAT: A type of enzyme that acetylates specific lysines of histones.

histone chaperone: A type of protein complex that binds to histones and facilitates their transactions in nucleosome assembly, disassembly, or histone exchange.

histone deacetylase HDAC: A type of enzyme that removes acetyl groups from acetylated lysines in histones.

histone variant: A protein closely related to one of the canonical histones that can replace it in a nucleosome to confer specific functions.

homeodomain: A conserved protein domain found in Hox proteins. It is a sequence-specific DNA-binding domain and is encoded by a recognizable DNA sequence called the homeobox.

homeotic genes (Hox genes): A set of genes related in sequence that direct the specific morphogenesis of body segments. Expression of specific Hox genes confer segmental identity in the antero-posterior axis; in vertebrates also proximo-distal identity in limbs.

Hoogsteen pairing: An alternative base-pairing scheme to that found in the canonical DNA double helix.

immunoprecipitation: Specific precipitation of a protein or protein complex using an antibody that specifically recognizes that protein.

imprinting control region: The site of an imprinted gene that bears the methylation signal determining the monoallelic expression of that gene.

Induced Pluripotent Stem Cell (iPSC): A pluripotent stem cell produced by reprogramming a differentiated cell.

inner cell mass: A clump of cells internalized within the hollow sphere of cells constituting the embryonic blastocyst. Gives rise to the embryo proper.

Intrinsically Disordered Region IDR: Protein domains that lack a defined structure but assume a variety of unstable conformations. They often include runs of the same or similar amino acids. They can participate in weak multivalent interactions and can lead to liquid-liquid phase separation.

intron: A part of a primary transcript that is spliced out of the mature mRNA and therefore does not encode a protein sequence.

ISWI (Imitation SWItch) nucleosome remodeling complex: A type of nucleosome remodeling complex whose catalytic ATPase subunit belongs to the ISWI family of helicase domains.

Jumonji C domain: A protein domain, also called JmjC domain, that binds Fe(II) and α-ketoglutarate and is associated with lysine demethylation activity.

kinetochore: A multiprotein structure that assembles on the centromere and links two chromatids. Attaches spindle fibers to segregate chromosomes at mitosis.

knock-down: Partial loss of function of a gene, usually by RNAi methods.

knock-out: Complete loss of function of a gene, usually by genetic deletion or insertion.

lamin: Intermediate filament protein that assembles into the nuclear lamina.

Lamin B Receptor (LBR): A protein that binds to lamins and chromatin and anchors them to the inner nuclear membrane.

Lamin-Associated Domain (LAD): Genomic regions associated with the nuclear lamina. Generally either heterochromatic or transcriptionally inactive.

Lamin-Associated Protein (LAP): A protein that binds to the nuclear lamina and mediates interactions with emerin and the cytoskeleton on one side and with heterochromatin on the other.

lamina: A stiff lining on the inner side of the nuclear envelope, formed by lamins. Provides attachment for heterochromatic or transcriptionally inactive chromatin.

leucine zipper: A α-helical protein domain containing leucines or similar hydrophobic amino acid at every seventh position, forming a hydrophobic surface on one side of the helix.

LINEs: Long Interspersed Nuclear Elements, a type of retrotransposon lacking LTRs (Long Terminal Repeats).

linker histone: The H1 histone. Not a component of the core nucleosome but binds to internucleosomal DNA as it enters and as it exits the nucleosome.

liquid phase condensation: Interactions among certain types of proteins that result in the formation of a separate liquid phase droplet.

lncRNA: Long non-coding RNA. A type of RNA longer than a few hundred nucleotides that does not code for a protein but is often used as a component of a regulatory complex, for example, by recruiting repressive Polycomb complexes.

LTR (Long Terminal Repeats): Terminal repeats found in tandem orientation at the two ends of a class of retrotransposon. Usually a few hundred nucleotides long, they contain a promoter that transcribes the retrotransposon.

MBD methyl binding domain: A set of factors that bind 5-methyl cytosine and serve as readers of methylated DNA.

MeCP2: The best known MBD factor that binds to 5-methyl cytosine. Mutated in Rett Syndrome.

Mediator: A large multisubunit complex that interacts with RNA polymerase II and the Pre-Initiation Complex on one hand and the enhancer factors on the other, mediating promoter activation.

miRNA, microRNA: A class of small RNA molecules, usually 22 nucleotides long, that produce post-transcriptional regulation by base pairing with corresponding mRNAs and regulate their function.

monoallelic expression: Expression of only one allele of a gene, typical of imprinted genes in mammals. See also allele-specific expression.

mismatch repair: Repair of non-canonical base pairs in DNA, produced by replication errors, mutations, chemical modifications.

mRNA cap: A cap structure added to the 5′ end of pre-mRNA transcripts, usually co-transcriptionally. It consists of a guanine attached to the 5′ end by a 5′-5′ triphosphate and then methylated at the 7 position. Essential for mRNA function.

nanopore: A passage of nanometer size through which a single molecule can be threaded. Often consisting of a pore-forming protein. In appropriate configurations it can be used to sense characteristic potential differences caused by the passage of individual nucleotides in a polynucleotide and therefore allow DNA sequencing.

NELF negative elongation factor: A protein complex that causes transcriptional pausing of RNA polymerase 20–50 nucleotides after the transcription start.

NGS, Next Generation Sequencing: A type of DNA sequencing methodology that has largely replaced the classical Sanger sequencing method. It usually refers to massively parallel sequencing techniques that sequence simultaneously millions of DNA fragments attached to a substrate.

nuclear envelope: The outer layer enclosing the nucleus. Consists of two lipid bilayers constituting the inner and outer nuclear membrane plus the nuclear lamina.

nuclear pore: An opening through the double nuclear membrane, framed by a large protein complex that mediates both active and passive transport of molecules between the nucleus and the cytoplasm.

nucleosome: The structural unit of chromatin, consisting of 147 nucleotides wrapped in two turns around a core of histone proteins H2A, H2B, H3 and H4.

nucleosome remodeling: A type of activity through which remodeling machines modulate the arrangement of the DNA and histones in a nucleosome or string of nucleosomes. Generally requires ATP hydrolysis.

Okazaki fragments: Short DNA sequences (~150 nucleotides) synthesized discontinuously from a short RNA primer and then linked to form the lagging strand in DNA replication.

ORF, Open Reading Frame: DNA sequence that, read in a specific triplet frame, contains no translation termination codon and therefore potentially encodes a continuous polypeptide.

P-TEFb: Positive Transcription Elongation Factor, a cyclin-dependent kinase complex that releases paused RNA polymerase and promotes transcriptional elongation.

PAF1: Polymerase-Associated Complex bound to transcribing RNA polymerase II. Helps recruit transcription factors, histone modification complexes and elongation factors.

palindrome: A symmetric sequence that reads the same in either direction.

paralog: an evolutionarily related gene that may have acquired different functions.

parental conflict model: Model proposed to account for allele-specifc expression of imprinted genes in mammals.

PcG, Polycomb Group: Genes belonging to the Polycomb Group because they participate in the Polycomb silencing mechanism.

PCNA, Proliferating Cell Nuclear Antigen: The central trimeric protein that clamps DNA at the replication fork and recruits a variety of other components involved in replication, chromatin assembly, histone modification and DNA damage repair.

pericentric: Usually referring to genomic regions on the border between centric heterochromatin and euchromatin.

persistence length: A measure of the stiffness of a filament. The characteristic length at which the filament can be considered freely flexible.

phase-separated condensate: Condensed state formed by multivalent interactions between molecules leading to the formation of a separate phase or liquid-droplet.

PHD finger: A type of zinc finger first found in a Plant HomeoDomain protein.

phenotype: Observable feature that can be altered by genetic mutation or alteration of gene expression.

phospho-switch: Reactivation of a repressed chromatin state induced by histone methylation of a lysine flanked by aan amino acid that can be phosphorylated. The presence of the phosphate prevents the recognition of the adjacent methyl lysine by a "reader" such as a chromodomain protein.

phosphodiester linkage: In DNA, this is the link mediated by a phosphate to the 5′ hydroxyl of a sugar on one side and the 3′ hydroxyl of another sugar on the other side.

pioneer factor: A type of DNA-binding protein that can access chromatin DNA sequences packaged in nucleosomes. Often able to open condensed chromatin regions and allow access of other DNA-binding factors.

piRNA: Piwi-interacting RNA. A class of small RNAs that binds to a complex formed by the Piwi type of Argonaute proteins and targets transcriptional silencing to repetitive DNA sequences.

Piwi proteins: A variety of Argonaute protein that mediates the processing and function of piRNAs and targets the silencing of repetitive DNA.

pluripotency: The ability of a cell to act as a stem cell that can enter multiple pathways of differentiation.

pluripotency factors: Transcription factors required for maintaining the pluripotent state of embryonic stem cells. The three principal pluripotency factors are considered to be OCT4, SOX2 and NANOG.

polyadenylation signal: A nucleotide sequence, usually AAUAAA, on an nascent RNA transcript that recruits a cleavage activity 10–30 nucleotides downstream, and the addition of a polyA tail to the 3′ cleavage site.

polytene chromosome: A chromosome produced by repeated DNA replication without cell division, in which the DNA copies remain precisely aligned giving rise to giant chromosomes.

Position-Effect Variegation (PEV): Variable state of heterochromatic silencing in which the target gene is repressed in some cells of a tissue but not others, producing a mosaic tissue.

POZ/BTB domain: A protein domain that mediates dimerization.

PRC1, PRC2: Polycomb Repressive Complex 1 and 2. PRC1 is assembled around a RING-domain ubiquitin transferase. PRC2 contains Enhancer of zeste (Ezh1 or Ezh2 in vertebrates), a histone H3K27 methyltransferase.

PRE: Polycomb Response Element, a DNA sequence usually a few hundred nucleotides long that in *Drosophila* recruits Polycomb complexes and can generate transcriptional silencing of a gene.

PIC, Pre-Initiation Complex: A multiprotein complex that assembles with RNA polymerase II at transcription start sites and permits transcription initiation.

progeria: A genetic syndrome that causes premature and greatly accelerated aging processes.

PROMPT, promoter upstream transcripts: Transcripts arising in the region of up to 2 kb upstream of the classical transcription start sites of genes. They arise from the nucleosome depleted region formed at a promoter, they are often antisense, and are usually rapidly degraded.

protamine: A type of small protein rich in arginine that coats and packages DNA in spermatozoa.

R-loop: Structure formed when an RNA transcript hybridizes with its template DNA strand, displacing the non-template DNA strand, which remains unpaired.

Reactive Oxygen Species (ROS): Free radicals or peroxides generally produced by electron transport mechanisms. Cause damage to proteins and DNA.

RdRP, RNA-Directed RNA Polymerase: An RNA polymerase that utilizes an RNA fragment to prime transcription of an RNA molecule, producing a double-stranded RNA. Used to replicate RNA viruses. Organisms that possess an RdRP can amplify RNA interference responses.

replication fork: A site on a double-stranded DNA molecule where the two strands are separated and replicative DNA synthesis takes place.

retrotransposon: a type of transposable element whose replication involves reverse transcription from an RNA molecule.

reverse transcriptase: An enzyme that synthesizes DNA on an RNA template.

RING finger: A type of zinc finger protein domain with a C3HC4 motif that mediates protein-protein interactions and is commonly found in E3 ubiquitin ligases.

RISC: RNA-Induced Silencing Complex that is targeted by short RNAs such as siRNAs or miRNAs to cleave or modify RNAs containing the complementary sequence.

RNA interference RNAi: A set of mechanisms triggered by double-stranded RNA molecules that result in transcriptional or post-transcriptional gene silencing

rRNA: Ribosomal RNA, RNA constituents of ribosomes.

S-adenosyl methionine, SAM: A small molecule in which the adenosyl group is attached to the sulfur of methionine. The resulting sulfonium ion is highly energetic and drives the ability of SAM to transfer the methionine methyl group to a large variety of potential acceptors.

satellite sequences: Genomic regions consisting of extensive tandem repeats of short sequences, ranging from half a dozen to 300 nucleotides.

SEC, Super Elongation Complex: A multifactor complex that includes ELL and P-TEFb. It allows elongation of transcription by RNA polymerase II past the pausing site.

SET domain: A protein domain that is the catalytic domain for methyl-transferases. Named after the first three proteins in which it was identified: Su(var)3–9, Enhancer of zeste and Trithorax.

shelterin: A protein complex that protects telomeres from DNA repair mechanisms and controls telomerase activity.

SINE (Short Interspersed Nuclear Element): A class of repetitive sequence elements generally derived by reverse transcription of short RNA species (a few hundred nucleotides) and able to transpose to new sites using transposases provided by longer elements. Alu elements are typical SINEs.

single nucleotide polymorphism (SNP): Small sequence variation arising in a population.

siRNA: Short interfering RNA. A class of short, mostly double stranded RNAs 20–24 base pairs long, produced by a Dicer enzyme. It has a gene silencing effect by targeting a RISC complex to cleave a homologous mRNA.

sirtuin: one of a class of enzymes related to yeast Sir2. Many sirtuins are deacetylases but act by transferring the acetyl to NAD^+, producing nicotinamide.

stem cell: An undifferentiated or incompletely differentiated replicative cell that can generate one or more cell lineages that proceed to differentiate.

stochastic: An adjective describing a random or probabilistic type of event or distribution.

Su(var): Suppressor of variegation gene (SUV in vertebrates). Generally a component of heterochromatin or a function important for heterochromatin formation.

SWI/SNF nucleosome remodeling complex: A family of nucleosome remodeling complexes whose catalytic subunit belongs to the SWI/SNF class of ATP-dependent helicases.

TAD, Topologically Associated Domain: A chromatin domain defined by preferentially internal contacts and infrequent contacts with adjacent chromatin regions. Formed by loop extrusion driven by cohesin.

TAF, TBP-Associated Factor: One of a set of protein complexes that associate with the DNA-binding TBP factor and are involved in transcription initiation by RNA polymerase II.

TBP (TATA-Binding Protein): A factor that binds to the TATA box, a TATA-rich short DNA sequence found about 30 bp upstream of many promoters. It is a constituent of the general transcription factor TFIID and helps to position RNA polymerase II on the transcription start site.

Telomerase: A protein complex with reverse transcriptase activity that includes a specific RNA molecule that serves as template to elongate telomeres.

telomere: The terminal region of chromosomal DNA. In most species it is a region of repetitive, short, G-rich motifs that recruit telomerase and other proteins that protect the DNA ends and permit terminal DNA replication.

TET (Ten-Eleven Translocation) protein: A class of proteins that demethylate 5 methyl cytosine through a series of oxidative steps that begin with hydroxymethyl cytosine.

topoisomerase: An enzyme that allows changes in the winding topology of DNA molecules by opening the sugar-phosphate backbone of one or both DNA strands and allowing the unwinding of helical turns.

transcription burst: The tendency of gene transcription to occur in bursts of transcriptional initiation followed by periods of inactivity.

transcription factories: Nuclear foci enriched in RNA Polymerase II where multiple genes are transcribed.

translocase: An activity that produces the progression of a protein along the DNA, generally associated with ATP hydrolysis.

transposase: A protein that mediates the insertion of a transposable element into a new genomic site.

transposon or transposable element: An invasive sequence element that can insert into a new genomic site.

transvection: A term derived from *Drosophila* genetics, referring to the ability of a regulatory sequence to control the activity of a gene elsewhere in the genome, usually through looping or pairing.

TSS: transcription start site

Tudor domain: A conserved protein domain forming an aromatic cage that binds methylated lysines or arginines.

UTR: Untranslated Region. A part of a mRNA sequence that is not translated into protein. Generally, a 5′ UTR is at the 5′ end and a 3′ UTR at the 3′ end.

van der Waals interactions: Weak electrostatic forces resulting from molecular dipoles or induced dipoles.

variegation: Uneven expression of a gene in different cells of a tissue, generally resulting from heterochromatic or Polycomb silencing effects.

WD40 domain: Protein domain of around 40 amino acids often ending in tryptophan (W) and aspartate (D). Most frequently found in seven repeats arranged as propeller blades in a circular protein structure.

Xic, X inactivation center: A region of the mammalian X chromosome that contains the *Xist* gene and other functions essential for X chromosome inactivation.

Xist RNA: X-Inactive Specific Transcript. A non-coding RNA species produced by the *Xist* gene on the mammalian X chromosome. Expressed only from the inactive X, it is associated with it and is essential for X inactivation.

zinc finger: A protein structural motif that uses cysteines and histidines to coordinate one or more zinc ions to produce a fold.

Subject Index

aberrant clonal expansion, 420, 421
  driver mutation, 420
acetylation, 426
Acetyl CoA, 53, 54, 346
A compartment, 296, 297
Active demethylation, 320, 361
Adenine Methylation, 108, 109
AEBP2, 245, 252, 256
aging, 407, 411
  aging of individuals, 411
  Chromatin and Aging, 425
  homeostatic mechanisms, 410
  organismal aging, 408
  replicative aging, 408
Ago, 173, 178
Airn lncRNA, 368–371, 377
Allele-Specific Expression, 357
alpha helix, 17, 19, 21
alternative splicing, 131, 133, 140,
  440–442, 444, 445
Alu element, 136, 143
Alzheimer's disease, 419
Angelman Syndrome, 372
ANRIL, 259, 260
Antennapedia, 214–216, 266

antisense RNA, 168, 464
antisense transcription, 369, 371
apoptosis, 409, 417, 432
Archaea, 32, 35
architectural proteins, 294
arginine methylation, 102
Argonaute protein, Ago, 170–172,
  174, 176, 177, 464
Ash1, 60, 266, 268, 269
Asx, 262
Asymmetric epigenetic inheritance,
  376
ATAC assay, 198, 447
  ATAC-seq, 450
  Tagmentation, 449
  Tn5 transposase, 447
  Tn5 transposon, 447
Aubergine, 177
axis of pseudo-symmetry, 36, 39, 79

band-interband pattern, 125–127,
  130, 275
Barr body, 390, 393
Base Excision Repair, 98
base pairing, 5, 12

base stacking interactions, 8, 9
B compartment, 296–298
Beckwith–Wiedemann Syndrome, 365
biotin tagging, 453
bisulfite sequencing, 91
bisulfite treatment, 89, 99
bivalent promoter, 256, 267, 269, 334, 335, 345, 353, 419
blastocyst, 320, 321, 325–329
blastomere, 321, 322
BLM helicase, 7
BMP, Bone Morphogenetic Protein, 323
body segments, 213
Bone Morphogenetic Protein, 323
bromodomain, 55, 56, 80, 85, 105, 188
BTB/POZ domain, 283, 286
burst frequency, 210
burst size, 210

3C, 291, 366, 367, 402, 452
3C methods, 450, 467
    4C method, 453
    5C method, 452
    Chromatin Conformation Capture, 450
    Hi-C method, 453
calico cats, 390, 391
Calypso, 262, 263
cancer frequency, 420
canonical PRC1, 257
Cas9, 472–475
CBP/p300, 195, 196, 262, 264, 270–272
CBX, 248, 249, 253, 256, 257, 262, 264
cell cycle, 412

Cell cycle checkpoint, 411
Cell cycle progression, 413
cell proliferation, 24, 57
cellular aging, 24
cellular senescence, 407, 422, 423, 428, 429, 432, 435, 446
    loss of heterochromatin, 425
    oncogene-induced senescence, 424
    senescence-associated heterochromatin foci, 424
    senescence-associated secretory phenotype, 424
centromere, 27, 28, 60, 73, 122, 134, 137, 141, 145, 146
    histone H3 variant CENP-A, 28
    kinetochore, 27
Chargaff's Rule, 3
ChIP, 240, 467
chromatid, 122
Chromatin Assembly Factor-1, 74
Chromatin compartments, 295, 297 301
    compartment A, 295
    compartment B, 295
Chromatin Conformation Capture, 290, 291, 310, 311, 477
    contact frequency, 292
chromatin fiber, 32, 38, 42, 84, 85, 114, 148, 261
    10 nm fiber, 41
    30 nm fiber, 42
    electron microscope visualization, 43
    Higher Order Structures, 41
chromatin immunoprecipitation, 130, 148, 161, 192, 226, 236, 237, 239, 298, 334, 429, 451, 454, 455, 459
    CUT&RUN, 456
    native ChIP, 456

chromatin loop, 193, 198, 280, 282, 283, 285, 286, 288–290, 300, 301, 304, 305, 308, 311, 367, 370
  loop anchor, 288, 293, 309
chromatin remodeling, 80, 84, 85, 105, 110, 270
chromatin replication, 68, 69, 241
chromocenter, 124, 149, 155
chromodomain, 61, 62, 66, 80, 157–159, 166, 174, 182, 225, 248–250, 252–254, 264, 273, 386, 388
chromoshadow domain, 158, 159, 166
Chromosome breakage, 410
chromosome condensation, 67
chromosome conformation capture, 290, 291, 310, 311, 477
chromosome painting, 114, 115
chromosomes, 43
chromosome territory, 114–116
CIZ1, 398
Clonal Expansion, 419
c-Myc, 332, 344, 345, 347, 348, 350, 394
coccid insects, 380
cognitive processes, 419
cohesin, 27, 28, 195, 198, 199, 271, 287–290, 304, 305, 309, 311, 378, 382–384, 404
  loop extrusion, 288
  loss of cohesin, 306
  Structural Maintenance of Chromosomes protein, 287
compartment A, 307
compartment B, 307
COMPASS, 267–269, 271, 273
COMPASS complex, 266

condensin, 28, 287, 382–384
core histones, 32–36, 39, 40, 45, 47, 68, 70
core promoter elements, 209
CpG island, 65, 90–92, 96, 97, 99–101, 189, 190, 195, 255–258, 266, 269, 334, 335, 363, 426
CRISPR, 176
CRISPR-Cas methods, 352, 354, 460, 465, 477
CRISPR-Cas genome editing, 474
CRISPR-Cas methods, 470
  CRISPR-Cas applications, 474
  CRISPR locus, 472
  CRISPR mechanisms, 471
  CRISPR versatility, 475
  guide RNA (sgRNA), 473
  Prime sequence editing, 475
  Proto-spacer Adjacent Motif (PAM), 473
CRISPR, guide RNA, 472
crRNA, 473
cryo-electron microscopy, 84, 457, 477
cryo-EM, 458, 459
CTCF, 19, 287–289, 293, 294, 299, 304–306, 308–310, 365–367, 377, 396, 403, 404, 444
cut&Run method, 456
CXXC domain, 106, 255, 269, 335, 336
CXXC motif, 95, 97, 99–101
cyclin, 411, 412
cyclin-dependent kinase, 411–414, 423
cytosine demethylase, 97
cytosine demethylation, 98
  5-hydroxymethylcytosine, 97

TET Demethylase, 97
cytosine methylation, 88, 110

DamID, 116, 118, 298, 430, 459,
  460, 467, 476, 477
  Dam methylation, 459
  Targeted DamID, 460
de novo DNA methylase, 362, 325
  Dnmt3A, 92
  Dnmt3B, 92
de novo DNA methyltransferase, 100
de novo DNMT, 102
de novo methylation, 95, 99
Dicer, 170–174, 181, 464
differentially methylated region, 360,
  361, 364
direct lineage conversion, 351, 352,
  355
DMR, 362
DNA adenine methyltransferase,
  Dam, 459
DNA-binding protein, 16, 17, 19, 28,
  44, 45, 46, 54, 80
DNA damage, 60, 75, 81, 167, 410,
  414, 423, 427, 432, 435, 442, 443,
  444, 446
DNA damage checkpoint, 414
DNA damage repair, 67, 167, 419
DNA demethylation, 319, 345, 362
  Active demethylation, 318
  passive demethylation, 316, 317,
    320, 361
DNA double helix, 2
  alternative DNA structures, 4, 6
  Base pairing, 3
  cooperativity, 10
  degrees of freedom, 11
  DNA helix twist, 8

DNA supercoil, 13
  major groove, 8
  melting, 9
  minor groove, 8
  persistence length, 11
  superhelical turns, 14
  Torsional Stress, 12
  writhe, 14
DNA methylation, 58, 87, 99, 101,
  105, 110, 116, 145, 155, 191, 207,
  269, 313, 314, 316, 331, 336, 337,
  339, 346, 349, 350, 360, 362, 363,
  375, 378, 396, 400, 404, 426, 444,
  446
  de novo methylation, 92
  DNA methylation in oocytes, 104
  DNA methylation in sperm, 103
  Effects of Histone Modifications,
    100
  gene body methylation, 101
  global DNA demethylation, 103
  hemimethylated CpG, 94
  maintenance methylation, 92, 94,
    96
  recruitment to transposable
    elements, 102
DNA methyltransferase, 92, 93, 109,
  110, 302
  de novo DNA methylase, 92
  DNMT1, 94
DNA polymerase, 20, 70
DNA replication, 6, 13, 16, 20, 24,
  60, 69, 74, 84, 85, 138, 175, 300,
  316, 376, 414, 419
  lagging strand, 21
  leading strand, 21
  Okazaki fragments, 21
  replication fork, 13

DNase 1 hypersensitive site, 197, 276
DNA sequencing, 127, 128, 465
DNMT1, 95, 96, 98, 99, 101, 102, 104, 108, 109, 155, 317, 337, 354, 361
DNMT3, 60, 99, 103–105, 108, 110, 317, 320, 336, 345, 361, 418
DNMT3A, 94, 418
DNMT3B, 94
dosage compensation, 384
dosage compensation complex, 384, 386–389
DOT1, 59
double helix, 3–5, 8–16, 36–38, 43–45, 69, 78
double-stranded RNA, 169, 172
DRB Sensitivity-Inducing Factor, 204
Drosophila, 26, 122, 249
DSIF, 205, 206, 209
DXZ4 domain, 403, 404
Dyskerin, 25
dystrophin, 184
dystrophin gene, 133, 443

E3 ubiquitin ligase, 68
E3 ubiquitin transferas, 246
ecdysone, 126, 128
EED, 273
electron microscopy, 31, 41, 43
  cryo-electron microscopy, 42, 456
Electron transport, 409
embryoid body, 330
embryonic stem cell, 24, 120, 128, 196, 197, 256, 257, 309, 320, 323, 327, 330, 329, 335, 338, 343, 353, 355, 391, 394, 404, 428, 435
EpiESC, 325
naïve embryonic stem cell, 325–328

primed embryonic stem cell, 325, 328
Emerin, 119, 120
endoplasmic reticulum, 117, 119
enhancer, 80, 185, 186, 188, 191–193, 195–198, 209–211, 226–230, 262, 270–272, 275, 277, 279, 280, 282, 284, 285, 288, 290, 293, 294, 304, 307, 309, 312, 365, 366, 367
  super-enhancer, 309
Enhancer of zeste, 156, 222, 225, 236
  Ezh2, 239
enhancer RNA, 194
epiblast, 322–327, 329
Epidermal Differentiation, 338, 339
epidermis, 415–418, 422
  keratinocytes, 417
erosion, 24
Esc, 238, 239, 241–245, 324, 325, 332, 334, 336, 340, 347
Esc/Eed, 62
euchromatin, 111
exon, 138–141, 208, 385
exosome, 194, 206, 424
extra sex combs, 222, 223
E(z), 58, 237–239, 241, 243

FAcilitates Chromatin Transcription, 207
FACT, 211
FANCJ, 7
farnesylation, 299, 436, 437
feeder layer, 324, 328
Fertilization, 314
fertilized egg, 316, 317, 318
FGF, 328
Fibroblast Growth Factor, 324

formaldehyde-assisted isolation of regulatory elements, 198
frameshift mutation, 16

G9a, 104, 105, 109, 110, 160, 336, 369, 370, 371
GAGA Factor, GAF, 232, 236
gene browser, 161
gene dosage, 379
General Transcription Factors, GTF, 55, 185, 187, 188, 189, 191, 199, 201
TFIIA, 200
TFIIB, 200
TFIID, 200
TFIIE, 200
TFIIH, 199, 200
TFII250, 55
TFIIIC, 55
genetic imprinting, 357, 358, 391
Evolution of Imprinting, 371
genetic recombination, 149
genome architecture, 123, 193, 275
genome browser, 118, 129, 130, 240
genome composition, 131
genome editing, 470, 475, 476
Genome size, 131
genomic imprinting, 377, 378
evolution of genomic imprinting, 378
genomic reprogramming, 391, 404
germ cell, 24
germ line, 90, 91, 99, 103, 104, 137, 175, 177–180, 362, 376
glucocorticoid receptor, 374
G-quadruplex, 5, 6, 7, 22, 28
guide RNA, 172, 173
gypsy insulator, 281, 284, 285

5hmC, 98, 99, 318, 419
H2A.X, 81
H2AZ, 76
H3.3, histone variant, 81, 84, 316
H3K4 methylase, 195, 273
H3K4 methylation, 102, 147, 148, 164, 268, 269, 271
H3K9 methylase, 102
H3K9 methylation, 23, 101, 102, 104, 105, 147, 156, 157, 159–163, 174–176, 178, 179, 298
H3K9 methyltransferase, 96, 107
G9a, 96
SETDB1, 96
SUV39, 96
H3K27 acetylation, 262, 269
H3K27 demethylase, 263
UTX, 263
H3K27 demethylation, 271
H3K27 methylation, 197, 225, 238, 240–242, 262, 265, 269
H3K27 methyltranferase, 239
H3K27 trimethylation, 256
H3S10 phosphorylation, 163, 164, 175, 264
H3S28 phosphorylation, 264, 265
H4K16 acetylation, 388
H4K20 methylation, 160
HAT, 55
Hayflick limit, 24, 422
HDAC, 119, 163
heat shock, 126, 127, 202, 235, 275–277
helicase, 7, 13, 69–71, 77, 200, 387
helix-turn-helix, 17–19, 29, 217, 218
hematopoietic cells, 24
hematopoietic stem cell, 340, 341, 415
hemimethylation, 95, 96, 108, 155, 337

hermaphrodite, 382, 384
heterochrmatin spreading, 161
heterochromatic genes, 161
heterochromatic silencing, 146,
  150–152, 154, 156, 163, 168, 181,
  260, 404, 426
heterochromatic spreading, 158, 163
heterochromatin, 23, 31, 42–44, 46,
  59–61, 88, 92, 102, 107–109, 111,
  113–115, 117, 121–123, 145, 148,
  296–299, 424–426, 455
  heterochromatin properties, 147
  heterochromatin spreading, 149,
  152
heterochromatin gene, 162, 182
HGPS, 437–440
Hi-C, 292–296, 300, 301, 305, 306,
  311, 477
High Mobility Group HMG proteins,
  81, 82, 85
  HMGA, 82
  HMGB, 82
  HMGN, 82
hippocampus, 419
HIRA, 75
histone acetylase, 163, 195
histone acetylation, 145, 298
histone acetyltransferase domain, 386
histone acetyltransferases, 54
  GNAT family, 55
  MYST family, 55
  p300/CBP, 55
  PCAF, 55
histone chaperone, 56, 68, 71, 73
  Chromatin Assembly Factor-1, 71
histone deacetylase, 57, 104, 107,
  121, 174, 262, 302
  inhibitors, 163

Histone Deacetylation, 163
histone demethylase nomenclature,
  65, 66
histone demethylases, 64, 65
histone fold, 38
histone genes, 46, 72
histone H2A variant, 197
H2A.Z, 81, 197
histone H3.3, 75
histone H3 variant, 197
histone acetylase, 167
histone lysine methyltransferase,
  58–60
histone mark, 54
histone methylases, 121
histone methylation, 59
histone methyltransferase, 156, 157,
  225, 302
  Set2, 101
histone modifications, 47, 50, 52,
  145, 147, 195
  Arginine methylation, 51
  histone code, 52
  histone modifications Table, 48
  Histone Phosphorylation, 65
  Histone Ubiquitylation, 67
  Lysine acetylation, 53
  Lysine methylation, 51, 57
  modification readers, 52
  modification writers, 52
  phospho-switch, 66
  ubiquitylation, 59
histone phosphorylation, 66, 67, 163
Histone Regulator A, HIRA, 74
histones, 31, 34, 38, 40
  Arginine Methylation, 61
  core histones, 31
  histone fold, 35

histone tails, 33
histone variants, 47
histone tails, 36–38, 47, 52–54, 56, 58–60, 62, 65
histone ubiquitylation, 68, 96, 109
histone variants, 72, 74, 85, 316, 425
  CENP-A, 73
  H2AX, 67, 75
  H2A.Z, 75
  Histone H3.3, 74
HK4 methylation, 265
HMGA protein, 83
HMGB proteins, 83
HMGN, 83
HMG proteins, 84
homeodomain, 217, 218
homeotic genes, 213, 214, 220, 221, 223, 262
  homeotic mutation, 214
  homeotic phenotype, 214, 215
  Hox gene cluster, 215, 217–219, 263, 272
Hoogsteen pairing, 3, 5
Hox, 18
Hox clusters, 220
Hox gene, 215, 217–219, 223, 226, 263, 230, 268
  evolutionary conservation, 218
HP1, 23, 29, 39, 61, 62, 103, 104, 107, 109, 119, 121, 147, 155, 157–161, 163, 164, 167, 168, 173–176, 179, 182, 248, 265, 299, 301–303, 361, 362, 426, 428, 433–436, 443, 444
HP1 hinge region, 158, 166, 167, 303
Hutchinson-Gilford Progeria, 435, 436
hypoblast, 322, 327

2i/LIF, 326–328

ICR, 363, 366–370
IDR, 166, 303, 304
Igf2 gene, 377
Igf2/H19, 367
Igf2/H19 locus, 364, 366, 372, 378
IGF2 receptor, 368
Igf2r, gene, 367–369
Igf2r locus, 368
Igf2r promoter, 369, 370
imaginal disc, 227–230
imprinted expression, 366, 377
imprinted gene, 350, 357–360, 371–373
Imprinting Control Region, 361, 362, 364, 365, 378
inactive X, 397, 398, 400, 401, 403, 438
inactive X chromosome, 390
  Architecture of the Inactive X, 402
induced pluripotent cell, 344
induced pluripotent stem cell, 344, 438
Ink4a/Arf, 259, 260, 339, 340, 413, 423
inner cell mass, 321–323, 325–327, 329
inner cell mass cell, 327
INO80, 81
insulator, 278–280, 282–286, 293–295, 305, 310–312, 365
  Tandem insulators, 282
insulator-binding proteins, 283
insulator body, 285, 286
insulators, 310
intercalating dyes 14
  ethidium bromide, 15
  proflavine, 15
  thalidomide, 15

intermediate filament, 118, 119, 121, 142
interphase, 31, 41, 43, 85, 111, 113, 116, 122, 123, 142
intestinal epithelium, 416, 422
crypts, 416, 417
villi, 416
intrinsically disordered region, 107, 164, 165, 199, 201, 210, 302, 310
intron, 131–133, 136, 138–141, 161, 162, 208, 227, 440, 441
inverted nuclear organization, 297
rod photoreceptor cells, 295
Ion Torrent sequencing, 21
iPSC, 348–350
iPS cell, 347, 439
ISWI, 78, 81, 387

Jarid2, 245, 252, 256
Jumonji domain, 64, 65

KAISO, 106
Kcnq1 promoter, 370, 371
Kcnqi locus, 370
Kcnq1 gene, 370, 373
Kcnqiot1 lncRNA, 370
Kcnq1ot1 promoter, 370, 371
KDM2B, 101, 255, 257, 345
keratinocyte, 338, 418
kinetochore, 28, 73
kleisin, 288
KLF4, 332, 344, 345, 347, 394
KMD2B, 335
kinases, 424

lac repressor, 18
LAD, 297, 299, 300, 332, 429, 430, 431

lagging strand, 22, 69–71
lambda repressor, 18
lamin, 116, 119–122, 142, 149, 295, 297–299, 423–425, 427–429, 431, 435–440, 444–446
farnesylation, 120
lamin-associated proteins, 433
lamina, 142, 143, 332, 426, 429, 432
Lamin-associated domain, 117, 118, 295, 298, 312
lamin associated protein, 119, 120
lamin B receptor, 120, 295, 297, 425, 434
lamins, 332
LAP, 428, 436
Late Replicating Region, 123
LBR, 299, 428, 436
leading strand, 22, 69, 70, 71
leucine zipper, 17, 18, 28, 29
Leukemia Inhibitory Factor, 323
2i/LIF, 325
LIF, 324, 325
ligase, 96
lineage-determining factors, 351
LINEs, long interspersed nuclear elements, 102, 103, 136, 137, 427
linker DNA, 82, 84
linker histone, 31, 38–41, 82, 84
liquid phase condensation, 164, 166, 182, 201, 301, 302, 310, 311, 400
liquid phase condensate, 107, 113, 164, 167, 182, 210, 260, 398
liquid phase separation, 165, 304, 310
liquid phase transition, 303
lncRNA, 367–370, 392, 393, 395, 396
longevity, 411, 441, 445
long non-coding RNA, 259

long terminal repeat, *see* also under
  transposable element, 102, 103,
  135
loop anchor, 306
loop extrusion, 195, 289, 304
loss of cohesin, 307, 308
lysine acetylation, 54, 58
lysine methylation, 58, 66

5mC, 88, 98, 99, 105, 108, 145, 316,
  318, 320, 419, 444
5mCpN, 108
5-methyl cytosine, 87, 97, 106, 354
  Detection of 5mC, 89
5-methylcytosine deamination, 90
6mA, 88, 108, 109
m6A RNA methylation, 210
m6A RNA methyltransferase, 399
macroH2A, 400
maintenance methylase, 95
major groove, 14, 16–19, 21, 218,
  315
marsupials, 372, 390
MBD proteins, 106
MeCP2, 98, 106–109, 302, 404, 405,
  444
Mediator, 193, 198–200, 202, 210,
  271, 288, 290, 458
melting, 10, 11
Mesenchymal stem cell, 433, 434
methylation imprint, 362, 363
methyl binding proteins, 105, 109
  KAISO, 105
  Methyl Binding Domain, 105, 106
methyl-C-binding proteins, 98
micrococcal nuclease, 32, 33, 197,
  295, 426, 456
minor groove, 14, 16, 17, 37
miRNA, 170–172, 333, 364

mitochondria, 408, 409
mitosis, 27, 31, 67, 121, 122, 134,
  146, 300, 411, 412
mitotic chromosome, 111, 112, 145,
  146, 148
mitotic spindle, 73
MLE, 386, 387
MLL, 60, 196, 206, 264, 266–272
MOF, 386–388
monoallelic expression, 357, 361,
  363–365, 375
monotremes, 372
morula, 320–322
mosaic tissues, 390, 420
mRNA capping, 202
MSL, 386
MSL1, 387, 389
MSL2, 385–387, 389, 390
MSL3, 387, 388
multipotent stem cell, 340
mutations, 420
  mutation frequency, 420
MyoD, 351

10 nm fiber, 42
30-nm chromatin, 84
30 nm fiber, 43, 148
N6-methyladenine, 87
NAD$^+$ (Nicotinamide Adenine
  Dinucleotide), 57
NADH, 409
naïve embryonic stem cell, 345, 349,
  350
naïve ESC, 346
naive pluripotency, 353
naïve state, 332
Nanog, 345
NANOG, 320, 332–334, 344, 375,
  394

nanopore sequencing, 89, 91, 468, 469, 476

Negative Elongation Factor (NELF), 204–206

Nesprin, 119, 120

N-terminal tails,37

Neural stem cells, 418, 419

neurogenesis, 419

next generation sequencing, 89, 188, 292, 449, 452, 453, 455, 466, 477
    Ion Torrent sequencing, 467
    massively parallel sequencing, 466
    pyrosequencing, 467

niche, 340, 376, 415

NMR, 458

non-coding RNA, 133

nuclear envelope, 23, 114, 116–120, 122, 149, 295, 296, 299, 300

nuclear lamina, 117–120, 122, 285, 286, 295, 297–299, 307, 309, 424, 425, 428, 430, 433, 435, 440

nuclear magnetic resonance, 456, 457

nuclear pore, 118, 119

nuclear speckle, 302

Nuclear transplantation, 319

nucleolus, 111–115, 117, 122, 127, 142, 149, 300, 302, 310, 425

nucleosomal DNA, 32, 36, 38, 45, 47, 59, 82, 207

nucleosome, 31, 38, 42
    DNA Accessibility, 45
    DNA-binding protein, 43
    dyad axis, 78
    linker DNA, 38
    nucleosome occupancy, 138
    reconstitution in vitro, 40

nucleosome assembly, 84

Nucleosome Destabilizing Factor, 208

nucleosome-free region, 193, 194, 196, 197

nucleosome occupancy, 139

nucleosome positioning, 190, 426

nucleosome remodeler, 195

nucleosome remodeling, 46, 54, 63, 75–78, 79, 83, 106, 191, 269
    INO80, 75
    SWI/SNF, 77
    SWR-C, 75

Nucleotide triphosphates, 1, 2

NuRD, 106

nurturing behavior, 374
    nurturing-induced epigenetic state, 374

OCT4, 320, 332–334, 336, 344, 345, 348, 375, 394

O-GlcNAc transferase, 263

Okazaki fragment, 22, 69, 70

oncogene-induced senescence, 425

oocyte, 103, 314, 315, 319, 343, 350, 351, 354, 362, 363, 375, 391, 404

oogenesis, 323

organismal aging, 411, 419, 427, 435, 440

organismal senescence, 432

organoid, 331, 354, 417, 446

OSKM factors, 344, 345–348, 351, 352

π electrons, 8, 15

p53, 39

p300/CBP, 61

PAF, 207, 211

pairing-dependent silencing, 222, 234, 236

Pairing effects, 233
    proximity effects, 233

palindromic sequence, 3, 5, 18
parental conflict, 368
parental conflict model, 358, 372
parental imprint, 357
   Methylation Imprint, 359
part, 24
pausing, 206
Pc, 236, 237, 264, 265
PCAF, 56
PcG, 221–224, 228, 230, 231,
   234–237, 239, 269, 334, 335
PCGF, 246–248, 250, 254–257
PcG proteins, 226
PcG repression, 338, 345
PcG silencing, 427
PCL, 245
PCNA, 69, 96
Polymerase Chain Reaction (PCR)
   methods, 460
pericentric, 122
pericentric heterochromatin, 124,
   125, 142, 145–147
pericentromeric heterochromatin, 161
persistence length, 12, 451
PEV, 152, 154, 159, 161, 163, 181
PGCF, 253
Ph, 251
PH, 253, 254, 260, 263
PHD finger, 63, 64, 96, 105, 188,
   192, 264
Pho, 232, 251, 252, 255
phosphodiester bond, 4, 184
phosphodiester linkage, 1
phospho-switch, 175, 264
PIC, 188, 191, 193, 194, 199–202, 458
ping-pong amplification, 103, 177
ping-pong mechanism, 178
Pioneer, 195
pioneer factor, 46, 195, 196, 270, 346

piRNA, 103, 170, 175, 176, 179–181
   piRNA production, 177
piRNA cluster, 175–177, 179
   Transcription of piRNA Clusters,
      178
piRNA production, 178
PIWI, 103, 104, 178, 179, 182
PIWI protein, 170, 176, 182
   Aubergine, 176
placental mammals, 372
Pleiohomeotic, 251
pluripotency, 322, 338, 343, 345,
   346, 348, 349, 352–355
pluripotency factor, 310, 320,
   332–334, 337, 339, 344, 347, 375,
   394, 404
pluripotent, 320, 323, 325–327
Pluripotent State, 331
pluripotent stem cell, 328, 329, 354
polar granules, 302
polyadenylation signal, 208, 209
Polycomb, 59–62, 68, 101, 109, 137,
   189, 197, 220–222, 224, 229, 231,
   233–235, 238, 248, 250, 256,
   260–263, 266–269, 272, 293, 303,
   304, 309, 339, 402, 405, 423, 446,
   454
   PcG Protein, 225
   Polycomb body, 235
   Polycomb Group Genes, 220
   Polycomb Mechanisms, 213
   Polycomb silencing, 230
Polycomb Group genes, 220
Polycomblike, 245
   PCL, 245
Polycomb repression, 337, 340, 355,
   418, 429
Polycomb repressive complex, 308,
   332, 333, 368, 455

Polycomb Repressive Complex 1
(PRC1), 62, 225
Polycomb Repressive Complex 2
(PRC2), 59, 62, 107, 225
polycomb response element, 311,
226–228, 279
PRE-dependent silencing, 231
Polycomb silencing, 244, 245, 257,
260–262
polydactyly, 220
Polyhomeotic, 249
Polymerase-Associated Factor 1, 206
polytene chromosome, 122–126, 130,
131, 142, 147–149, 155, 275, 389,
294
chromocenter, 122
puffs, 126
band–interband pattern, 124
position-effect variegation, 150, 151,
179, 182
variegated eye color, 151
Positive-Transcription Elongation
Factor b, 204, 205
Posterior sex comb, 222, 236
POZ/BTB domain, 105, 106
Prader–Willi Syndrome, 372
PRC1, 60, 226, 236–238, 240, 246,
248–252, 255, 256, 258–263, 272,
334, 369–371, 399, 400
Canonical PRC1, 249
non-canonical PRC1, 250, 254
variant PRC1, 254
PRC2, 60, 67, 226, 236–242,
244, 245, 249, 252, 256–260,
262, 268–270, 272, 334, 335,
339, 369–371, 398, 400, 458
PRE, 229–236, 238, 240, 244, 251,
252, 255, 261, 266, 268, 269, 272

Pre-Initiation Complex, 186, 192,
198, 200, 211
Primase, 21, 69
primed ESC, 346
primed state, 327, 332
progeria, 439
progeria syndromes, 432
Hutchinson–Gilford Progeria
Syndrome, 432
Werner Syndrome, 432
Progerin, 437, 439, 440, 444
proliferative advantage, 420
promoter, 185, 186, 192, 193
Promoter access, 191
promoter elements, 187, 262
promoter motifs, 186, 187, 188,
190
Promoter regulation, 186
promoter types, 188
promoter upstream transcripts,
194
Type III promoters, 189
Type II promoters, 189
Type I promoters, 189
pronucleus, 315, 317, 318, 319
Protamine, 314–316, 353
proteasome, 67, 247
protein arginine N-methytransferase,
61
proteostasis, 407
protospacer-adjacent motif (PAM),
474
proximity effect, 260
proximo-distal axis, 219
PR-Set7, 60
PSC, 237, 246, 331
P-TEFB, 332
puffs, 127, 128, 276

quantitative real-time PCR, 462, 464
    quantification cycle, 462

random X inactivation, 391, 394
reactive oxygen species, 409, 410
repetitive sequence, 131–133, 145,
    147, 149, 161, 162, 168
replication fork, 22, 68–71, 74, 81,
    191, 241
replicative senescence, 414, 427
reprogramming, 340, 341, 343–350,
    352–355, 446
retinoblastoma protein Rb, 412, 413
retrotransposon, 28, 142
retrovirus, 103
Rett Syndrome, 107, 108, 405
reverse transcriptase, 24, 26, 102,
    103, 136, 137, 462, 475
REX1, 396, 405
REX1 factor, 395
Rhino, 179
Rhino protein, 178
ribosomal RNA, 111, 113, 115, 183
RING, 247, 248, 250, 253, 255, 272
RING domain, 96, 246, 386, 387
RISC, 172, 173
RITS, 174
R-loop, 138
RMB15, 399
RNA capping, 178, 205
    mRNA 5' cap, 205
RNA-dependent RNA polymerase,
    174
RNA-directed RNA polymerase, 173
RNA guide, 170
RNAi, 168, 169, 173, 182, 464
RNAi knockdown, 464, 465
RNA-Induced silencing complex,
    170, 171, 464

RNA-interference, 181
RNA Pol I, 115, 183
RNA Pol II, 59, 60, 74, 139, 148,
    183–187, 191, 194, 198, 199, 201,
    203, 204, 206, 208, 256, 258, 261,
    266, 267, 269, 303, 332, 335, 399,
    458
RNA Pol II C-terminal domain, 199,
    200–202
    CTD, 203, 205–207, 211
    C-terminal domain, 184
RNA pol III, 183
RNA polyadenylation, 178
RNA polymerase, 46, 80, 127, 154
RNA polymerase II, *see also* RNA
    Pol II, 101, 126, 178, 210
RNA polymerase III, *see also* RNA
    Pol III, 136
RNA splicing, 139, 172, 178, 202,
    385, 436, 442
    alternative splicing, 120
    cryptic splice site, 439
    effect of DNA methylation
        splicing, 443
    splice donor, 140
    splice site, 140, 440
RNA splicing factors, 167
RNF2 ubiquitin ligase, 395
RNF12, 396, 405
rod photoreceptors, 297
roX, 387, 388, 389
roX RNA, 386
rRNA, 300
RYBP, 254

S-adenosyl methionine, 51, 58, 156,
    157, 346
SAM domain, 249, 251, 260, 263
SAM motif, 249

sarcopenia, 407
satellite sequence, 132–134, 145, 146, 168, 181, 427, 435
SCM, 251–255, 261
SCNT, 347, 350, 351
scs, 277, 310
senescence, 24, 430, 431, 433
senescence-associated heterochromatin foci, 425
senescence-associated secretory phenotype, 427
separate liquid phase, 115
SET1, 207, 206, 211
SETD2 methyltransferase, 59, 104, 207
SETDB1, 102, 103, 105, 160, 332, 361, 362
SET domain, 58–60, 105, 156, 157, 225, 266, 269
sex comb, 221, 224
Sex Comb on Midleg, 249
sex determination, 381–385, 382, 406
Sex-lethal gene, 384, 385
sgRNA, 475
Shelterin, 23
Short Interspersed Nuclear Element, 136
SINEs, short interspersed nulcear elements, 102
single molecule sequencing, 467
nanopore sequencing, 468
Pacific Biosciences, 468
Single Nucleotide Polymorphisms, 360
siRNA, 170, 172–175, 181, 464, 465
sister chromatid, 27, 28
SMC, 310, 311, 383

somatic cell nuclear transfer, 355
somatic cell nuclear transplantation, 342, 343
Somatic Mutations, 419
SOX2, 332–334, 344, 345, 348, 354, 394
Special Chromatin Structure, 276, 277, 310
SPEN, 399, 405
sperm, 316, 362, 363, 375
spermatogenesis, 323
spermatozoon, 314, 315
sperm DNA, 320
spindle, 27
splice donor site, 141
spliceosome, 140–142
splice site, 441, 442, 444
splicing, 140–142
alternative splicing, 138
splicing body, 302
SRY gene, 381
stress granule, 302
Structural Maintenance of Chromosomes protein, 287
Su(3)-9, 176
Su(Hw), 283–286, 310
supercoil, 14
super-enhancer, 310
superoxide dismutase, 410
Suppressor of Hairy wing, 281
Suppressor of zeste2, 222, 246
Suppressor of zeste12, 222
suppressors of variegation, 153, 164
SUV4-20, 160
SUV4-20H1, 60
SUV39, 105
SUV39H, 119, 433–435
SUV39H1, 102, 156, 160

Su(var)3-9, 58, 154, 156, 158–160, 168, 174, 179, 225
Su(var) gene, 154, 157, 221
Su(z)12, 238, 239, 241, 242, 244
SWI/SNF, 78, 80, 81, 261, 266, 269
SWR1, 81
SXL, 390

T3 promoter, 452
T7 promoter, 452
TAF, 188, 191, 192, 200
TATA box, 187–189, 200
TATA-box binding protein, TBP, 17, 178, 187, 200
TBP-associated factor, 187
telomerase, 7, 24–26, 422, 440
telomerase RNA TERC, 29
telomere, 7, 20–24, 26–29, 112, 137, 141, 155, 181, 439, 445, 451
    D-loop, 23
    dyskerin, 24
    Shelterin, 22
    telomerase RNA TERC, 24
    telomere shortening, 23, 24
    T-loop, 22
telomere shortening, 23, 407, 414, 422, 423, 432, 434, 435, 440, 444
telomeric repeat, 22– 24, 26
teratoma, 323, 328
TERC, 25
TERT, 25
Tet, 345
TET, 317–320, 325, 336, 343, 354, 419
TET demethylase, 98, 99, 101
TET enzymes, 110
tetraploid cell, 329
TFIIA, 178

TFIID, 188, 192, 206
TFIIH, 202, 204
thermostable DNA polymerase, 461
tissue renewal, 415
    Loss of Tissue Renewal, 421
tissue stem cells, 415, 416, 420–422, 432
    senescent stem cells, 426
T-loop, 23, 29
Tn5 transposase, 448–450
Tn5 Transposon, 448
topoisomerase, 13, 14, 28, 69
Topologically Associating Domain, TAD, 292, 293–298, 300, 301, 304–309, 396, 402–404, 406
torsional stress, 13
totipotency, 316, 354
totipotent, 322, 326, 327
transcription factory, 201, 308
Transcription, 183
transcriptional bursting, 209
    burst frequency, 209
    burst size, 209
transcriptional gene silencing, 179
transcriptional pausing, 202, 204, 210
transcriptional silencing complex, 173
transcription burst, 301
transcription elongation, 138, 206, 207, 208, 211, 442
transcription start site, TSS, 80, 185
Transcription termination, 208, 209
translocase domain, 77, 78
transposable element, 26, 102, 103, 109, 131, 132, 134–138, 143, 145–147, 161, 168, 175, 176, 178, 180, 427
    long terminal repeat, LTR, 26
    retrotransposons, 26, 28, 135

retroviruses, 135
transposon mobilization, 427
transposase, 135, 136, 198, 427
transposon, 129, 137
transvection, 235
trichostatin A (TSA), 57
Trithorax, 58, 60, 157, 206, 222, 225,
    265, 266, 273
Trithorax Group, 266
Trithorax-related (Trr), 266, 267
trophectoderm, 321–323, 326, 327
trophoblast, 321, 322, 375
Trr, 195, 268, 270
Trx, 267, 268, 269
Trithorax Group genes, 222
trxG, 222
Tsix, 394, 396, 406
Tsix RNA, 393
TSS, 186, 188–191, 193, 198, 200,
    206
Tudor domain, 63, 66, 85
Type II promoters, 190

Ubiquitin, 67, 247, 248
ubiquitin ligase, 95
ubiquitylation, 206–208, 246–248,
    250, 252, 254, 256, 257, 261, 262,
    265, 272
deubiquitylation, 263
Ubx, 217, 220–222, 226, 227, 229,
    237, 263
UHRF1, 96, 97, 101, 317
Ultrabithorax, 216
Utx, 404
UTX, 264, 268, 271–273

variant PRC1, 255–257, 272
villi, 417

WD40 domain, 62, 242, 243
Werner syndrome, 433–435, 446
white gene, 150–152, 154, 159, 179,
    231–234, 236
winged helix domain, 46
writers, 53
WRN helicase, 7, 432–435

X chromosome choice, 392, 394, 396
X chromosome counting, 392, 394,
    395, 396
X chromosome dosage, 380
X chromosome dosage compensation,
    376, 380–382, 385, 406
dosage compensation complex,
    383
X Dosage Compensation in C.
    elegans, 382
X Dosage Compensation in
    Drosophila, 384
X chromosome genes, 379, 380
X chromosome inactivation, 350,
    390, 405
escaper genes, 404
imprinted X inactivation, 390, 391
random X inactivation, 390, 391
X chromosome reactivation, 404
X dosage compensation in
    C. elegans, 383
X inactivation, 393–395, 398, 403,
    404
X inactivation center, Xic. 392, 393,
    395, 406
Xist, 394–398, 400, 404–406
Xist RNA, 392, 393
Xist-dependent Silencing, 397, 398
Xist RNA localization, 401
Xist RNA repeat elements, 397

X-ray crystallography, 456, 458
X to autosome ratio, 381–382

Y chromosome, 382
YY1, 251, 255, 396, 398

ZFP57, 361–363, 378
zinc finger, 17–21, 29, 99, 246, 283, 284, 287, 386

www.ingramcontent.com/pod-product-compliance
Lightning Source LLC
Chambersburg PA
CBHW070740220326
41598CB00026B/3712